Assessing Listening and Spoken Language in Children With Hearing Loss

Assessing Listening and Spoken Language in Children With Hearing Loss

Tamala S. Bradham, PhD, CCC-A
K. Todd Houston, PhD, CCC-SLP, LSLS Cert. AVT

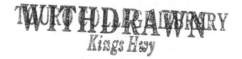
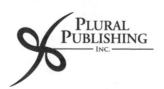
PLURAL
PUBLISHING
INC.

12069

KH

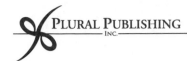

5521 Ruffin Road
San Diego, CA 92123

e-mail: info@pluralpublishing.com
website: http://www.pluralpublishing.com

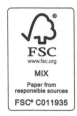

FSC
www.fsc.org
MIX
Paper from
responsible sources
FSC® C011935

Typeset in 10.5/13 Palatino by Flanagan's Publishing Services, Inc.
Printed in the United States of America by McNaughton and Gunn, Inc.

Library of Congress Cataloging-in-Publication Data

Assessing listening and spoken language in children with hearing loss / [edited by] Tamala S. Bradham, K. Todd Houston.
      p. ; cm.
  Includes bibliographical references and index.
  ISBN 978-1-59756-576-9 (alk. paper) — ISBN 1-59756-576-8 (alk. paper)
  I. Bradham, Tamala S., editor. II. Houston, K. Todd, editor.
  [DNLM: 1. Child. 2. Hearing Loss. 3. Auditory Perception. 4. Language Development. WV 271]
  RF290
  617.8—dc23
                                        2014039337

4/3/23

Contents

Preface

Over the past few decades, we have seen medical treatments described as "miracles" become standards of care. The widespread adoption of universal newborn hearing screening (UNHS) has opened the doors for so many children with hearing loss and their families. Because of earlier identification of hearing loss, these children can receive advanced hearing technology—such as digital hearing aids—within the first days or weeks of life. Digital hearing aids allow access to environmental sounds and spoken language unlike ever before. And when digital hearing aids cannot provide enough benefit, cochlear implants can take children from a world of mostly silence to hearing laughter, music, and, most importantly, their parents' or caregivers' voices. All of these advances are taking place within the framework of a very complex healthcare system that can be challenging for everyone involved. However, one advantage that the management of pediatric hearing loss has over other healthcare areas is the collaborative nature that most professionals support and the range of resources available.

THE NEED FOR THIS BOOK

Our goal in writing this book is to equip you with the knowledge, insights, strategies, and tools that will enable you to provide evidence-based practices when assessing the communication abilities of children with hearing loss. To adequately assess any child with hearing requires the cooperation of the child's family and col-laboration with a range of professionals. While most of healthcare practices today reside in "silos" where each discipline practices its area of expertise with little or no awareness of what others are doing, pediatric hearing loss is different. We are ahead of the curve in working collaboratively with other disciplines, but there is always room for improvement.

This book evolved out of the 2010 OPTION*Schools*, Inc. meeting in Memphis, Tennessee in which there were teachers of the deaf and hard of hearing, speech-language pathologists, audiologists, lawyers, and psychologists present. A survey was conducted on the assessments completed by all of the schools. The survey revealed that these programs used a total of 66 measurements to assess listening, speech, language and cognition in the children they were serving. It was surprising, to say the least, that such a variety of instruments was used. This survey also raised many questions! Programs wanted to know why certain measures were being used, what the measures assess, whether the measures were valid, and so forth. From these questions, a resource guide was created. OPTION*Schools*, Inc., has graciously agreed to share this wonderful resource in this book (see Appendix A).

Another reason for this book is that we often hear: "Is it necessary to have all these tests, assessments, and evaluations?" "Why does my child have to be re-evaluated so frequently?" "We already have the diagnosis of hearing loss, why do we need to go to _____ ?" [Fill in the blank—genetics, ophthalmology, psychologist, family support group, early intervention, etc.]. So, we answer with a question: "How do you start, or modify, intervention if you don't have an assessment that drives the plan?"

Finally, university training programs, especially those in deaf education, speech-language pathology, and audiology, have not changed quickly enough in light of the increased complexity of hearing health care. It is nearly impossible to cover all of the topics relevant to our areas of study as evidence-based practices, service delivery models, and treatment approaches continue to evolve due to new advancements in technology, systems, and research. Our university training programs continue to be 1, 2, or 4 years—depending on the discipline. Curricula have changed but not the number of credit hours. One noted difference is that audiology changed from a 2-year master's program to a 4-year clinical doctorate as the terminal degree. Perhaps speech-language pathology will follow and will soon—within the next decade—require a clinical doctorate prior to licensure and certification. We hope that this text will help to augment the training of new graduates who are starting their careers as well as add to the knowledge of seasoned professionals who now find themselves serving children with hearing loss who are learning to listen and use spoken language.

TO OUR AUDIENCE

Assessing Listening and Spoken Language in Children With Hearing Loss is relevant to administrators, government agencies, university training programs, teachers of the deaf and hard of hearing, special needs teachers, regular education teach-

ers, audiologists, speech-language pathologists, psychologists, and physicians. The content is applicable to multiple settings, including but not limited to, community speech and hearing centers, university training programs, hospitals, outpatient practices, private practices, state agencies, and most importantly, early intervention, preschools, and elementary through high school educational programs. The wide applicably of this book's content is in keeping with the principle that care is provided through a complex system of sites, services, and relationships, and that we must work together to ensure the best possible outcome for the child and family we are serving.

DESCRIPTION OF CONTENTS

The book is divided into three parts: Foundations in Assessments, Assessments, and Beyond the Assessments: Components to Consider. We are grateful to the outstanding contributing authors who gave their time to share their knowledge and expertise about best practices, which are based on the research and evidence available at this time of publication. For each chapter, there are key points to guide the reader, words that are bold can be found in the glossary, and resources mentioned are listed in the back of the book.

- Chapter 1: Assessing a Child With Hearing Loss: Past, Present, and Future
  The focus of this chapter sets the stage for the various evaluations that a child will have and the importance of having a multidisciplinary, interprofessional team.

■ Chapter 2: Assessment Tools: Evaluating Our Measurements
This chapter covers standardized and norm referenced tests, criterion referenced tests, reliability, validity, and questionnaires. This chapter helps the reader understand how to select a test that assesses what he or she needs based on the child's functioning at the time.

■ Chapter 3: Medical Assessment
This chapter provides an overview of the medical workup that a child may undergo following the diagnosis of hearing loss, including genetics, ophthalmology, and otolaryngology.

■ Chapter 4: Auditory Assessments
The auditory assessments chapter covers objective and behavioral testing, understanding the audiogram, assessing functional listening, and provides suggestions for monitoring hearing status.

■ Chapter 5: Speech Production Assessment
Evaluating speech production is critical to developing spoken language. This chapter discusses an effective process for evaluating vocalizations and a child's development of speech, and the chapter also includes, for the first time in print, a new tool for assessing speech production, *The Paterson-Cole Phonologic Evaluation Procedure, (PC-PEP)*.

■ Chapter 6: Language Assessment of Children With Hearing Loss
This chapter provides an overview of the process of selecting receptive and expressive language assessments, how some can be modified without invalidating the results, specific adaptations that may be used—in some cases—that may be necessary. The chapter ends with a comprehensive assessment protocol that can be used to accurately evaluate the language performance of any child with hearing loss.

■ Chapter 7: Psychoeducational Assessment
Understanding the psycho-educational component is essential in setting realistic expectations with the family and educational programming. This chapter provides an overview of psychoeducational assessments provided to children with hearing loss.

■ Chapter 8: Literacy Assessment
Reading is an auditory task. This chapter provides the framework in which a child needs to develop literacy skills and how to assess the child with hearing loss in mastering these skills.

■ Chapter 9: Assessment of the Listening Environment
Assessing the listening environment in the home, child care setting, and/or educational environment is critical to ensure that the child has auditory access to spoken language. In adverse listening environments, children exert more energy trying to listen and may be accused of being distracted and "not listening" when the environment is not conducive to auditory learning.

■ Chapter 10: Hearing Aid Assessment
Assessing the functioning of the hearing aids is key to ensuring the child has access to environmental

sounds and spoken language. This chapter focuses on how hearing aids should be programmed based on evidence-based practices and red-flags for when the hearing aids may not be performing as needed.

- Chapter 11: Cochlear Implants Assessment
  As FDA guidelines continue to change, more people are electing to receive cochlear implants to improve their hearing. This chapter addresses candidacy, assessments of the cochlear implant system, and red flags for when the cochlear implant may be not performing as expected.
- Chapter 12: Supporting Families Through the Assessment
  Family-centered care is paramount to the success of the child learning to listen and use spoken language. This chapter discusses how professionals can provide appropriate family support through a family-centered care perspective and what that looks like in today's practice.
- Chapter 13: Assessment Considerations for Children With Hearing Loss Who Are Culturally and Linguistically Diverse
  Although the most prominent language in the United States is English, the US is not a monolingual country. This chapter describes special considerations speech-language pathologists, audiologists, and educators should take into account when evaluating the speech and language of non-English-speaking children.
- Chapter 14: From Assessment to Intervention
  Putting the pieces together in the development of an intervention or treatment plan is always a difficult task. This chapter provides general guidelines for professionals to consider when interpreting their test results and formulating appropriate short and long term goals.

EVOLVING TERMINOLOGY

How do you describe a child who has additional needs and/or diagnoses? We all have been taught that we are a person first before anything. Through the years, we have heard terms like *deaf child or deaf and hard of hearing child,* and more recently—a child who is deaf or hard of hearing, a child with hearing impairment, or a child with hearing loss. By taking a lesson from Dr. Karen Anderson, we chose to use the term *child with hearing loss* for this book. As Dr. Anderson has shared, the terms *deaf* and *hard of hearing* do not necessarily relate to audiometric thresholds (mild, moderate, severe, or profound). Functional hearing varies regardless of what the unaided thresholds or real ear measurements reveal. A person's identity comes from within that person and their supporting environment. Kent (2003) revealed that the majority of students with hearing loss (55.8%) did not self-identify as having a hearing disability. The choice of wording of *children with hearing loss* for this book was not a trivial matter. We acknowledge that the Deaf Community has experienced no loss, and we also do not wish to reinforce the notion that we are trying to "fix" a child with hearing loss. In light of research revealing that more children are born into a family with normal hearing (Mitchell & Karchmer, 2004), more families are choosing listening and spoken language (Alberg, Wilson & Roush, 2006), and how children are identifying themselves only as persons with a "hearing problem" (Kent, 2003), we elected to use the term, *child with hearing loss.*

Another terminology note is that we also elected, in most cases, to use the word *family* instead of *parent* or *parents.* This is an attempt to include all the significant people who care for the child: aunts, uncles, cousins, grandparents, parents, adopted parents (i.e., forever parents), foster parents, siblings, and neighbors. There are a few places where parent is used due to the context of the sentence. Please note that we still mean to include all the people who care for and support the child with hearing loss.

In closing, we are pleased to share this incredible resource with you. While it is focused on assessment of children with hearing loss, many of the diagnostic principles and strategies discussed apply to other children with special needs or unique diagnoses. While it is impossible to provide all of the information needed on the topic of assessment of listening and spoken language in a single text, we do know that the information provided will be invaluable to those professionals who are serving children with hearing loss and their families. Assessment guides intervention, and without comprehensive diagnostic processes, children with hearing loss may not receive the appropriate intervention, treatment, or educational support that meet their specific communicative or learning needs. Through assessment and ongoing data collection and performance tracking, professionals can ensure that each intervention or treatment session is designed to facilitate the child's listening, speech, language, cognition, and conversational competence. Intervention tailored to individual learning needs maximizes outcomes; and, as professionals, we all want the children with hearing loss we are serving to reach their fullest potential. It all starts with assessment.

REFERENCES

Alberg, J., Wilson, K., & Roush, J. (2006). Statewide collaboration in the delivery of EHDI services. *The Volta Review, 106*(3), 259–274.

Anderson, K. (2014). *Supporting Success for Children with Hearing Loss.* Retrieved from http://successforkidswithhearingloss.com/

Kent, B. (2003). Identity issues for hard of hearing adolescents aged 11, 13, and 15 in mainstream setting. *Journal of Deaf Studies and Deaf Education, 8*(3), 315–324.

Mitchell, R. E., & Karchmer, M. A. (2004). Chasing the mythical ten percent: Parental hearing status of deaf and hard of hearing students in the United States. *Sign Language Studies, 4*(2), 138–163.

Acknowledgments

The journey to create a best practice model for assessing children with hearing loss has been paved with many efforts over the past two decades to establish a system that defines screening, identification, use of appropriate hearing technology, and the provision of family-centered early intervention to children with hearing loss. We wish to acknowledge all of the pioneers that have contributed to current service delivery models. We are humbled by your tireless commitment to children with hearing loss and their families. Also, for all the innovators of tomorrow who will continue to navigate these waters, we look forward to the new discoveries, tools, and other resources that you will bring to improving these services. The future for children with hearing loss remains bright because of your efforts.

We wish to thank all of our contributing authors who unselfishly shared not only their knowledge and expertise but their passion for serving children with hearing loss and their families. This book would not have been possible without your willingness to share your work. Similarly, we wish to thank our reviewers who provided feedback and valuable insights on every chapter. You helped us to strengthen the content, and we will remain grateful for your efforts. This book is better because of you!

We also extend our gratitude to Valerie Johns, Gem Rabanera, Taylor Eaton, Megan Carter, and Rachel Singer at Plural Publishing. Your encouragement, guidance, and gentle reminders kept us focused and on track throughout the writing and editing processes. Thank you for everything!

And finally, on a personal note, we'd also like to thank Tami's family: Bill, Caroline, William, and Camden; and Todd's family: Maria, Kaitlyn, and Jordan. We couldn't do this without your love, support, and patience.

Contributors

Joni Alberg, PhD
Executive Director
BEGINNINGS for Parents of Children
    Who are Deaf or Hard of Hearing, Inc.
Board of Directors
AG Bell Association
Adjunct Assistant Professor
School of Medicine, Division of Speech
    and Hearing Sciences
University of North Carolina at Chapel Hill
Raleigh, North Carolina
Chapter 12

Andrea Bell, BA
Graduate Student Clinician
University of Akron
Akron, Ohio
Chapter 14

Tamala S. Bradham, PhD, CCC-A
Quality Consultant
Vanderbilt University Medical Center
Center for Quality, Safety, and Risk
    Prevention
Nashville, Tennessee
Chapters 1, 4, 11, 12, and 14

Stephen Camarata, PhD
Professor
Department of Hearing and Speech
    Sciences
Professor
Department of Psychiatry
Vanderbilt University School of Medicine
Nashville, Tennessee
Chapter 2

Janet DesGeorges
Executive Director
Hands & Voices
Boulder, Colorado
Chapter 12

Allan O. Diefendorf, PhD
Professor
Department of Otolaryngology-Head
    and Neck Surgery
Indiana University School of Medicine
Indianapolis, Indiana
Chapters 1 and 4

**Michael Douglas, MA, CCC-SLP, LSLS
Cert AVT**
Principal
Mama Lere Hearing School
Vanderbilt University
Nashville, Tennessee
Chapter 13

**Hannah Eskridge, MSP, CCC-SLP, LSLS
Cert. AVT**
Assistant Professor
Department of Otolaryngology
University of North Carolina
NCFI Barnhardt CASTLE Director
Chapel Hill, North Carolina
Chapter 6

**K. Todd Houston, PhD, CCC-SLP, LSLS
Cert. AVT**
Professor
School of Speech-Language Pathology
    and Audiology
College of Health Professions
The University of Akron
Akron, Ohio
Chapters 1, 11, and 14

Carol Flexer, PhD, CCC-A, LSLS Cert. AVT
Distinguished Professor Emeritus
School of Speech-Language Pathology
  and Audiology
College of Health Professions
The University of Akron
Akron, Ohio
Chapter 9

Dana Kan, MA, NBCT
Doctoral Student
Department of Hearing and Speech
  Sciences
Vanderbilt University
Nashville, Tennessee
Chapter 2

Hope Lancaster
Doctoral Student
Department of Hearing and Speech
  Sciences
Vanderbilt University
Nashville, Tennessee
Chapter 2

Patti Martin, PhD
Director
Audiology and Speech Pathology
Arkansas Children's Hospital
Adjunct Assistant Professor
Audiology and Speech Pathology
University of Arkansas for Medical
  Sciences/University of Arkansas at
  Little Rock
Little Rock, Arkansas
Chapter 12

Ryan McCreery, PhD
Director of Audiology
Boys Town National Research Hospital
Omaha, Nebraska
Chapter 10

Marietta M. Paterson, EdD, CED
Associate Professor

Director of Education of the Deaf
Department of Speech and Hearing
  Sciences
The University of Southern Mississippi
Hattiesburg, Mississippi
Chapter 5

Christina Barris Perigoe, PhD, CCC-SLP, CED, LSLS Cert. AVT
Coordinator
Early Oral Intervention Graduate
  Program
Department of Speech and Hearing
  Sciences
The University of Southern Mississippi
Hattiesburg, Mississippi
Chapter 5

Susan Randich, PhD
Psychologist
St. Joseph Institute for the Deaf
St. Louis, Missouri
Chapter 7

Donna Fisher Smiley, PhD, CCC-A
Audiology Supervisor
EARS Program
Arkansas Children's Hospital
Little Rock, Arkansas
Chapter 4

Carrie Spangler, AuD
Educational Audiologist
School of Speech-Language Pathology
  and Audiology
College of Health Professions
University of Akron
Akron, Ohio
Chapter 9

Pon Trairatvorakul, MD
Fellow, Developmental and Behavioral
  Pediatrics
Division of Developmental and
  Behavioral Pediatrics

Cincinnati Children's Hospital Medical
  Center
University of Cincinnati
Cincinnati, Ohio
Chapter 3

Krystal L. Werfel, PhD, CCC-SLP
Assistant Professor
Department of Communication Sciences
  and Disorders
University of South Carolina
Columbia, South Carolina
Chapter 8

Susan Wiley, MD
Professor
Developmental Pediatrician

Co-Director of the Division of
  Developmental and Behavioral
  Pediatrics
Cincinnati Children's Hospital Medical
  Center
University of Cincinnati
Cincinnati, Ohio
Chapter 3

**Kathryn Wilson, MA, CCC-SLP, LSLS
Cert. AVT**
Director of Embedded Practice
Professional Learning Initiative
Oberkotter Foundation
Philadelphia, Pennsylvania
Chapter 6

This book is dedicated to all the families who have a child with hearing loss. You have taught us how to listen, and you inspire us to be voices in shaping early intervention, educational, and healthcare practices today and in the future.

PART I

Foundations in Assessments

CHAPTER 1

Assessing a Child With Hearing Loss: Past, Present, and Future

Tamala S. Bradham, K. Todd Houston, and Allan O. Diefendorf

KEY POINTS

- Assessments are completed based on the family's concerns, to provide a diagnosis, and to develop treatment options for the family to consider. Assessments are necessary to formulate appropriate intervention models.
- Hearing and hearing-related conditions are a healthcare priority.
- To move forward in the new era of health care, understanding the evolution of early hearing loss detection and intervention (EHDI) is essential. Learning from the past moves the profession forward in providing efficient, evidence-based care.
- Transformational changes occurring in health care today as a result of changes in reimbursement are striving to be more patient-centered, equitable, timely, safe, effective, and efficient.
- Tomorrow's healthcare system will be transparent, accessible, and innovative. If you can dream it, then it can happen.
- The assessments for children with hearing loss require an interdisciplinary team to assess medical factors, developmental, hearing, speech, language, listening/speech perception, conversational competence/pragmatics, cognition, and literacy.

Think about the last time you took a test. Maybe it was a college final exam, a test for state licensure, or a recent medical evaluation. Recall how you felt about taking that test, or being examined: are you like Hermione Granger from *Harry Potter* who was disappointed when final exams were cancelled or do you get anxious or worry about how well you did? For most individuals, it is probably the latter. Then, on top of it, after you take the test, you have to wait for the grade or results. So, why are there tests and assessments? What is the purpose? What are we trying to achieve?

INTRODUCTION

To effectively address the concerns a family has about their child, an assessment is the necessary first step. An **assessment** is

3

the act of making a judgment about something (Merriam-Webster, 2014). In this case, professionals complete assessments to determine a diagnosis and to make a prognosis. When making a diagnosis, the professional is identifying a disease, illness, or condition by examining someone (Merriam-Webster, 2014). Understanding the nature of the concerns, the signs and symptoms, and, if possible, the etiology of the condition, the professional can provide the family with information about treatments and prognosis. If an assessment is not completed, treatment options cannot be explored, concerns cannot be addressed, and hope cannot be instilled.

In March 2001, the Institute of Medicine (IOM) released "Crossing the Quality Chasm: A New Health System for the 21st Century" report. In this report, IOM describes the immense divide between current service delivery practices and what we know to be best evidence-based practices. This report states that people "should be able to count on receiving care that meets their needs and is based on the best scientific knowledge . . . " (IOM, 2001, p. 1). While more than a decade has passed since this report was published, many would argue that this report remains true today. There is still much work to be done to ensure that all people receive the care that meets their unique needs, that is delivered efficiently, and is safe and effective. In order to deliver high quality care, it is essential to complete an assessment to obtain a baseline of performance and determine the appropriate plan of care.

This chapter provides an overview of hearing and hearing loss and the evidence of hearing loss as a national priority. The past, present, and a snapshot of the future are shared. Finally, an overview of the necessary assessments for children with hearing loss and the importance of having an interdisciplinary team are provided.

HEARING AND HEARING LOSS

The auditory system has two primary functions: hearing and balance. Additionally, the auditory system is made up of four parts: the outer ear, the middle ear, the inner ear, and the auditory cortex. Hearing sensitivity is measured across several speech **frequencies** (250 through 8000 Hz) and loudness is measured using a **decibel (dB) hearing level (HL)** scale ranging from −10 to 115 dB HL in 5 dB HL increments. In the United States (U.S.), a child is said to have a hearing loss if the measured thresholds are 15 dB HL or greater across the speech frequencies in at least one ear. The World Health Organization (WHO) defines disabling hearing loss in adults (15 years and older) with a pure tone average (PTA) of 41 dB HL or greater for the better ear (WHO, 2014). In children, disabling hearing loss is defined as PTA of 31 dB HL or greater for the better ear (WHO, 2014). There are different *degrees* of hearing loss ranging from slight to profound and *variations* of hearing loss that include temporary, fluctuating, permanent, or progressive hearing loss. There are many causes of hearing loss, including nongenetic factors, genetic factors, syndromes associated with hearing loss, and acquired hearing losses.

Permanent hearing loss associated with nongenetic factors can often be prevented and include: (a) anoxia; (b) atresia, stenosis, or microtia; (c) birth injuries; (d) complications associated with the Rh factor in the blood; (e) inner ear malformations (e.g., Mondini's malformation or large vestibular aqueduct); (f) low birth weight; (g) maternal diabetes; (h) maternal infections (e.g., rubella, cytomegalovirus, toxoplasmosis, syphilis, and herpes simplex virus); (i) prematurity; (j) toxemia during pregnancy; and/or (k) toxins (i.e., drugs and alcohol consumed by the mother during pregnancy) (American Speech-Language-Hearing Association [ASHA], 2014).

Approximately 60% of children identified with hearing loss have a genetic component that caused their hearing loss (Smith, Kochhar, & Friedman, 2009). The hearing loss may be present at birth or may develop later in life. Genetic hearing losses are described as autosomal recessive (e.g., Connexin 26), autosomal dominant, X-linked, or mitochondrial inheritance patterns. Many genetic syndromes are also associated with hearing loss: (a) Alport syndrome, (b) CHARGE syndrome, (c) Crouzon syndrome, (d) Down syndrome, (e) Goldenhar syndrome, (f) Pendred syndrome, (g) sickle cell disease, (h) Tay-Sachs disease, (i) Treacher Collins syndrome, (j) Usher syndrome, and (k) Waardenburg syndrome (ASHA, 2014).

Hearing loss can be acquired at any time. Examples of conditions that cause acquired hearing loss include: (a) chicken pox, (b) encephalitis, (c) head injury, (d) measles, (e) mumps, (f) meningitis, (g) noise exposure, (h) otitis media, (i) ototoxic medications (i.e., cancer treating agents), and (j) presbycusis (ASHA, 2014).

DETERMINING IF HEARING LOSS IS A HEALTHCARE PRIORITY WORTH ASSESSING

To determine if a condition is a healthcare priority, the following parameters should be considered: (1) the condition is an important health problem, (2) adequate knowledge about the condition is available in order to establish evidence-based protocols, (3) acceptable and valid screening tools, diagnostics tests, and treatments are available, (4) resources (i.e., facilities, equipment, people) are available for screening, identification, and treatment, (5) early screening detection, and intervention result in improved outcomes, and (6) the cost-benefit ratio is appropriate (American Academy of Pediatrics, 1999; Mausner & Kramer, 1985).

Is Hearing Loss an Important Health Issue?

Prevalence rates vary depending on the population tested, the type and degree of hearing loss, the tests used to measure hearing, and the ages at which the hearing tests were administered (Bess & Paradise, 1994). With this in mind, there are 360 million people with hearing loss representing over 5% of the world's population (328 million adults and 32 million children) (WHO, 2014). The majority of people with hearing loss live in low- and middle-income countries (WHO, 2014). In the United States, permanent hearing loss is the most common birth defect, affecting approximately 3 newborns per 1,000 births (White, 2004). One in 1,000 (0.1%) infants are born with severe to profound hearing loss (NIH, 1993; Northern & Downs, 2002). Prevalence is higher (5% of the pediatric population) for children with milder forms of **sensorineural hearing loss** (<40 dB HL), and 11.3% for school-aged children for all types of minimal to moderate hearing losses (Bess, Dodd, & Parker, 1998).

One of the most common types of temporary hearing loss in children is caused from **otitis media**. The WHO reported a global burden of 65 to 330 million individuals with otitis media with effusion and accounted for 28,000 deaths (Acuin et al., 2004). In the United States, between 50% and 85% of children under the age of three years experience at least one episode of acute otitis media (Klein, 1989). Otitis media with effusion can affect as many as 80% of children with approximately 2.2 million cases of otitis media identified annually in the United States (American Academy of Family Physicians & American Academy of Otolaryngology-Head & Neck Surgery, 2004; van Zon, van der Heijden, van Dongen, Burton, & Schilder, 2012). Acuin et al. (2004) estimated that chronic otitis media may contribute to more than half of the global burden of children with hearing loss.

Hearing is critical to speech and language development, communication, literacy, and learning. Children with hearing loss have increased difficulties with communication skills, increased behavioral and pragmatic problems, decreased psychosocial well-being, and lower educational accomplishments compared with children with normal hearing (Calderon & Low, 1998; Davis, 1990; Davis, Elfenbein, Schum, & Bentler, 1986; Wake, Hughes, Collins, & Poulakis, 2004). Early identification of hearing loss resulting in timely family-centered early intervention, though, can lessen the impact on a child's development (Sininger, Grimes, & Christensen, 2010; Yoshinaga-Itano, Baca, & Sedey, 2010). Several case control and cohort studies have suggested that intervention improves children's use of residual hearing and their speech-language skills, social and emotional status, and academic performance (Geers, Strube, Tobey, Pisoni, & Moog, 2011; Greenberg, Calderon, & Kusche, 1984;

Moeller, Tomblin, Yoshinaga-Itano, Connor, & Jerger, 2007; Ramkalawan & Davis, 1992). With early access to audition and intense habilitation, children with hearing loss often can be educated alongside hearing peers in their neighborhood schools instead of requiring years of expensive special education placements, which generates substantial cost benefit for society (Barton, Stacey, Fortnum, & Summerfield, 2006; Bond et al., 2009; Francis, Koch, Wyatt, & Niparko, 1999).

In 1993, the U.S. Surgeon General, Dr. C. Everett Koop, issued a challenge to the U.S. healthcare system to reduce the age congenital hearing loss was identified. He acknowledged the harmful effects of childhood hearing loss when so few people recognized this largely invisible disability. In 1995, the World Health Assembly passed a resolution on the prevention and control of major causes of hearing loss and for early detection of hearing loss in "babies, toddlers, and children, as well as in the elderly, within the framework of primary health care" (section 1, para. 1).

Is Knowledge About Hearing Loss Available to Establish Evidence-Based Protocols?

Many important professional and advocacy groups, such as the National Institute for Health (NIH), American Academy of Pediatrics (AAP), the March of Dimes, the American Academy of Audiology (AAA), American Speech-Language-Hearing Association (ASHA), the Joint Committee on Infant Hearing (JCIH), and the Alexander Graham Bell Association for the Deaf and Hard of Hearing (AG Bell), have created position papers, held conferences, and convened working groups focused on childhood hearing loss and intervention

(Nation Center for Hearing Assessment and Management [NCHAM], 2010). As such, the U.S. Preventive Services Task Force (USPSTF) concluded "that there is moderate certainty that the net benefit of screening all newborn infants for hearing loss is moderate" (USPSTF, 2008, para. 5).

identified hearing loss should receive appropriate intervention, including hearing aids if appropriate, by a qualified professional at no later than 6 months of age (AAP, 2007). A child can be screened and tested for hearing loss at any time with valid, evidence-based protocols.

Are Acceptable and Valid Screening Tools, Diagnostics Tests, and Treatments Available?

There are valid, safe, and cost-effective screening tools available to determine the presence or absence of hearing loss within hours of birth. The JCIH recommends the **1-3-6 model**. That is, hearing should be screened by 1 month of age, audiological evaluation should be completed no at later than 3 months of age (for those who did not pass the screening), and infants with

Are Resources (i.e., Facilities, Equipment, People) Available for Screening, Identification, and Treatment?

During the past two decades, newborn hearing screening, diagnosis, and intervention programs have expanded dramatically (Figure 1–1). In the United States, each state and territory has an established early hearing detection and intervention (EHDI) program, typically housed within the State Department of Education or the

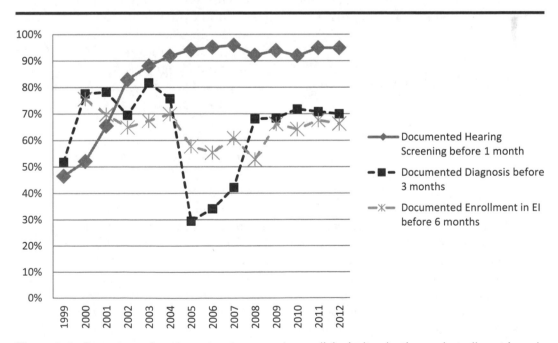

Figure 1–1. Percentage of newborns hearing screening, audiological evaluation, and enrollment in early intervention in the U.S. from 1999–2012 (CDC, 2014).

State Department of Health. EHDI programs are "responsible for establishing, maintaining, and improving the system of services necessary to screen newborns for hearing loss, providing timely and appropriate diagnostic assessments for those who do not pass the screen, enrolling children identified with permanent hearing loss in appropriate early intervention programs, coordinating these services with the child's primary healthcare provider, and delivering appropriate family education and support" (White & Blaiser, 2011, p. 84). With mandated and voluntary **universal newborn hearing screening** for newborns in all 50 states, more than 97% of all newborns today receive a hearing screening before they leave the hospital or birthing center (ASHA, 2014; Centers for Disease Control and Prevention [CDC], 2012). Most importantly, the age of hearing loss identification has decreased from an average of 2 to 3 years of age to an average of 2 to 3 months of age (White, Forsman, Eichwald, & Muñoz, 2010).

Does Early Detection and Intervention Result in Improved Outcomes?

Without appropriate opportunities to learn language, children will fall behind their hearing peers in language, cognition, social-emotional development, and academic achievement (Sininger, Grimes, & Christensen, 2010; Yoshinaga-Itano, Baca, & Sedey, 2010). Research demonstrates that when hearing loss is identified early (prior to 6 months of age) and followed immediately (within 2 months) with appropriate intervention services, outcomes in language development, speech development, and social-emotional development are significantly better compared with children with later identified, **congenital** hearing loss (Carney & Moeller, 1998; Moeller, 2000; Yoshinaga-Itano et al., 1998).

What Is the Cost–Benefit Analysis, If Any?

When children with hearing loss are not identified and do not receive early intervention, special education for a child with hearing loss costs schools an additional $420,000, and has a lifetime cost of approximately $1 million per individual (Honeycutt et al., 2004; Johnson et al., 1993; Mohr, Feldman, & Dunbar, 2000). Most individuals with severe to profound hearing loss are poorer than other Americans, with 53% having family income of less than $25,000 compared to 35% of the general U.S. population (Blanchfield, Feldman, Dunbar, & Gardner, 2001). Based on incidence data, it is estimated that there will be slightly over 15,000 new cases each year with societal losses amounting to $4.6 billion over the lifetime of the child (Mohr et al., 2000). Earnings also have been reported to be less. According to Mohr and colleagues (2000), 50% to 70% of people with severe to profound hearing loss before retirement age are expected to earn only 50 to 70% of their peers with normal hearing. Depending on when the hearing loss occurred, an adult will lose between $220,000 and $440,000 in earnings (Mohr et al., 2000).

For conductive hearing losses associated with otitis media, the total cost in the United States exceeds five billion dollars per year when both direct costs (e.g., antibiotic therapy and surgery) and indirect costs (e.g., parental time caring for child and transportation for doctor visits) are considered (Stool et al., 1994). Other intangible costs include the economic consequences associated with the number of school days missed and the problems associated with speech and language delays.

An infant with a hearing loss is generally healthy looking and develops relatively normally during the first year of life. When hearing loss goes undetected in that first year, however, it will interfere tragically with the child's ability to learn to speak and read, access the mainstream curriculum, and to contribute productively to society.

HISTORICAL PERSPECTIVE OF EVOLVING QUALITY CARE IN IDENTIFICATION OF HEARING LOSS IN CHILDREN

The underlying rationale for universal early detection of hearing loss is that early detection followed by early intervention maximizes developmental outcomes to the child and family, and impacts society in beneficial ways. Undetected hearing loss in infants and young children compromises optimal language development and personal achievement.

When hearing loss is not detected through early hearing detection and intervention (EHDI) programs, it often goes undetected until the child is a toddler or older, especially in children who have no medical conditions and/or other disabilities. In 1988, while C. Everett Koop was serving as Surgeon General of the United States, the Congressional Commission on Education of the Deaf issued an alarming report: the average age at which permanent hearing loss among infants and young children was being identified in the United States was 2½ to 3 years of age. In response, Dr. Koop stated, "Given the importance of language development and communication during those early years,

this is unacceptable" (Koop, 2010). Subsequently, in 1989 Dr. Koop issued a challenge to researchers, educators, healthcare providers, and parents to work together to find better ways of identifying very young children who are deaf or hard of hearing. He also set a goal that by the year 2000 all infants with permanent hearing loss would be identified before 12 months of age (Koop, 2010).

In the 1990s, three important initiatives stimulated efforts for universal early detection of hearing loss in infants. First, by 1990 a coalition of 300 national organizations and state and territorial health departments had designed the **Healthy People 2000** initiative (U.S. Department of Health and Human Services, 1991). As part of the initiative related to hearing, a goal was established to "reduce the average age at which children with significant hearing impairment are identified to no more than 12 months of age by the year 2000" (based on the baseline estimation of 24 to 30 months declared by C. Everett Koop). Second, in 1993 the *NIH Consensus Statement on Early Identification of Hearing Impairment in Infants and Young Children* recommended that "universal screening be implemented for all infants (both well babies and babies from the neonatal intensive care unit) within the first 3 months of life." Finally, in 1994, the JCIH issued their position statement that endorsed "the goal of universal detection of infants with hearing loss as early as possible. All infants with hearing loss should be identified by three months of age, and receive intervention by six months of age."

In the latter half of the decade, the NIH, the Bureau of Maternal and Child Health (MCHB), and the Centers for Disease Control and Prevention (CDC) individually and collectively sought solutions to achieve the JCIH goals. The NIDCD

(1997) developed recommended guidelines for newborn hearing screening, and grants from MCHB established the Marion Downs National Center for Infant Hearing and later the National Center for Hearing Assessment and Management (NCHAM), focusing on newborn hearing screening, follow-up assessment, and intervention services. The CDC provided essential leadership for the development of uniform state and national database systems to ensure that newborns and infants identified with, or at risk for, hearing loss have access to screening, follow-up, and intervention services. As a partner in most of these advocacy efforts and in concert with mounting evidence supporting universal early detection of hearing loss, the JCIH issued their 2000 position statement advocating "early detection of, and intervention for infants with hearing loss through integrated, interdisciplinary state and national systems of universal newborn hearing screening, evaluation, and family-centered intervention" (JCIH, 2000, p. 9). The JCIH Year 2000 Position Statement was certainly facilitated by the AAP endorsement of early detection of hearing loss through universal newborn hearing screening (AAP Task Force on Newborn and Infant Hearing, 1999).

Recent accomplishments demonstrate essential ongoing efforts to sustain and improve early detection of hearing loss outcomes. A supplement to the JCIH 2007 Position Statement has been published, providing comprehensive guidelines for EHDI programs on establishing strong **early intervention** (EI) systems with appropriate expertise to meet the needs of children with hearing loss (JCIH et al., 2013). In addition, several organizations —including but not limited to, AAA, ASHA, CDC, and NCHAM—established

Early Hearing Detection and Intervention-Pediatric Audiology Links to Service (EHDI-PALS), a Web-based link to information, resources, and services for children with hearing loss. The primary focus of EHDI-PALS is to provide a national Web-based directory of facilities that offer pediatric audiology services to children younger than five years of age (see Appendix A).

Today, universal early detection of hearing loss is a public health priority and a primary healthcare standard due to a concatenation of historical, political, and technological factors that have evolved over the past 50 years in the United States. Thus, children and families are accessing and receiving appropriate services meeting their family desires and expectations. Yet, to achieve improved outcomes in service for all children, early intervention systems must continue partnering with all stakeholders (families, service providers, researchers) to document what works for children and families and to strengthen the evidence base supporting these practices.

CURRENT PERSPECTIVE OF QUALITY CARE IN IDENTIFICATION OF HEARING LOSS IN CHILDREN

Health care is in need of fundamental change (IOM, 2001). Services rendered should meet the patients' needs, be based on the best scientific knowledge available, and be provided in an efficient manner that minimizes costs, resources, and time. Yet there is strong evidence that this frequently is not the case (Berwick, & Hackbarth, 2012). Many patients, doctors, nurses, and healthcare leaders are concerned that the care delivered is not, essentially, the care that should be received (IOM, 2001).

In spite of the widespread recognition of the importance of effective newborn hearing screening, diagnosis, and intervention programs, progress has been gradual and much work remains to be done (Bradham & Houston, 2011). Although UNHS has proven to be effective, nearly 60% of infants referred from newborn hearing screening do not receive a timely diagnosis (Russ, White, Dougherty, & Forsman, 2010) and many are lost to follow-up (CDC, 2012). While approximately 77% of children confirmed to have a permanent hearing loss enroll in early intervention by the age of 6 months, not all of these children have access to the services they need for speech and language development (Russ et al., 2010). Although EHDI programs have become more robust, considerable work remains to ensure that all children who do not pass a hearing screening receive the appropriate follow-up services (Bradham & Houston, 2011). In a systematic review of the EHDI system, Bradham and Houston (2011) identified several issues related to lost to follow-up and lack of access to services by qualified professionals which included the need for Web-based data management systems, interagency collaboration and data sharing, and preservice and in-service educational opportunities for physicians, nurses, audiologists, speech-language pathologists, early interventionists, and teachers.

To survive the transformational changes occurring in health care today, service delivery models must change. The service models should be innovative to facilitate access to care, and to initiate plans of care that ameliorate the consequences of late-diagnosed hearing loss. When professionals are designing ways to deliver hearing services, the following dimensions of health care should be considered:

- **Patient-centered**—providing care that is respectful of and responsive to individual patient preferences, needs, and values and ensuring that patient values guide all clinical decisions. Hearing healthcare programs should be able to accommodate differences in patient preferences and encourage shared decision making.
- **Equitable**—providing care that does not vary in quality because of personal characteristics such as gender, ethnicity, geographic location, and socioeconomic status. Hearing healthcare programs should be designed to respond to patients' choices and preferences based on their needs and values.
- **Timely**—reducing sometimes harmful delays for both those who receive and those who give care. Patients should receive their hearing health care when they need it and in the form necessary.
- **Safe**—avoiding injuries to patients from the care that is intended to help them.
- **Effective**—providing services based on scientific knowledge to all who could benefit and refraining from providing services to those not likely to benefit. The hearing health care provided should not vary substantially from provider to provider or from place to place.
- **Efficient**—avoiding waste, including waste of equipment, supplies, ideas, and energy (IOM, 2001).

The professional who can achieve major gains in these six dimensions will be far better at meeting the patient's need as well as being able to keep their practice more viable than their peers who have not incorporated these dimensions. With the implementation of these dimensions, patients should experience care that is safer, more reliable, and more integrated (IOM, 2001).

FUTURE PERSPECTIVE OF QUALITY CARE IN IDENTIFICATION OF HEARING LOSS IN CHILDREN

With the overall quality of care guiding changes in proposed healthcare reimbursement models and with consumers being more knowledgeable about their needs, the healthcare model of the future will be very different. Hearing healthcare programs will be responsive at all times, and access to care will no longer be an issue. Services rendered will be provided over the Internet, by telephone and texting, using telepractice in addition to in-person visits. The service delivery model of the future will follow these guiding principles as outlined by IOM (2001):

1. Care is based on continuous healing relationships. Patients should receive care whenever they need it and in many forms, not just face-to-face visits. This implies that the healthcare system must be responsive at all times, and access to care should be provided over the Internet, by telephone, and by other means in addition to in-person visits.
2. Care is customized according to patient needs and values. The system should be designed to meet the most common of needs, but should have the capability to respond to individual patient choices and preferences.
3. The patient is the source of control. Patients should be given the necessary information and opportunity to exercise the degree of control they choose over healthcare decisions that affect them. The system should be able to accommodate differences in patient preferences and encourage shared decision making.
4. Knowledge is shared and information flows freely. Patients should have unfettered access to their own medical information and to clinical knowledge. Clinicians and patients should communicate effectively and share information.
5. Decision making is evidence-based. Patients should receive care based on the best available scientific knowledge. Care should not vary illogically from clinician to clinician or from place to place.
6. Safety is a system priority. Patients should be safe from injury caused by the care system. Reducing risk and ensuring safety require greater attention to systems that help prevent and mitigate errors.
7. Transparency is necessary. The system should make available to patients and their families information that enables them to make informed decisions when they are selecting a health plan, hospital, or clinical practice, or when they are choosing among alternative treatments. This should include information describing the system's performance in terms of safety, evidence-based practice, and patient satisfaction.
8. Needs are anticipated. The system should anticipate patient needs, rather than simply react to events.

9. Waste is continuously decreased. The system should not waste resources or patient time.

10. Cooperation among clinicians is a priority. Clinicians and institutions should actively collaborate and communicate to ensure an appropriate exchange of information and coordination of care (pp. 3–4).

Tomorrow's hearing healthcare delivery model will follow a new model 1-3-6 weeks (Burk, Burns, Earley, & Gatzemeyer, 2009) in which the hearing screening is completed within 1 week after birth, assessments are completed within 3 weeks, and treatments and intervention can start by 6 weeks. The medical treatments for hearing loss also will be more sophisticated. Based on the child's DNA, the physician will be able to provide customized medical treatments that may preserve the child's residual hearing. Families will have access to a pediatric audiologist and well-trained early interventionists, teachers of the deaf, and speech-language pathologists. Through distance service-delivery models—such as telepractice—parents will no longer have to drive hours for weekly intervention or habilitation, because they will get real time feedback about their child's communication development. These diagnostic sessions will modify and reformulate intervention providers, service frequency, and shared goal setting.

TYPICAL DOMAINS OF ASSESSMENT IN CHILDREN WITH HEARING LOSS

As stated by Shipley and McAfee (2009), assessment is the process of collecting valid and reliable information, integrating it, and interpreting it to make a judgment or decision about communicative behaviors of interest. Assessments usually lead to a diagnosis, greater confirmation about a child's present level of performance, the presence or absence of delays or disorders, and the assignment of a diagnostic category.

For an assessment to be meaningful and useful, it must have foundational integrity. This integrity may be ensured if each assessment adheres to these five principals (Shipley & McAfee, 2009):

■ *A good assessment is thorough.* It should incorporate as much relevant information as possible so that an accurate diagnosis and appropriate recommendations can be made.

■ *A good assessment uses a variety of assessment modalities.* It should include a combination of interview and case history information, formal and informal testing, and client observation.

■ *A good assessment is valid.* It should truly evaluate the intended skills.

■ *A good assessment is reliable.* It should accurately reflect the client's communicative abilities and disabilities. Repeated evaluations of the same client should yield similar findings, provided there has been no change in the client's status.

■ *A good assessment is tailored to the individual client.* Assessment materials that are appropriate for the child's age, gender, skill levels, and ethnocultural background should be used.

Hearing is crucial for the acquisition of spoken language. For a child suspected of demonstrating a hearing loss, a thorough assessment that targets the child's abilities across multiple communication domains will be vital to accurately measure the present level of performance, diagnose any communication delays or disorders, render a prognosis, and plan for appropriate treatment, intervention, or habilitation. Those domains are as follows:

Hearing

The assessment of hearing falls within the scope of practice of the pediatric audiologist. The audiologist assesses the hearing function and quantifies the hearing loss, if one is present. Depending on the age of the child, the audiologist will use a range of instrumentation and test batteries.

Speech

The speech-language pathologist typically assesses a child's speech production in the areas of articulation and phonology. The speech assessment describes the articulatory or phonological development and status of the child. The assessment: (a) determines whether the child's speech sufficiently deviates from normal expectations to warrant concern or intervention, (b) identifies factors that relate to the presence or maintenance of the speech disorder, (c) determines the direction of treatment, (d) makes prognostic judgments about change with and without intervention, and (e) monitors changes in articulatory or phonological abilities and performance across time (Shipley & McAfee, 2009).

Language

Assessing the receptive and expressive language abilities of children with hearing loss is not complete without fully evaluating the child's present level of performance in the following areas (Shipley & McAfee, 2009):

- **Semantics:** the meaning of language;
- **Syntactic:** the rules governing grammatical constellation of language units;
- **Morphologic:** units of meaning;
  - **Free morphemes:** units that can stand along (most words);
  - **Bound morphemes:** units that cannot stand alone; they must be attached to a **free morpheme** (e.g., pre-, -ing);
- **Pragmatic:** the social aspects of language (e.g., eye contact, turn-taking); and
- **Phonologic:** speech sounds, sound patterns, and rules of sound organization.

Listening/Functional Speech Perception

While the audiologist may evaluate the child's use of hearing technology within the sound booth by administering a battery of speech perception measures, other measures of audition and how the child is responding auditorily to environmental sounds as well as speech should be assessed. These measures help determine whether a child is benefitting from specific hearing technology or whether modifications to the current technology strategy should occur. Also, tracking functional speech perception over time determines whether alternative amplification needs exist (e.g., whether the child should be referred for an evaluation for cochlear implantation).

Cognition/Psychoeducational

Usually given by a school psychologist, the psychoeducational assessment provides estimates of the child's intellectual or cognitive abilities and educational achievement levels. It also yields recommendations relevant for educational planning. Sources of assessment data include background information, educational history and records, and results from tests of intelligence and educational achievement. In addition, rating tests of attention, behavior/emotions, and adaptive behavior also may be included in the assessment.

Literacy

The assessment is used to determine the presence of any reading or written language deficits. Children with oral language deficits are at high risk of developing written language deficits in their school years. Early identification and remediation of deficits in oral language, **phonological awareness**, print awareness, and **metalinguistics** can significantly increase the child's potential for academic success later in life (Shipley & McAfee, 2009).

CONCLUSION

Assessment is a critical first step in determining the communicative and academic needs of children suspected of having hearing deficits. Once the hearing loss has been diagnosed, the full range of assessments—across several domains—will formulate interventions, which also should correlate with the parents' desired outcomes for their child. As more children

with hearing loss are identified earlier —often as newborns—professionals must have the necessary knowledge and skills to assess young children and to deliver family-centered, evidence-based services that are timely, safe, effective and efficient. As these children grow and learn, assessments will remain intertwined with their developmental, communicative, psychosocial, and academic lives. Professionals must remain focused and administer the correct assessments at the appropriate times to diagnose, to ascertain a prognosis, to track performance, or to develop new intervention or habilitation strategies. With appropriate assessment, evidence-based treatment can be delivered, resulting in the best possible outcomes for children with hearing loss. As professionals, this is our ultimate goal and responsibility.

REFERENCES

Acuin, J., Department of Child and Adolescent Health, & Development, & the Team for Prevention of Blindness and Deafness. (2004). *Chronic suppurative otitis media: Burden of illness and management options.* Geneva, Switzerland: World Health Organization. Retrieved from http://www.who.int/pbd/publications/Chronicsuppurativeotitis_media.pdf

American Academy of Family Physicians, American Academy of Otolaryngology-Head & Neck Surgery, & American Academy of Pediatrics Subcommittee on Otitis Media With Effusion (AAFP, AAO, AAP). (2004). Otitis media with effusion. *Pediatrics, 113*(5), 1412–1429.

American Academy of Pediatrics. (1999). Task Force on Newborn and Hearing. Newborn and infant hearing loss: Detection and intervention. *Pediatrics, 103*(2), 527–530.

American Academy of Pediatrics (AAP). (2007). Joint committee on infant hearing. Year 2007 position statement: Principles and guidelines for early hearing detection and intervention programs. *Pediatrics, 120*(4), 898–921.

American Speech-Language-Hearing Association (ASHA). (2014). *Professional issues: Newborn infant hearing screening.* Retrieved from http://www.asha.org/PRPSpecificTopic.aspx?folderid=8589935234&section=Key_Issues

Assessment. (n.d.). In *Merriam-Webster's online dictionary.* Retrieved from http://www.merriam-webster.com/dictionary/assessment

Barton, G. R., Stacey, P. C., Fortnum, H. M., & Summerfield, A. Q. (2006). Hearing-impaired children in the United Kingdom, IV: Cost-effectiveness of pediatric cochlear implantation. *Ear and Hearing, 27*(5), 575–588.

Berwick, D. M., & Hackbarth, A. D. (2012). Eliminating waste in U.S. health care. *Journal of the American Medical Association, 307*(14), 1513–1516. doi:10.1001/jama.2012.362

Bess, F. H., Dodd-Murphy, J., & Parker, R. A. (1998). Children with minimal sensorineural hearing loss: Prevalence, educational performance, and functional status. *Ear and Hearing, 19*(5), 339–354.

Bess, F. H., & Paradise, J. (1994). Universal screenings for hearing impairment: Not so simple, not risk free, not necessarily beneficial and not presently justified. *Pediatrics, 93*(2), 330–334.

Blanchfield, B. B., Feldman, J. J., Dunbar, J. L., & Gardner, E. N. (2001). The severely to profound hearing-impaired population in the United States: Prevalence estimates and demographics. *Journal of the American Academy of Audiology, 12*(4), 183–189.

Bond, M., Mealing, S., Anderson, R., Elston, J., Weiner, G., Taylor, R. S., . . . Stein, K. (2009). The effectiveness and cost-effectiveness of cochlear implants for severe to profound deafness in children and adults: A systematic review and economic model. *Health Technology Assessment, 13*(44), 1–330.

Bradham, T. S., & Houston, K. T. (2011). Future directions for EHDI programs: Recommendations from a strategic analysis. *The Volta Review, 111*(2), 281–288.

Burk, P., Burns, J., Earley, D., & Gatzemeyer, M. (2009). *Oklahoma follow-up: Changing 1-3-6 months to 1-3-6 weeks.* 8th Annual National EHDI Meeting Presentation, Dallas, TX.

Calderon, R., & Low, S. (1998). Early social-emotional, language, and academic development in children with hearing loss: Families with and without fathers. *American Annals of the Deaf, 143*(3), 225–234.

Carney, A., & Moeller, M. P. (1998). Treatment efficacy: Hearing loss in children. *Journal of Speech and Hearing Research, 41*, S61–S84.

Centers for Disease Control and Prevention (CDC). (2012). *Documented status of infants not passing hearing screening United States, 2007–2010.* Retrieved from http://www.cdc.gov/ncbddd/hearingloss/2010-data/ehdi_lfu_2007_2010.pdf

Centers for Disease Control and Prevention (CDC). (2014). *Annual data early hearing detection and intervention (EHDI) program.* Retrieved from http://www.cdc.gov/ncbddd/hearingloss/ehdi-data.html

Davis, J. (Ed.). (1990). *Our forgotten children: Hard-of-hearing pupils in the schools.* Washington, DC: U.S. Department of Education.

Davis, J. M., Elfenbein, J. L., Schum, R. L., & Bentler, R. A. (1986). Effects of mild and moderate hearing impairments on language, educational, and psychosocial behavior of children. *Journal of Speech and Hearing Disorders 51*(1), 53–62.

Francis, H., Koch, M., Wyatt, J., & Niparko, J. (1999). Trends in educational placement and cost-benefit considerations in children with cochlear implants. *Archives of Otolaryngology-Head and Neck Surgery, 125*(5), 499–505.

Geers, A. E., Strube, M. J., Tobey, E. A., Pisoni, D. B., & Moog, J. S. (2011). Epilogue: Factors contributing to long-term outcomes of cochlear implantation in early childhood. *Ear and Hearing, 32*(Suppl. 1), 84S–92S. doi:10.1097/AUD.0b013e3181ffd5b5

Greenberg, M., Calderon, R., & Kusche, C. (1984). Early intervention using simultaneous communication with deaf infants: The effect on communication development. *Child Development, 55*(2), 607–616.

Honeycutt, A., Grosse, S., Dunlap, L., Schendel, D., Chen, H., Brann, E., & Homsi, G. (2003). Economic costs of mental retardation, cerebral palsy, hearing loss, and vision impairment. *Research in Social Science and Disability, 3*, 207–228.

Institute of Medicine (IOM). (2001). *Crossing the quality chasm: A new health system for the 21st century.* Washington, DC: National Academy Press. Retrieved from http://www.iom.edu/~/media/Files/Report%20Files/2001/

Crossing-the-Quality-Chasm/Quality%20 Chasm%202001%20%20report%20brief.pdf

Johnson, J. L., Mauk, G. W., Takekawa, K. M., Simon, P. R., Sia, C. C. J., & Blackwell, P. M. (1993). Implementing a statewide system of services for infants and toddlers with hearing disabilities. *Seminars in Hearing, 14*(1), 105–119.

Joint Committee on Infant Hearing (JCIH). (1994). Position statement. *American Speech-Language-Hearing Association (ASHA), 36,* 38–41.

Joint Committee on Infant Hearing (JCIH). (2000). Year 2000 position statement: Principles and guidelines for early hearing detection and intervention programs. *American Journal of Audiology, 9,* 9–29.

Joint Committee on Infant Hearing (JCIH), Muse, C., Harrison, J., Yoshingaga-Itano, C., Grimes, A., Brookhouser, P. E., . . . Martin, B. (2013). Supplement to the JCIH 2007 position statement: Principles and guidelines for early intervention after confirmation that a child is deaf or hard of hearing. *Pediatrics, 131*(4), e1324–e1349.

Klein, J. O. (1989). Epidemiology of otitis media. *Pediatric Infectious Diseases Journal, 8*(S1), S9.

Koop, C. E. (1993). We can identify children with hearing impairment before their first birthday. *Seminars in Hearing, 14*(1), Foreword.

Koop, C. E. (2010). Foreword: Pursuing excellence in early hearing detection and intervention programs. *Pediatrics, 126*(Suppl. 1), S1–S2.

Mausner, J. S., & Kramer, S. (1985). *Epidemiology: An introductory text.* Philadelphia, PA: W. B. Saunders.

Moeller, M. P. (2000). Early intervention and language development in children who are deaf and hard of hearing. *Pediatrics, 106*(3), E43. Retrieved from http://www.pediatrics.org/ cgi/content/full/106/3/e43

Moeller, M. P., Tomblin, J. B., Yoshinaga-Itano, C., Connor, C. M., & Jerger, S. (2007). Current state of knowledge: Language and literacy of children with hearing impairment. *Ear and Hearing, 28*(6), 740–753.

Mohr, P. E., Feldman, J. J., & Dunbar, J. L. (2000). The societal costs of severe to profound hearing loss in the United States. *International Journal of Technology Assessment in Health Care, 16*(4), 1120–1135.

National Center for Hearing Assessment and Management (NCHAM). (2010). Position state-ments. Retrieved from http://infanthearing .org/resources_home/positionstatements/ index.html

National Institute of Health (NIH). (March 1–3, 1993). Early identification of hearing impairment in infants and young children. *NIH Consensus Statement, 11*(1), 1–24. Retrieved from http://consensus.nih.gov/1993/1993Hearing InfantsChildren092html.htm

National Institute on Deafness and Other Communication Disorders [NIDCD]. (1997). *Recommendations of the NIDCD working group on early identification of hearing impairment on acceptable protocols for use in state-wide universal newborn hearing screening programs* [Document developed as part of the NIDCD workshop on universal newborn hearing screening]. Chevy Chase, MD: Author.

Northern, J. L., & Downs, M. (2002). *Hearing in children.* Baltimore, MD: Lippincott Williams & Wilkins.

Ramkalawan, T., & Davis, A. C. (1992). The effect of age of intervention and hearing loss on some language metrics in young hearing-impaired children. *British Journal of Audiology, 26,* 97–109.

Russ, S. A., White, K., Dougherty, D., & Forsman, I. (2010). Preface: Newborn hearing screening in the United States: Historical perspective and future directions. *Pediatrics, 126*(S1), S3–S6. doi:10.1542/peds.2010-0354D

Shipley, K. G., & McAfee, J. G. (2009) *Assessment in speech-language pathology: A resource manual* (4th ed.). Clifton Park, NY: Delmar Cengage Learning.

Sininger, Y. S., Grimes, A., & Christensen, E. (2010). Auditory development in early amplified children: Factors influencing auditory-based communication outcomes in children with hearing loss. *Ear and Hearing, 31*(2), 166–185.

Smith, R. J. H., Kochhar, A., & Friedman, R. A. (2009). Hereditary hearing impairment. In J. B. Snow, Jr. & P. A. Wackym (Eds.), *Ballenger's otorhinolaryngology-head and neck surgery* (17th ed., pp. 289–303). Shelton, CT: B. C. Decker.

Stool, S. E., Berg, A. O., Berman, S., Carney, C. J., Cooley, J. R., Culpepper, L., . . . Sisk, J. E. (1994). Managing otitis media with effusion in young children. Quick reference guide for clinicians. *AHCPR Publication 94-0623.* Rockville, MD: Agency for Health

Care Policy and Research, Public Health Service, U.S. Department of Health and Human Services.

U.S. Department of Health and Human Services, Office of Disease Prevention and Health Promotion. (1991). *Healthy People 2000: National health promotion and disease prevention objectives*. Washington, DC: U.S. Government Printing Office. Retrieved from http://odphp.osophs.dhhs.gov/pubs/hp2000/hppub97.htm

U.S. Preventive Services Task Force. (2008). *Universal screening for hearing loss in newborns: U.S. Preventive Services Task Force Recommendation Statement* [AHRQ Publication No. 08-05117-EF-2]. Retrieved from http://www.uspreventiveservicestaskforce.org/uspstf08/newbornhear/newbhearrs.htm

van Zon, A., van der Heijden, G. J., van Dongen, T. M., Burton, M. J., & Schilder, A. G. (2012). Antibiotics for otitis media with effusion in children [Review]. *Cochrane Database System Review, 9*, CD009163.

Wake, M., Hughes, E. K., Collins, C. M., & Poulakis, Z. (2004). Parent-reported health-related quality of life in children with congenital hearing loss: A population study. *Ambulatory Pediatrics, 4*(5), 411–417.

White, K. R. (2004). Early hearing detection and intervention programs: Opportunities for genetic services. *American Journal of Medical Genetics, 130A,* 29–36.

White, K. R., & Blaiser, K. M. (2011). Strategic planning to improve EHDI programs. *The Volta Review, 111*(2), 83–108.

White, K. R., Forsman, I., Eichwald, J., & Munoz, K. (2010). The evolution of early hearing detection and intervention programs in the United States. *Seminars in Perinatology, 34*(2), 170–179.

World Health Organization (WHO). (1995). *Prevention of hearing impairment. Resolution of the 48th World Health Assembly, WHA, 48(9).* Geneva, Switzerland: Author. Retrieved from http://www.who.int/pbd/publications/wha_eb/wha48_9/en/

World Health Organization (WHO). (2014). *Deafness and hearing loss fact sheet.* Retrieved from http://www.who.int/mediacentre/factsheets/fs300/en/

Yoshinaga-Itano, C., Baca, R. L., & Sedey, A. L. (2010). Describing the trajectory of language development in the presence of severe to profound hearing loss: A closer look at children with cochlear implants versus hearing aids. *Otology & Neurotology, 31*(8), 1268–1274.

Yoshinaga-Itano, C., Sedey, A., Coulter, D. K., & Mehl, A. L. (1998). Language of early and later identified children with hearing loss. *Pediatrics, 102*(5), 161–1171.

CHAPTER 2

Assessment Tools: Evaluating Our Measurements

Stephen Camarata, Hope Lancaster, and Dana Kan

KEY POINTS

- This chapter covers standardized and norm referenced tests, criterion referenced tests, reliability, validity, and questionnaires.
- This chapter helps the reader understand how to select a test that assesses what is needed based on the child's abilities at that time.

INTRODUCTION

Teachers and clinicians are best able to meet the needs of their students when an accurate assessment of that child's abilities has been completed. Although this would seem to be a rather straightforward endeavor, in reality there are many factors that must be considered. The topic of this book, assessing listening and spoken language in children with hearing loss, illustrates this point. From the outset, the clinician must be mindful of the impact that reduced auditory abilities may have on their child's performance. Stated simply, to what extent does the child's hearing level confound my results? What things should I be testing and what do the scores mean? Each of these issues is addressed in this chapter.

Sadly, there has been a tragic history of misdiagnosing people with hearing loss with other kinds of disabilities, such as low intellectual functioning, because of a misunderstanding of the impact of the hearing loss on testing. Although this problem has long been known (Grinker et al., 1969) aspects are still challenging (Camarata, 2013) even though misdiagnoses as intellectually disabled are much rarer (Carvill, 2001). Because of this, the chapter will include fundamental aspects of test properties, known as **psychometrics** and will also include a section on how to interpret these kinds of tests that may not have been developed for people who are deaf or hard of hearing. The final section will also include a way of linking information from speech and language testing to cognitive and achievement testing as well, which is of particular importance for teachers and clinicians serving children who are deaf or hard of hearing in school or other educational settings.

The science of psychometrics has a venerable history; intelligence testing for example has been employed for more than 100 years following its origins in France under the research of Binet (Binet & Simon, 1916). The intelligence test arising from this original research is currently in its fifth edition (Roid, 2003) and is still widely used today, including on children with hearing loss. Since the original efforts to measure mental abilities, there has been a plethora of instruments designed to measure intelligence as well as specific skills including speech and language. However, early errors in testing in children with disabilities such as hearing loss as well as other inaccurate assessments resulted in the development of scientific principles to evaluate the accuracy of these tests. This science of test development is called psychometrics, and specific principles to evaluate each kind of test have been developed (Nunnally, 1978; Salvia, Ysseldyke, & Bolt, 2009). Because these principles are crucial for any kind of psychological or educational testing, including speech and language testing, a description of these principles is provided.

PSYCHOMETRICS OF ASSESSMENT

Reliability

There are a number of foundational elements that every assessment should include in the examiner manual or test information. Foremost among these is **reliability**. This is the ability to repeat or replicate the measures included in the test. If someone else tests the same child a few days later, will the same results be observed? If two different examiners give the same test to the child, will the results be the same? These are but two of the kinds of reliability that are crucial for teachers and clinicians to properly interpret testing outcomes.

Stated simply, reliability measures the precision of the assessment tool. If a microscope is out of focus, it will be difficult to accurately measure an amoeba or other single-celled creature, because the image will be blurry. In the same way, if a test result is not repeated across observers, or even worse, within the same observer, then that skill is being measured with a fuzzy microscope. The test manual will include a section on reliability. It is worthwhile to carefully review the reliability information to determine exactly how fuzzy this test is with the students being tested. There is some common sense involved. For example, toddlers and preschool children generally are much more inconsistent in their behavior than older students, so it is not surprising that the replicability of the test may be lower in younger children even when it is a very good test. Also, if a test has fairly stringent administration guidelines, it will be more repeatable than a test with less specific guidelines.

The domains, however, being tested may require less specific materials and instructions. For example, autism assessments need to be conducted in "real life" social situations, which by nature are a bit open-ended. So, the test requirements may include interview questions that allow the child latitude in his or her responses. In contrast, a receptive vocabulary test may require that the examiner say a single word or the child simply point to a picture from an array of three or four choices. One can imagine that the reliability for the vocabulary test will be much higher than for the autism interview but that pointing to a picture would not be a good assessment platform for diagnosing autism. It is important always to bear in mind the purpose of the assessment and the age of the participants when judging whether or not a test has sufficient reliability.

Correlation and Percent Agreement

Generally, there are two primary ways that reliability is reported: **correlation** and **percent agreement**. Each of these is a reasonable metric but they serve different purposes. A **correlation coefficient** measures the degree of association between two sets of numbers. For reliability, this translates to the test scores each child received on the test when it was repeated. A correlation coefficient ranges from –1 to 1, with the numbers closest to one indicating a strong association between the two sets of test scores. The negative numbers refer to an inverse relationship: that is as the score on one measure increases, the other decreases. For reliability, a negative correlation is an indication of very poor reliability. As an example of an inverse correlation, consider amount of time watching TV, exercise time, and school performance in high school students. Barr-Anderson, Van Den Berg, Neumark-Sztainer, and Story (2008) reported that adolescents with a TV in their room spent more time watching TV, exercised less, and had poorer school performance. As amount of TV time increased, exercise time decreased. Similarly, as TV time increased, school performance decreased. These are both examples of an inverse correlation where the correlation coefficient is negative. For speech and language tests, clinicians should look for high positive correlation coefficients. This means that the scores from the first administration of the test are strongly associated with the

second administration of the test. In short, the results were stable when repeated. By general convention a correlation of 0.5 is considered fair, a correlation of 0.7 is considered good, and a correlation of 0.8 is considered excellent (Hemphill, 2003).

Another type of reliability score that is sometimes reported is percent agreement. This metric is employed when qualitative aspects of the tests require replicability. For example, in a speech test measuring articulation errors (pronunciation errors), it is important to specify whether the same errors were reported when the test was repeated. Did the score sheet include an /r/ error both times? It is possible for a test to have a high correlation for overall score and have relatively poor percent agreement. In the speech example, if the first administration included the same number of errors as the second administration, but a different pattern of errors, the correlation coefficient would be very high but the percentage agreement would be quite low. In general, tests report correlation coefficients because clinicians are interested in the overall score. But if the error patterns are important, clinicians also should pay attention to the percent agreement for classifying these errors.

Inter–Judge/Intra–Judge Reliability

Inter-judge reliability is defined as the extent to which the test yields the same results when two or more clinicians administer the test. One can imagine that this is a very important measure because what good is a test if different examiners do not get the same results? When test makers generate test normative data, they will usually also evaluate inter-judge reliability by having several judges administer the test. In the reliability section of the test manual, this will usually be reported as a correlation coefficient. Again, a high positive correlation is what should be sought. For most purposes, correlation coefficients should be above 0.8 with correlation coefficients of 0.9 being desirable.

Intra-judge reliability refers to the degree that the same clinician will get the same results when administering the test repeatedly. One can imagine that if the same clinician does not replicate his or her own findings, the test will be of very limited utility. Certainly, percentage agreement measures of reliability should be very high for intra-judge evaluations. Again using the speech example, if a clinician scores the tape for an articulation test and generates error patterns, to what extent does she generate the same error patterns when coming back to that tape a few days later? If that percentage agreement is fairly low, then the test is unreliable. Broadly, a test must have high intra-judge reliability to be useful. It is logical that if an individual reviewer cannot replicate his or her findings, it is unlikely that inter-judge reliability will be acceptable. If the same person cannot repeat observations, how can another clinician repeat those unstable observations?

Standard Error of Measurement

Because test scores are not 100% precise, it is useful to establish a probability range for a score. Pollsters do this when they say that a particular result, such as who will win the next election, has a ± margin of error. In standardized testing, in the space for recording the score in the test record, there is often a **confidence interval** or a range for what this score actually represents. For example, the Woodcock-Johnson Tests of

Achievement, Third Edition (Woodcock, McGrew, & Mather, 2001) printout of the score report includes the "age equivalency" for the child being tested, but the next column includes a range. This range is based on the reliability of that particular test.

The mathematics of this is to multiply the standard deviation of the test by the square root of one minus the reliability coefficient or $[SD * \sqrt{1 - r}]$. For example, if the reliability correlation on a test is 0.84, then $1 - 0.84 = 0.16$ and the square root of this is 0.4. If the test is scaled like a traditional IQ test so that the standard deviation of the test is 15, then the standard error of measure is $15 \times 0.4 = 6$. This means that any standard score on a test is plus or minus 6 points. So, if the score is 84, that means the child's true or real score is somewhere between 78 and 90 on that test. The margin of error is ±6 points.

The concept that any score represents a range rather than a precise number is important because when a test is used to measure progress, the score on the retest must be higher than the range from the margin of error in order to be sure that the child actually made improvement. In the above example, if the child's score moved from an 84 to an 88, this "gain" may have been simply due to chance rather than an actual improvement in his or her performance. Also, if the score declined from 84 to a 79, this may not have reflected a real decline or deterioration in the child's performance; it simply may have been a fuzzy microscope instead. This shows why it is important to use tests that are highly reliable, if possible. What happens when the reliability improves to 0.96? In this case, $1 - 0.96$ equals 0.04 and the square root of 0.04 is 0.2. Now the **standard error of measure** is

0.2 × 15 which is equal to 3. The margin of error has been cut in half so that the range for that same observed score of 84 is now 81 to 87. Now an increased score to 88 is actually evidence that the child actually did gain because it is beyond the margin of error by ±3 points! Clinicians always need to be aware of the reliability of a test in order to understand how precise the scores are and how variable they are and under what conditions.

In addition, the reliability coefficients in the test manual are usually derived from children who do not have hearing loss. One can hypothesize that children with hearing loss may have more variable results that other children, such as those used in the reliability studies. For example, an expressive vocabulary test requires that the test administrator reliably understand the words that the child says as he or she names each picture or photo in the test manual. Because children with hearing loss often have speech/articulation errors, their answers could be less intelligible to examiners. This is turn, could reduce the intra- and inter-judge reliability. One examiner may hear the child's answer as correct, whereas another may not comprehend the answer and mark it as incorrect. Because of this, the reliability estimates published in the manual may be higher than what is actually observed in the field when testing children with hearing loss.

Validity

Validity is defined as the extent to which a test measures what it is designed to assess (Nunnally, 1978). If the test is designed to measure speech, does it actually do this in a way that reflects the child's speaking ability? Does the intelligence test accurately measure a child's ability to learn new information? Does the receptive language test measure comprehension of vocabulary, morphology, and syntax? In short, do the results accurately inform the teacher or clinician regarding the child's abilities in the domains tested?

It should also be noted that high reliability does not necessarily ensure that a test is actually a good one. For example, a clinician could, with the proper instrumentation, measure an 8-year-old's head circumference very accurately. And these measurements would have very high intra-judge and inter-judge reliability. Indeed, the correlation between these measurements would probably approach +1.00! But even with this high reliability, if the purpose of these measurements is to generate an estimate of a child's IQ, the validity of this measure would be very poor. Head circumference, even when measured precisely and reliably, does not accurately assess IQ. For example, Gale, O'Callaghan, Bredow, and Martyn, (2006) reported that the association between head circumference and IQ was quite low in 8-year-olds.

Thus, validity is whether the test actually measures the skill or domain that it purports to measure. This is extremely important in hearing-impaired children because tests that normally measure a particular domain may not work as designed in this population. For example, mistakes have been made when a test that purports to measure intelligence but in reality measures receptive language ability is applied to these children because language comprehension skills may be much lower than thinking ability in children with hearing loss. The test is then actually not a valid test of intelligence even though it may have high reliability and validity in children without hearing loss.

Scientists studying test development have conceptualized validity into a number of different domains (Salvia et al., 2009). For the purposes of this chapter, the most relevant are construct, content, and predictive validity. **Construct validity** refers to whether the domain is real. In order to be real, the domain has to both capture the trait being sampled and be independent of another well-established domain. That is the problem with applying verbal IQ tests to populations with limited language abilities (Camarata & Swisher, 1990). In hearing children, verbal ability is a reasonable construct for estimating intelligence. But in children with hearing loss, whose verbal abilities may be attenuated due to the hearing loss rather than due to any general lack of intelligence, verbal IQ can in fact act as a proxy for receptive language ability and therefore an improper "construct" for intelligence.

Another example is auditory processing disorder (APD) or central auditory processing disorder (CAPD) (ASHA, 2005). Although it is certainly true that auditory discrimination, sequencing, and auditory working memory are impaired in a number of clinical populations (including children who are deaf or hard of hearing), it is unclear whether this construct is independent of language abilities (Caccace & McFarland, 1998). That is, because typically developing children show similar deficits in discrimination, sequencing, and auditory working memory, it is unclear whether this is a casual element in the disability. Also, because measures of a well-established construct, language ability, are highly correlated with APD or CAPD test results, the con-

struct validity of this domain is not well established. From a psychometric standpoint, in order to be accepted as a unique domain or construct, the correlation coefficients with other measures of well-established domains, such as language ability, must be relatively low. From a conceptual standpoint, this means that the items on the test are not confounded with language, or another related construct.

And this leads to the concept of **content validity**. This is defined as the extent to which the items on the test actually measure the target domain. The test items or contents should be conceptually and statistically related to the domain. For example, if a test is measuring receptive vocabulary, the test items should all sample this domain. If the test is designed to measure articulation, or speech, then the test should include items that sample a child's ability to pronounce the phonemes in the target language (e.g., English). Test makers evaluate content validity by determining to what extent items or sets of items predict the overall test score. As with construct validity, the test manual should provide evidence that the test in fact has reasonable items that sample the target domain, such as speech and language.

Specificity and Sensitivity

Additional aspects of validity that are of particular importance to clinicians and teachers serving children with hearing loss are **sensitivity** and **specificity**. These aspects refer to the extent that a test that is used for diagnostic purposes actually identifies the diagnostic typology without making mistakes. Sensitivity refers to how well the test identifies those with a particular condition. Specificity refers to whether the test actually separates the condition from other conditions. For example, if universal hearing screening in infants catches a high percentage of children who end up actually having a hearing loss, then this procedure is considered to be highly sensitive to hearing loss. On the other hand, if along with the children who actually have a hearing loss, the universal hearing screening also catches a large number of children who do not have hearing loss, then the test is not very specific.

Another example of high sensitivity with low specificity can be seen in autism. If one uses late talking, that is late onset of words, to screen for autism in two-year-olds, all, or nearly all, would be a hit for autism, but very few would actually have autism (Camarata, 2014). So, the test would catch virtually all children with autism and thus would be highly sensitive. But, because there would also be many false positives, the test would have low specificity (Williams & Brayne, 2006). Tests can also be highly specific and not very sensitive. It should be reasonably clear that for diagnostic purposes clinicians would like for test to be both sensitive and specific.

From a practical standpoint, clinicians testing children with hearing loss should have a firm view of the purpose of the tests being administered. If it is to qualify the student for services in an area associated with the hearing loss, such as autism spectrum disorder, learning disability, intellectual disability, and so on, the sensitivity and specificity of the instrument for children with hearing loss must be considered. Otherwise, there is a high probability the child will be mislabeled, especially if the assessment has high sensitivity and low specificity.

TYPES OF ASSESSMENTS

The level of information that a test provides varies according to the structure of the test. Some tests are relatively narrow in focus and measure a specific domain in great detail. Other tests survey broader domains, or multiple domains, but in less detail. For example, the Structured Photographic Test of Expressive Language (SPELT; Werner & Krescheck, 1983) exclusively provides a detailed examination of grammatical morphology in the expressive language modality. The Woodcock-Johnson Tests of Achievement, on the other hand, tests many aspects of school related skills such as reading, writing, and mathematics. But each of these domains is broadly sampled (Woodcock et al., 2001). Another aspect of test construction is the nature of the standardization and the nature of the information provided by the test. For example, tests can be **norm-referenced** or **criterion referenced**. Each of these procedures can yield useful information for clinicians, and each has strengths and weaknesses that should be considered when interpreting test results.

Norm–Referenced

A test is considered "norm-referenced" if it has been constructed and standardized using a set of "normative" procedures. This means that the test items have been selected so that the results conform to a "normal distribution" or bell-shaped curve in typical populations. Also, the extent to which the test actually fits a "normal" bell-shaped curve is evaluated in the general population. This process, called standardization, includes administering the test to representative samples of children (and adults) selected from the target population. A representative sample means that appropriate age levels, ethnicity, and gender were properly selected and included in the sample. The data from these norming samples are then used to construct the norming tables in the test manual. That is, the test scores are mathematically transformed in the normally distributed test quotients, percentile ranks, and/or age equivalencies in the manual.

Quotients are scaled scores that inform a clinician or teacher how far a child is above or below the "average" level in their age group. Quotients are often reported wherein the mean score is 100 and the standard deviation is 15. A typical range on this scale is often thought to be the mean ± one standard deviation: 85 to 115. A child scoring below 85 would be performing below the typical range and a child with a score above 115 is thought to be performing above average on that test. Often, performance more than two standard deviations below the average is considered evidence of a significant disability. In the case of an intelligence test, scores below 70 (the average of 100 minus 30 which is two times the standard deviation of 15) are interpreted as evidence of a significant intellectual disability.

The standard scores can also be used to calculate a child's percentile rank. Conceptually, this score informs a teacher or clinician about a child's relative standing on a hypothetical group of 100 children at the same age level. For example, a quotient of 100 means that score is at the 50 percentile: the child scored exactly in the middle of the range for her age level. A quotient of 70 is at the 3rd percentile, which means that 97% of the children in the norming sample got a higher score. Age equivalency is an estimate of the child's ability on the test relative to a developmental level. That is, age equivalency tells a clinician or teacher the comparable age performance for that test score. For example, a 40-month-old preschooler may have the expressive vocabulary of a 5-year-old (60 months). This means that the 3½-year-old received a higher score than other children her age and, in fact, received a score that is "average" for a five 5-year-old. In contrast, it is also possible for a child to be developing more slowly that her peers and receive an age equivalency that is below her actual age. For example, a child with hearing loss may have difficulty with auditory comprehension so that at age five (60 months), his ability to understand what others say is more like what is seen in 3½-year-olds (40 months).

When using age equivalencies, caution is advised since they are general estimates and not precise. Furthermore, age equivalencies can be misleading when used improperly due to reliability (margin of error) and the inherent test score variability at each age level. For example, a 6-year-old child receiving a quotient of 92 on a test, which is solidly in the normal range, could be six months or even a full year "behind" based on age equivalency if there is high variability around the median score in the 6-year-old standardization sample. Stated directly, age equivalencies are based on the average score at a particular age level and do not take into account where the children at that age level are highly variable in their performance. Although teachers and parents appear to prefer age equivalencies as an estimate of a child's skill level, it is important to understand, and to communicate to teachers and parents, that these scores are not precise (Salvia et al., 2009) and should not be used when determining eligibility for services.

Broadly, norm-referenced tests are useful for comparing a child performance to that of other children at the same grade level or at the same age level. These tests allow a clinician or teacher to gain insight into how well a particular child performs on a particular set of items relative to the standardization sample. In addition, norm-referenced tests are ideal for comparing relative strengths and weaknesses in an individual child on a variety of tests because all will be scaled the same way. For example, a child's relative standing on mathematical achievement can be compared to his or her relative standing on writing ability, reading achievement and so on. Also, if the achievement test is conormed with a cognitive test, as in the Woodcock-Johnson series of tests (Woodcock et al., 2001), then a child's intellectual abilities can be compared to how well he or she does on school-based achievement tasks.

On the other hand, norm-referenced tests are relatively insensitive to individual learning over time. The reason for this is that the norms are benchmarked at a particular age and that even when a child learns quite a bit in a particular year, this may not be reflected again in the standard score. For example, assume a typically developing child that is average for his or her age and thus gets a quotient, or standard score, of 100. If this child learns about as much as the other children over a year, his or her quotient the next year will be 100 once again. So gain scores in norm-referenced tests reflect how much the child has learned relative to the standardization sample. It is fairly possible that the child learned quite a bit while also

declining in terms of his or her standard score. A practical example may be useful to illustrate this point. The MacArthur scale (MacArthur-Bates Communicative Development Inventories, 2007) provides percentile ranks for expressive vocabulary levels in toddlers. An 18-month-old who says about 9 words on the standardized word set of 36 items will be at the 50th percentile for productive vocabulary on this test. If that same child learns another 10 words on the item list over the next six months, he or she will actually decline to the 25th percentile because the other children in the cohort for the standardization sample learn, on average 12 additional test words (Fenson et al., 2000). The point here is that the standardization sample includes the amount of gain the average child makes so that even when a child has learned quite a great deal, there may be a decrease in his or her standard score, because the other children learn *more* over the same time period. In terms of quotients, the above child would have declined from an initial score of 100 at age 18 months to approximately 89 at age 24 months even though the child learned quite a few words.

Because norm-referenced tests have to be administered in a standardized way, repeated administrations may artificially inflate the scores on the second, third, and fourth administration of the test as the child essentially learns the test items. Test makers try to avoid this problem by issuing different forms such as form A and form B of the Peabody Picture Vocabulary Test (Dunn & Dunn, 2007); the teachers and clinician should be cognizant of the pitfalls of a repeated short-term test administration, nonetheless. Finally, as described above, the reliability coefficient also indicates the magnitude of a gain that can be reliably detected on a particular test. Lower reliability means that observing a real gain on a test requires that: (a) the child gains more than the other children in the normative sample and (b) the gain is sufficient to overcome a test's standard error of measure (margin of error). All of these factors collectively limit the utility of norm-referenced tests for measuring progress in an individual child.

Criterion–Referenced (Questionnaires and Developmental Inventories)

Another kind of approach to testing is to generate "criterion" that are benchmarked at a particular age. For example, most children begin saying their first words at about 12 months of age. So a criterion-referenced instrument—such as a questionnaire used for a parent interview or a developmental inventory (checklist) such as the aforementioned communication development index (MacArthur Inventory, 2007) for measuring expressive vocabulary—would chart the age at which a child said his or her first word. These inventories are referred to as criterion-referenced because they provide specific behaviors or targets that are being surveyed. These often take the form of questionnaires that can be answered by teachers or parents regarding a child's developmental milestones such as sitting up, walking, talking, and so on. Or, they can be employed as standard observational checklists. For example, the Denver Developmental Screening Test is a survey employed by clinicians to assess developmental level in toddlers and preschoolers (Frankenburg, Dodds, Fandal, Kazuk, & Cohrs, 1975).

Criterion-referenced tests—including checklists, developmental inventories, and questionnaires—are particularly useful when specific testing is not possible, for example if the child is too young to actively respond to particular test items, or when seeking information about behaviors that occur in the natural environment such as at home in classrooms which clinicians may have restricted access. The advantage of **criterion-referenced measures** is that they can be used to benchmark progress: a clinician can identify the new behaviors a child has learned. Criterion-referenced measures also are useful for comparing teacher and parent reports of child developmental milestones. A child may provide a completely different profile at home versus at school. An example of a widely used criterion-reference measure is the autism diagnostic observation schedule (ADOS; Lord et al., 2000) wherein a clinician specially trained to look for autism symptoms administers a series of play activities and/or interview questions in order to observe the child's performance in quasi-naturalistic but structured activities. After observing the child in these scenarios, the clinician then rates the child's performance on a series of social and communication criteria, as well as behavioral criteria associated with autism.

Although criterion-referenced measures are quite useful for indexing skills such as expressive vocabulary, play behaviors, social interaction and so on, these are not "norm-referenced" in the same manner as other kinds of standardized test such as traditional intelligence measures. Also, criterion-referenced measures are not normally distributed in the same way as quotients derived from norm-referenced tests. For example, the aforementioned ADOS criteria are useful for distinguishing children with autism from typically developing children and children with global intellectual disabilities; it does not yield quotients, standard scores, or age equivalency scores. Indeed, the criterion measures on this assessment are benchmark to a child's developmental level rather than his or her age level or grade level. The four "modules" correspond to whether a child is nonverbal, just beginning to speak, uses phrase speech or is conversational, regardless of his or her age.

Teachers and clinicians should certainly use criterion-referenced measures in their assessment of children with hearing loss. These measures are particularly useful when they sample a skill set that is predictive of future learning or yields insight into deficit areas that require additional training. Additionally, as with the ADOS or the Denver Developmental Screening Test, it can be used to determine whether a child with hearing loss is learning or meeting the same developmental criteria as other children. On the other hand, one must be cautious in administering these kinds of scales if they have not been employed with children with hearing loss. For example, there are no data available for the ADOS on children with hearing loss and their sense impairment could potentially misleading examiners if they are unfamiliar with the "usual" social and behavioral skills of children with hearing impairment. This is especially true if some of these "typical behaviors" in hearing loss overlap with key markers for autism in children without hearing loss.

For example, in school-age children and adolescents, repetitive rocking and unusual hand movements are markers for autism and are correctly sampled using the ADOS. However, people with severe blindness often display these kinds of movements even when they don't have autism. Because of this, the criterion measure of repetitive rocking and unusual hand movements should not be used to diagnose autism in children who are blind. Similarly, caution must be used when assessing children with hearing loss for conditions such as autism or intellectual disability (Camarata, 2013).

Another example of a criterion-referenced assessment measure is Cottage Acquisition Scales for Listening, Language, and Speech (Wilkes, 1999). In this instrument, the areas evaluated include listening, speech, language and cognition. Each of these content areas is divided into ordered "steps" for scaling a child's performance. A child's abilities place him or her on this scale regardless of age level. These criteria are then used as a teaching sequence in each domain. Normative information is not provided.

SAMPLING

This leads to a discussion of the sampling properties of the test, regardless of whether it is norm-referenced or criterion-referenced. That is, the test manual should describe how the items were developed and who was included in the standardization **sample** for a norm-referenced test or in the comparison sample for a criterion-referenced instrument. A clinician or teacher should review the test manual to determine the age levels of the children included in the standardization sample, the racial makeup of the standardization sample, the demographic characteristics of the sample, as well as gender representation. It should be borne in mind that nearly all tests, regardless of whether they are norm-referenced or criterion-referenced, are developed and "standardized" on typically developing samples. Because of this, these measures are useful in identifying potential "deficit areas" but are of very limited utility for comparing children within a group such as children with hearing loss. Likewise, it is critically important that clinicians and teachers be familiar with the normal traits of the population so that criteria that are different are not mistakenly interpreted incorrectly, and with regard to norm-referenced tests, interpreted with caution if nonstandard administration procedures are needed because of the specific features of the target population.

Also, because standardized test generally include representative "typical" samples from the general population, they may under sample minority populations. For example, representativeness of sampling procedures of previous editions of the Peabody Picture Vocabulary Test has been discussed in the literature (Champion, Hyter, McCabe, & Bland-Stewart, 2003). Practically speaking, this means that in addition to considering the impact of the hearing loss on test results and test interpretation, clinicians and teachers must also consider cultural factors as well. Although it may appear that these caveats render norm-referenced standardized tests and criterion-referenced measures virtually useless with children with hearing loss, in fact, they are highly useful if administered and interpreted properly. That is, criterion-referenced tests will provide insight into a child's developmental level on a variety of practical skills and norm-referenced tests can provide insights into relative performance in children with hearing loss. However, the nature of the sample used to standardize and norm the tests must be reviewed to properly employ these measures.

Another aspect of sampling has to do with test construction. Both criterion-referenced and norm-referenced tests are essentially "samples" of target behaviors thought to yield insights into a child's development. A test of mathematical achievement includes a pool of items selected from the overall construct of mathematical ability. Clearly, a test cannot possibly include every kind of mathematical knowledge taught in schools or that students possess. Rather, a sample of the knowledge base is surveyed in order to estimate an individual child's mathematical knowledge. Because of this, another sampling consideration is whether the items on the test are actually reflective of the domain being assessed in the target population. As an example, "applied problems" includes a combination of mathematical reasoning and, because the items are presented verbally, receptive language ability. In typically developing children, this is not a problem because the items actually sample a child's ability to solve word problems. But, if the child doesn't know English or has a receptive language problem that is sufficiently extensive to limit his or her ability to comprehend the instructions or the questions on the test (which is presented verbally), then this test may not actually be sampling mathematical ability. Again, clinicians and teachers are urged to think through the validity of the test for this population and whether the items are actually sampling the target domain being assessed.

INFORMAL ASSESSMENTS AND DATA COLLECTION

By now it is probably apparent that all standardized test information, regardless of whether it is criterion-referenced or norm-referenced, must be augmented with informal assessments and data collection. These generally take the form of teacher- and/or clinician-constructed assessments. It is to be hoped that these assessments reflect skills that are appropriate for children with hearing loss. For example, a teacher may be interested in how well a student with hearing loss is learning vocabulary words that are specific to a particular reading lesson. The teacher could construct an informal word list from the reading materials and conduct an informal assessment prior to the instruction module in order to determine how much of the vocabulary the child knows. After instruction, this teacher could then use the informal assessment to chart a child's progress on reading vocabulary for this lesson.

Similarly, a standardized test can be augmented with individually constructed informal assessments. A clinician may administer a standardized articulation test such as the Arizona Articulation Proficiency Scale (Fudala & Reynolds, 1986) —which provides norm-referenced information on a child's speech production—to a child with hearing loss. The clinician may wish to augment this with an informal speech assessment of the child's articulation in spontaneous language samples (Shriberg, Austin, Lewis, McSweeny, & Wilson, 1997), or the clinician may wish to sample specific speech sounds in syllable contexts that are not included in the standardized test. The point here is that the clinician can assess articulation skills in a much wider variety of contexts than is provided in the standardized tests and can do so with considerable flexibility when constructing informal sampling contexts.

From a practical standpoint, the standardized assessments should be viewed as a starting point for more in-depth evaluation using informal assessments that shed additional light on an individual child's capabilities, especially in domains or skills that are particularly important for the target population. For example, one could imagine that understanding the extent to which an individual child can use environmental auditory information is important in this population and that this can be sampled individually in the classroom or in other relevant contexts. Naturally, this can take the form of individually constructed informal measures. The key here is that the teacher or clinician must have a clear perspective on what kinds of information are needed to teach this child and, what kinds of individually constructed measures will best capture that child's abilities and chart their learning.

Perhaps the strongest argument for using informal assessments is the need for individualized data collection in order to measure a particular child's progress. For example, a standardized test such as the Peabody Picture Vocabulary Test can provide a norm-referenced look into whether a child's receptive vocabulary is below expected levels relative to the standardization sample. But this test is not sufficiently sensitive to measure whether a particular child is learning a particular set of vocabulary words that the teacher and/or the clinician are targeting. Charting this kind of progress requires construction of an informal assessment that is specific to that child. Generally, clinicians and teachers of children with hearing loss will have to rely upon these kinds of assessments to determine whether a child is learning his or her individual personalized goals. As a matter of accountability, teachers and clinician should be probing and charting progress on a regular basis, such as weekly or biweekly. Data collection of this nature will be directly focused on informal measures of the target domain.

Case History/Parent Interview

Another example of informal measurement is the case history. Generally, a teacher or clinician will benefit from knowing about the child's background. In this case, parents can provide a written summary of their child's developmental history. This can include when a child achieved developmental milestones such as sitting up, walking, and so on; when the hearing loss was first detected; whether it was treated with hearing aids or a cochlear implant or some other intervention; and whether the child has had a significant illness or history of illnesses that may have impacted development. From a testing standpoint, clinicians and teachers should be providing parents with a standard form of the case history so that written information can be elicited.

Often, this information can be augmented with a parent interview wherein a set of standard questions is asked to validate what is written in the case history. In addition, the case history can be reviewed and areas that require additional information can be probed during the interview process. Although these take the form of informal assessments, clinicians will find that standard questions about illnesses and other health information as well as requesting more details about developmental milestones yields helpful additional information. As with any kind of an assessment, whether standardized or informal, a parent interview process benefits from a "game plan" or a predetermined set of interview questions so that the clinician or teacher can guide the interview process and ensure that all the relevant topics are covered during the interview. From a technical standpoint, parent interviews yield criterion-referenced information, but this is even less "standardized" than published criterion-referenced checklist or inventories. Because of this, clinicians and teachers should interpret this information with caution and without bias or judgmental perspectives.

SUGGESTED DOMAINS

Although this may seem to be an intuitive topic, clinicians should be thoughtful about the domains they are going to assess in children with hearing loss and what kind of information is needed to generate a comprehensive view of the child's strengths and weaknesses. The following domains are an essential part of any assessment.

Speech

First and foremost, after the audiologist has completed a thorough hearing evaluation so that a child's hearing status is known, the clinician should assess a child's speech production. This includes articulation of individual speech sounds but should also include estimates of overall intelligibility as well as performance in informal language samples. This will provide an overview of the child's current competence for speech production, errors, as well as an evaluation of how well the child performs in real-life speaking situations. It should be noted that intelligibility is not necessarily the sum total of the articulation errors. Rather, two different children could have the same number of errors with regard to misarticulations, but one child could be much less intelligible then the other due to the nature of the errors. As a simple example, consider the differences in whether a listener could understand a child who only makes one error per word. If this error is a predictable substitution at the ends of words, the child's speech will be much more understandable than if the error is to omit the first consonant from all words. This is because initial consonants have a much higher contribution two overall intelligibility. For example, a child who says "tat" for the word "cat" is much more understandable then a child who says "at" for "cat." Both children got exactly 50% of the consonants in the word *cat* correct, but the nature of the errors changes the intelligibility.

Because of this, the clinician should be cognizant of how intelligible the child is in spontaneous speech and when the clinician is working on improving speech production, should prioritize targets that are both developmentally appropriate and contribute the most acoustic information for intelligibility. It is also important to bear in mind that many children with hearing loss make vowel errors; these are a high priority both because vowels are developmentally earlier than most consonants, and because they contribute dramatically to overall intelligibility. It should be noted that a speech assessment of children with hearing loss should be completed on vowel sounds as well as consonants.

Expressive Language

In addition to speech, the clinician should assess expressive language ability. This includes words (vocabulary); word endings such as plurals, possessives and other grammatical markers (grammatical morphology); as well as sentence production (syntax) (see Camarata, 1992). Examples of standardized tests of these domains include the Clinical Evaluation of Language Fundamentals (CELF; Semel, Wiig, & Secord, 2003), the Test of Language Development (TOLD; Newcomer & Hammill, 2008), Preschool Language Scale (PLS; Zimmerman, Steiner, & Pond, 2002), and the Structured Photographic Elicited Language Test (SPELT; Werner & Kreschek, 1983). As with all testing, the standardized assessments should be augmented with informal assessments such as language sampling and assessment of narrative abilities. It is also important to bear in mind that testing may be impacted and/or require modification based on the child's hearing profile. For example, elicited imitation may be adversely affected by a child's ability to hear word endings such as grammatical morphemes (i.e., contracted auxiliary). If a child can read, it may be useful to validate production by presenting items in the written modality as well as by listening. Clinicians should complete a comprehensive inventory of the child's expressive language skills and think through the intervention plan in light of the child's overall needs. Clearly, because words are the foundation of spoken language, expressive vocabulary should be a high priority.

Receptive Language

The domains that are assessed in the expressive language ability set should also be assessed in terms of listening comprehension. That is, receptive vocabulary, comprehension of grammatical morphemes, and of syntax, including complex sentences should be tested. The aforementioned measures—CELF, TOLD and PLS—include receptive items and the Test of Auditory Comprehension of Language (TACL; Carrow-Woolfolk, 1998), which only tests receptive ability, all can be used to assess receptive language ability. Naturally, a child's ability to understand what is said to him or her is foundational to learning and is a key skill in children with hearing loss. Clinicians may also want to know to what extent the child can perform both with and without visual information. Studies of multisensory processing indicate that visual input improves auditory processing in children without hearing loss. This is also true in children with hearing loss; however, the auditory channel alone is often much worse then in other populations. Because of this, clinicians should think through the functional environments in which the child will be expected to understand spoken language. If the child has access to visual information that is simultaneous with the auditory (i.e., lipreading), performance will improve relative to when the child is unable to have access to visual input. Clinicians should assess language comprehension in both auditory only and in auditory plus visual contexts. Naturally, the same version of a test cannot be administered twice within a certain time period due to reliability and test-retest learning conditions. However, tests with different versions (form A and form B) can be used, such as the Peabody Picture Vocabulary Test (4th ed., Dunn & Dunn, 2007). It is important to review the test instructions to know how often a test can be administered to ensure validity of the measures gathered.

In addition, because language comprehension is the foundation upon which literacy and other forms of achievement rely, these abilities should be a very high priority in any clinical remediation program. Naturally, informal assessments such as vocabulary lists, lists of grammatical morphemes, question forms, and complex syntax should all be included in the assessment as well as in the data collection for progress monitoring. In addition, because conversational skills are directly founded upon receptive language ability, the clinician should consider the relationship between the child's understanding and his or her ability to carry on conversations so that the latter skill can also be targeted as needed.

Literacy

Perhaps because of the long-standing deficits in language acquisition in children with hearing loss, the reading skills of these children have also been relatively poor when compared to children without hearing loss, including those with language disorders (Brisco, Bishop, & Norbury, 2001). This is intriguing because children with hearing loss often receive fairly intensive instruction on phonological awareness as a part of their aural rehabilitation. Of course, reading includes not only the ability to decode the phonemes included in the words as letters, but comprehension as well. So, a child with limited language ability would have poor reading outcomes even if he or she were proficient at spelling and reading decoding such as "sounding out words" or phonics. Naturally, these decoding skills are often weak in children with hearing loss because they may not have sufficient auditory acuity to discriminate individual phonemes or they may not have these phonemes stored in their lexical representations. Stated simply, the phonemic structure of individual words may be problematic for children with hearing loss.

Regardless, it is clear that a comprehensive assessment of a hearing-impaired child should include literacy. Measures of phonics and phonological awareness should be administered as well as tests of reading comprehension. Both domains will yield estimates of overall literacy (Woodcock et al., 2001). Because reading comprehension is a very high priority for children with hearing loss, a thorough assessment of these domains should be completed. As with language assessment, the impact of the child's hearing status also must be taken into consideration when administering and interpreting the results of any standardized test. Also, ample informal criterion-referenced assessments should be completed in order to yield a comprehensive perspective on the child's literacy.

Cognitive Abilities and Achievement

As mentioned previously in this chapter, cognitive ability should be assessed with caution due to potential confounds (see Chapter 7). It is particularly important that in addition to the usual standard assessments (such as the Stanford-Binet, Weschler, or Woodcock-Johnson) the clinician administer estimates of fluid reasoning that are either completely nonverbal or with a very low verbal load so that language ability secondary to hearing loss does not yield an underestimate of the child's thinking abilities. It is also important that clinicians be aware that multiple broad abilities are needed to yield a fair estimate of the child's thinking ability.

In order to consider the implications of hearing impairment on cognitive abili-

ties and achievement, it is important to determine how cognitive abilities and achievement are modeled and tested, as a means of then reviewing potential impacts. The starting point for this analysis is the speech and language abilities of children with hearing loss, which of course, is the primary ramification of having reduced speech and language input into the developing brain.

Although such a view properly focuses on the primary weaknesses associated with hearing loss (speech and language), there may be advantages to taking a more comprehensive view of psychoeducational testing in this population. Moreover, it is not surprising that speech and language-learning problems can also be associated with other learning that relies on linguistic competence. For example, because reading is, essentially, decoding and comprehending language information represented using text rather than verbal communication (Hulme & Snowling, 2013), children with hearing loss are often at risk for reading disabilities as well. Similarly, there has also been an effort to understand any relative weaknesses in cognitive abilities that are associated with speech and language-learning deficits. For example, researchers have long hypothesized that speech and language disorders are associated with a relative weakness in auditory processing abilities. But, more broadly, there is a general sense that thinking abilities are relatively independent of speech and language abilities in hearing impairment.

This view perhaps arises from a two-factor model of intellectual ability, with cognitive skills grossly being classified as verbal and performance, with any weaknesses in cognitive abilities being limited to the verbal domain in children with hearing impairment. Using this view, performance intelligence is preserved, whereas verbal intelligence may be lower and commensurate with the poor speech and language skills (Camarata & Swisher, 1990). But, more recent models of general intellectual abilities include more than two factors. For example, Cattell-Horn-Carroll theory (CHC theory; Carroll, 1993; Horn, 1988) includes nine broad abilities that contribute to estimates of overall intellectual ability. Although this model has been available for more than two decades (Carroll, 1993), studies of cognitive abilities are primarily based on two factor analyses of intellectual abilities in the field of speech and language disorders (Tomblin et al., 1997).

CHC Theory: Broad and Narrow Abilities

It may be useful to provide a brief review of Cattell-Horn-Carroll (CHC) theory as a prelude to using the WJ Tests of Cognitive Abilities and Achievement to examine cognitive abilities and achievement in children with hearing loss (Table 2–1). In this model, the goal of cognitive testing is to estimate an individual's General Intellectual Ability (abbreviated as GIA or simply as *g*). General Intellectual Ability is hypothesized to consist of nine broad intellectual abilities that ultimately relate to general cognitive level. These nine broad abilities include fluid reasoning (Gf), visual spatial reasoning (Gv), processing speed (Gs), auditory processing (Ga), short-term memory (Gsm), long-term retrieval (Glr), comprehension knowledge (Gc), quantitative skills (Gq) and reading and writing ability (Grw). These latter two skills, Gq and Grw, are commonly examined using achievement tests rather than tests of cognitive abilities. The following brief descriptions of each of these broad abilities may be helpful.

Fluid reasoning is the ability to generate inferences from known information. For example, a classic fluid reasoning task is to predict what comes next in a series. That is, the first few items in a series are presented and the individual is asked to then provide the next item in the series. Visual spatial reasoning is defined as the ability to integrate and interpret visual information. Processing speed is a measure of the "cognitive clock," or the efficiency one can quickly and accurately complete items of moderate difficulty. Auditory processing within CHC theory is analogous to visual spatial ability and not the more narrow forms of auditory processing sometimes studied in language disorders (Tallal, 1990). Rather, auditory processing is viewed as the ability to rapidly and efficiently decode, encode, and mentally operate on auditory information. Short-term memory is a measure of the ability to quickly store and retrieve information (within a few seconds), whereas long-term retrieval reflects this retrieval ability over a much longer time period. Comprehension knowledge is defined as the depth and breadth of knowledge including verbal communication, information, and reasoning related to stored information and verbal abilities. Quantitative skills are precisely what the name implies: the ability to comprehend quantitative concepts and relationships and the facility to manipulate numerical symbols. Finally, reading and writing ability includes basic reading and writing skills and the associated skills needed to decode and interpret text.

Estimates for these broad abilities are generated using tests of narrow abilities. For example, the broad cognitive ability of auditory processing (Ga) can be estimated by having an individual integrate a series of individual sounds into words (Sound

Table 2–1. Nine CHC Broad Abilities

Broad Ability	Acronym	Description
Stores of Acquired Knowledge		
Comprehension Knowledge	*Gc*	Breadth and depth of knowledge including verbal communication, information, and reasoning when using previously learned procedures.
Quantitative Ability	*Gq*	Ability to comprehend quantitative concepts and relationships, the facility to manipulate numerical symbols.
Reading–Writing	*Grw*	An ability associated with both reading and writing, probably including basic reading and writing skills and the skills required for comprehension/expression.
Thinking Abilities		
Long-Term Retrieval	*Glr*	Ability to efficiently store information and retrieve it later, often through association.
Visual-Spatial Thinking	*Gv*	Spatial orientation and the ability to analyze and synthesize visual stimuli. The ability to hold and manipulate mental images.
Auditory Processing	*Ga*	Ability to discriminate, analyze, and synthesize auditory stimuli. Includes phonological awareness.
Fluid Reasoning	*Gf*	Ability to reason, form concepts, and solve problems that often Involve unfamiliar information or procedures. Manifested in the reorganization, transformation, and extrapolation of information.
Cognitive Efficiency		
Processing Speed	*Gs*	Ability to rapidly perform automatic or simple cognitive tasks.
Short-Term Memory	*Gsm*	Ability to hold information in immediate awareness and use it within a few seconds. Includes working memory.

Source: Adapted from Camarata and Woodcock, 2006. Used with permission.

Blending on the WJ III), mentally "fill in" a missing phoneme to identify a word (Incomplete Words on the WJ III) or identify patterns in speech or in music (Sound Patterns-Voice and Sound Patterns-Music in the WJ III) are narrow abilities related to overall (broad) auditory processing ability. Clearly, these cognitive "narrow abilities" for auditory processing are of high importance for measuring abilities in children with hearing impairment. Narrow abilities in the achievement area of quantitative knowledge (Gq) can include math

computation, which is the ability to solve numeric problems; math fluency, which is the ability to solve math problems of moderate difficulty rapidly and accurately; and applied problems, which is the ability to solve problems presented verbally.

These are included in the WJ III as Calculation, Math Fluency, and Applied Problems respectively. All broad cognitive abilities are sampled using sets of narrow abilities shown to relate to these broad abilities. In this way, a comprehensive view of cognitive abilities will include multiple estimates using narrow abilities to sample each broad ability. Such an approach for assessing cognitive abilities (and achievement) provides important advantages over applying a two-factor approach to investigating the relationship between language disorders and potentially related aspects of cognitive ability and achievement. Figure 2–1 includes a depiction of the relationship between a broad ability (Reading), associated narrow abilities, and the WJ III tests associated with these narrow abilities.

The Woodcock-Johnson Tests of Cognitive Abilities and Tests of Achievement are constructed to examine the broad abilities contributing to overall intellectual ability (GIA) and key aspects of achievement. Although language disorders will probably include a number of abilities that are at relatively typical levels of performance, using the Woodcock-Johnson will permit study of relative strength and weakness across and within broad abilities to yield additional information beyond a two-factor model or models

of specific narrow deficit (such as poor discrimination of formant transitions in auditory processing).

Broad and Narrow Abilities—CHC Theory and Links to Achievement (Gq and Grw)

A comprehensive, conormed instrument is required to simultaneously examine cognitive and achievement and to validly assess patterns of relative strengths and weakness in these areas. In addition, the assessment battery must accurately sample the domains under consideration. The WJ series of tests were specifically developed using CHC theory to construct tests that sample relevant narrow abilities to estimate each subject's relative performance on the broader cognitive or achievement domain being assessed. For example, the broad ability of auditory processing (Ga) is sampled using the narrow abilities of Incomplete Words, Auditory Attention, Sound Patterns Voice, Sound Patterns Music, and Sound Blending. These five narrow abilities can then be

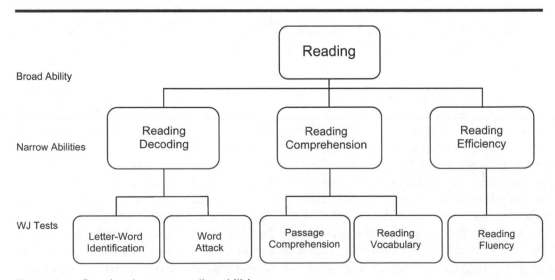

Figure 2–1. Broad and narrow reading abilities.

used to estimate overall auditory processing ability (Ga). It should be noted that best practice includes using at least two narrow abilities to estimate performance on broad ability. Thus, the first binder in WJ III tests of cognitive abilities includes Sound Blending and Incomplete Words as two narrow abilities that estimate broader Ga. In this way, performance on more than one narrow abilities test can contribute to a broader estimate of an individual's overall cognitive performance.

Teachers and clinicians can then examine achievement in light of the results from the cognitive testing. Academic skills such as mathematics, reading, and writing can be evaluated in order to identify patterns of strengths and weaknesses and to construct a relevant curriculum for that child. Although a speech language pathologist or deaf educator may requests that a school psychologist or other clinician administer the cognitive and achievement tests, it is important that the teacher and the clinician work together to gain a fuller understanding of the implications of the test results.

INTERPRETING AND INTEGRATING TESTING RESULTS

The product of all this testing should be an individual comprehensive view of the child with hearing loss. His or her speech and language abilities, literacy, cognitive abilities, hearing profile, and academic skills (achievement) should all be evaluated with norm-referenced, criterion-referenced and informal assessments in order to identify and prioritize instructional goals. At the very foundation should be language and literacy skills

as these provide access to educational and later on, employment opportunities. In addition, language skills are the very foundation of the child's development. It is also vitally important that a reasonably accurate assessment of the child's cognitive abilities be completed. On the one hand, it is all too easy to underestimate a child's thinking abilities and academic potential if an improper assessment has been completed; on the other hand, if a child does have intellectual disabilities or other cognitive limitations, this is also important information for instructional planning. In general, no clinician or teacher should assume that the child is incapable of learning and should employ criterion-referenced and data-driven informal assessments to benchmark the speed of learning for targets during intervention. This in turn will yield more accurate assessments of the child's ability to learn new material particularly in different modalities such visual and listening.

In addition, this kind of multifactual interpretation of the child's test information will identify patterns of strengths and weaknesses that are extremely useful in intervention and in teaching. For example, if a child's literacy decoding skills are much stronger than his or her reading comprehension, this would suggest that instruction should focus on reading comprehension until it comes up to the same level as the phonemic awareness abilities. Similarly, no clinician should assume that teaching reading decoding will automatically generate generalized reading comprehension: both domains should be taught, and looking at the relative strengths and weaknesses will inform the teacher and clinician as to the priority for the child at any particular point in development.

Similarly, if the testing indicates that auditory processing is a relative weakness while visual spatial thinking is a relative strength, the teacher and clinician should consider how visual supports can be integrated with auditory cues. Of course, this is precisely what happens in lip-reading where the visual information augments the understanding the articulation process and supports listening comprehension. But this can also be useful for other kinds of instruction. The visual domain may prime the auditory domain. And, instructional situations that require high levels of listening comprehension may be less effective then auditory plus visual or using visual priming as a way of preparing the child for the verbal instructions. That is, providing written instructions if a child knows how to read can prime upcoming auditory information. These are but a few examples of how skilled clinicians and teachers can "connect the dots" for an individual child to tailor intervention and instruction to the nuances of their individual profile. This will also allow for predicting speed of learning and provide a means for charting progress.

SUMMARY

The purpose of this chapter is to provide an orientation to assessment in children with hearing loss. The information herein is crucial for administering, interpreting, and using testing data as a means of diagnosing concomitant conditions and for constructing effective intervention and instructional programs for these children. The various levels of testing were discussed and described, including norm-referenced, criterion-referenced, and informal assessments, as well as examples of when these types of assessments can be used. In addition, clinicians and teachers should use multiple sources of information when evaluating and teaching children with hearing loss.

Factors such as the validity and reliability of the assessments, the standardization samples, and the adaptations of these measures to the particular aspects of hearing loss that may impact administration and interpretation of these tests, were described. In addition, this chapter included a discussion of the specific domains that should be assessed in order to provide a comprehensive and accurate view of the cognitive, academic, and speech and language abilities of these children. Finally, ways that these different strands of information can be woven into a proper interpretation to guide instruction and intervention were provided. In general, clinicians and teachers should not blindly administer tests without considering the strengths and weaknesses of these assessments for the hearing-impaired population. Used properly, these yield important data that provide unique insights into an individual child. Used improperly, they can underestimate a child's potential as well as result in incorrect treatment and classroom placement. The key focuses on individualizing interpretation of the various sources of information while considering the strengths and limitations of these measures.

REFERENCES

American Speech-Language-Hearing Association (ASHA). (2005). *(Central) Auditory processing disorders* [Technical report]. Available from http://www.asha.org/policy. Retrieved from http://www.asha.org/policy/TR2005-00043/#sec1.3

Barr-Anderson, D. J., Van Den Berg, P., Neumark-Sztainer, D., & Story, M. (2008). Characteristics associated with older adolescents who have a television in their bedrooms, *Pediatrics, 121*(4), 718–724.

Binet, A., & Simon, T. (1916). *The development of intelligence in children: The Binet-Simon Scale* (No. 11). Baltimore, MD: Lippincott Williams & Wilkins.

Briscoe, J., Bishop, D. V., & Norbury, C. F. (2001). Phonological processing, language, and literacy: A comparison of children with mild to moderate sensorineural hearing loss and those with specific language impairment. *Journal of Child Psychology and Psychiatry, 42*(3), 329–340.

Cacace, A. T., & McFarland, D. J. (1998). Central auditory processing disorder in school-aged children: A critical review. *Journal of Speech, Language, and Hearing Research, 41*(2), 355–373.

Camarata, S. (2013). Pediatric hearing impairment, autism, and autism spectrum disorder: Implications for clinicians. *SIG 9 Perspectives on Hearing and Hearing Disorders in Childhood, 23*(1), 4–12.

Camarata, S. (2014). Early identification and early intervention in autism spectrum disorders: Accurate and effective? *International Journal of Speech-Language Pathology, 16*(1), 1–10.

Camarata, S., & Swisher, L. (1990). A note on intelligence assessment within studies of specific language impairment. *Journal of Speech, Language and Hearing Research, 33*, 205–207.

Carroll, J. B. (1993). *Human cognitive abilities.* New York, NY: Cambridge University Press.

Carrow-Woolfolk, E. (1998). *Test of auditory comprehension.* Austin, TX: Pro-Ed.

Carvill, S. (2001). Sensory impairments, intellectual disability and psychiatry. *Journal of Intellectual Disability Research, 45*(6), 467–483.

Champion, T. B., Hyter, Y. D., McCabe, A., & Bland-Stewart, L. M. (2003). "A matter of vocabulary": Performances of low-income African American Head Start children on the Peabody Picture Vocabulary Test–III. *Communication Disorders Quarterly, 24*(3), 121–127.

Dunn, L. M., & Dunn, D. M. (2007). *Peabody Picture Vocabulary Test–4 manual.* Bloomington, MN: NCS Pearson.

Fenson, L., Bates, E., Dale, P., Goodman, J., Reznick, J. S., & Thal, D. (2000). Reply: Measuring variability in early child language: Don't shoot the messenger. *Child Development, 71*(2), 323–328.

Frankenburg, W. K., Dodds, J. B., Fandal, A. W., Kazuk, E., & Cohrs, M. (1975). *Denver Developmental Screening Test.* Denver, CO: Denver Developmental Materials.

Fudala, J. B., & Reynolds, W. M. (1986). *Arizona Articulation Proficiency Scale: Manual.* Torrance, CA: Western Psychological Services.

Gale, C. R., O'Callaghan, F. J., Bredow, M., & Martyn, C. N. (2006). The influence of head growth in fetal life, infancy, and childhood on intelligence at the ages of 4 and 8 years. *Pediatrics, 118*(4), 1486–1492.

Grinker, R., Vernon, M., Mindel, E., Rothstein, D., Easton, H., Koh, S., & Collums, L. (1969). *Psychiatric diagnosis, therapy and research on the psychotic deaf* [Research Grant number RD-2407-S]. Washington, DC: U.S. Department of Heath, Education, and Welfare.

Hemphill, J. F. (2003). Interpreting the magnitudes of correlation coefficients. *American Psychologist, 58*(1), 78–79.

Horn, J. L. (1988). Thinking about human abilities. In J. R. Nesselroade & R. B. Cattell (Eds.), *Handbook of multivariate psychology* (pp. 645–685). New York, NY: Academic Press.

Hulme, C., & Snowling, M. J. (2013). The interface between spoken and written language: Developmental disorders. *Philosophical Transactions of the Royal Society Biological Sciences, 369*(1634), Article #20120395. http://dx.doi.org/10.1098/rstb.2012.0395

Lord, C., Risi, S., Lambrecht, L., Cook, E. H., Jr., Leventhal, B. L., DiLavore, P. C., . . . Rutter, M. (2000). The Autism Diagnostic Observation Schedule–Generic: A standard measure of social and communication deficits associated with the spectrum of autism. *Journal of Autism and Developmental Disorders, 30*(3), 205–223.

MacArthur-Bates Communicative Development Inventories: User's guide and technical manual. (2007). Baltimore, MD: Paul H. Brookes.

Newcomer, P., & Hammill, D. (2008) *Test of Language Development–Primary* (4th ed.). Austin, TX: Pro-Ed.

Nunnally, J. (1978). *Psychometric methods.* New York, NY: McGraw-Hill.

Roid, G. H. (2003). *Stanford-Binet Intelligence Scales (SB5).* Rolling Meadows, IL: Riverside.

Salvia, J., Ysseldyke, J., & Bolt, S. (2009). *Assessment: In special and inclusive education.* Clifton Park, NY: Delmar Cengage Learning.

Semel, E., Wiig, E. H., & Secord, W. H. (2003) *Clinical Evaluation of Language Fundamentals*

(4th ed.). Toronto, Canada: The Psychological Corporation/A Harcourt Assessment Company.

Shriberg, L. D., Austin, D., Lewis, B. A., McSweeny, J. L., & Wilson, D. L. (1997). The percentage of consonants correct (PCC) metric extensions and reliability data. *Journal of Speech, Language, and Hearing Research, 40*(4), 708–722.

Tallal, P. (1990). Fine-grained discrimination deficits in language-learning impaired children are specific neither to the auditory modality nor to speech perception. *Journal of Speech and Hearing Research, 33*, 616–617.

Tomblin, J., Records, N., Buckwalter, P., Zhang, X., Smith, E., & O'Brien, M. (1997). Prevalence of specific language impairment in kindergarten children. *Journal of Speech-Language-Hearing Research, 40*, 1245–1260.

Werner, E. O. H., & Kresheck, J. (1983). *SPELT-II: Structured photographic expressive language test.* DeKalb, IL: Janelle.

Wilkes, E. M. (1999). *Cottage acquisition scales for listening, language & speech: User's guide.* San Antonio, TX: Sunshine Cottage School for Deaf Children.

Williams, J., & Brayne, C. (2006). Screening for autism spectrum disorders: What is the evidence? *Autism, 10*, 11–35.

Woodcock, R. W., McGrew, K. S., & Mather, N. (2001). *Woodcock-Johnson Tests of Achievement.* Itasca, IL: Riverside.

Zimmerman, I. L., Steiner, V. G., & Pond, R. E. (2002). *Preschool language scales* (4th ed.). San Antonio, TX : The Psychological Corporation.

PART II

Assessments

CHAPTER 3

Medical Assessment

Pon Trairatvorakul and Susan Wiley

KEY POINTS

- Accurate and early identification of hearing loss along with early and effective intervention are critically important to maximize a child's potential. The premise of 1-3-6 (screen by 1 before 1 month, diagnose before 3 months, and intervene before 6 months) serves as a guide for providers to support the Early Hearing Detection and Intervention (EHDI) System.
- Etiology may help us recognize risks for other health or developmental problems, understand recurrence risk, and can impact aspects of management, such as guiding the frequency of monitoring for hearing levels and developmental progress.
- For children with hearing loss, ensuring empowered family members partnering with an interdisciplinary approach to care with strong communication across settings will provide a foundation to support the unique needs for the child.

Vignette 1

A family just had a newborn baby boy. As part of the usual newborn nursery care, their son had a hearing screen by a hospital screener. The screener discusses the results of the screening. The baby did not pass his hearing screening. The family asks what they should do next.

IMPORTANCE OF EARLY DIAGNOSIS AND MANAGEMENT OF HEARING LOSS

Successful implementation of Universal Newborn Hearing Screening (UNHS) has transformed our care model for children with hearing loss. Prior to UNHS, children with hearing loss were identified at much later ages, often due to concerns about language delays (Fitzpatrick, Whittingham, & Duriuex-Smith, 2014; Sininger et al., 2009; Uus & Bamford, 2006; Young

& Reilly, 2011). It was a rare child who was identified early with hearing loss. In our current care model, that scenario has fortunately shifted such that it is much less common for children to have a delayed identification of hearing loss. In 2012, the Centers for Disease Control and Prevention (CDC) indicated 96.6% of infants in the United States (U.S.) and territories had completed a newborn hearing screen (CDC, 2014); however, loss to follow-up continues to be an issue. Late identification can occur if children are not followed effectively from screening to diagnosis or in the setting of a late-onset or progressive hearing loss.

The main purpose of UNHS was to identify children as newborns to positively impact language development. In fact, UNHS has made a striking difference for children with hearing loss. Children who are identified in infancy and receive early and effective interventions have language levels that fall in the average range of skills as compared to hearing peers (Kennedy et al., 2006; Meinzen-Derr, Wiley, & Choo 2011; Moeller, 2000; Pimperton & Kennedy, 2012; Vehaert, Willems, Van Kerschaver, & Desloovere, 2008; Yoshinago-Itano, Sedey, Coulter, & Mehl 1998). These language levels are still in the low average range, but this accomplishment is a marked improvement from the outcomes of children born before UNHS.

These are precisely the improved outcomes hoped for by **Early Hearing Detection and Intervention (EHDI)** programs across the United States. The importance of early diagnosis and management of hearing loss was championed by the Joint Committee on Infant Hearing (JCIH) through their position statement (JCIH, 2007) and guide the concept of "1-3-6." The 1-3-6 guidelines state that newborns' hearing should be screened no later than 1 month of age, hearing loss diagnosed no later than 3 months of age, and family-centered early intervention initiated no later than 6 months of age. Semantics are important in this statement. This guideline is not intended to indicate that all children should wait until 3 months for a diagnosis or wait until 6 months to receive intervention, but rather to guide the outside limits of the standard of care. If diagnosis and intervention can occur before these outside timelines, better outcomes are anticipated for young children in the areas of language, social-emotional skills, academic performance, and thus improved opportunities for adults with hearing loss.

Another potential benefit of earlier identification of hearing loss is the allowance of more time for families to gain an understanding of their child's needs and feel less anxiety in needing to "make up for lost time" for a late identified language-delayed toddler. With early identification, families can begin to address how children will need to learn and process information differently because of their hearing loss. As most parents of children with hearing loss are hearing, early intervention programs can be very important in guiding parents' journey in building communication and language with their infant. Parents with hearing loss also benefit from this service as their experiences growing up may be different from those of their child. Early interventions services provided in a culturally sensitive manner can be particularly powerful in supporting families in this new journey. Strong early intervention programs (JCIH, 2013) include timely intervention by specialized expertise providers, culturally accessible services, regular monitoring of child progress, inclusion of families as active participants (i.e., family-centered early intervention), availability of family-to-family support, access to guidance and involvement of adults with hearing loss, and guidance of the EHDI program with input from adults with hearing loss and families of children with hearing loss, and supports for children who have additional disabilities.

Limitations Inherent in UNHS

It is important to recognize the limitations inherent in UNHS. The United States is still struggling with high rates of loss to follow-up (LTF) of infants who did not pass their hearing screening. In 2011, 35% of infants were considered lost to follow-up as state systems were not able to determine the child's hearing status (CDC, 2013). This is one of the greatest barriers to the success of UNHS and EHDI. Furthermore, some children with milder degrees of hearing loss are not identified due to the standards set for determining screening pass/refer results. UNHS also will not identify late-onset hearing loss; therefore, a child who passes his hearing screening but has language delays or concerns about hearing as relayed by the family should still be referred for a full audiological evaluation.

There is also great variability in screening and intervention programs among the states. Supporting families through the various systems of care for optimal completion of the EHDI process from screening to intervention for those identified with a hearing loss is complex. Each provider should accept responsibility in providing appropriate care, supporting families effectively through the process, and ensuring an effective transition of care across systems (birth hospitals, audiology centers, pediatricians, pediatric otolaryngologists, early intervention systems, state EHDI programs).

> **Vignette 2**
>
> Our family with their infant son has completed their outpatient re-screening and is now in the pediatric audiology center for a diagnostic evaluation. They ask a number of questions about why their child has a hearing loss and what this means for their son.

NORMAL ANATOMY

Understanding basic anatomy guides our classification of types of hearing loss. Classification of the types of hearing loss guides our approach to appropriate management strategies.

The anatomy of the ear is divided into three main sections: the outer ear, the middle ear, and the inner ear (Figure 3–1). The outer ear includes the external ear (pinna or auricle), external auditory meatus, and ends at the outer surface of the tympanic membrane. The middle ear includes the inner surface of the tympanic membrane, the inner ear bones (ossicles, named malleus, incus, and stapes), the eustachian tube, and the superior border of the mastoid bone. The inner ear includes the cochlea (which houses the organ of Corti), the vestibular system (labyrinth and semicircular canals and is responsible for balance), and the eighth cranial nerve. The organ of Corti lies within the cochlea and is lined with one row of inner hair cells (IHC) and three rows of outer hair cells (OHC). There are approximately 3,500 IHCs and about 12,000 OHCs. The hair cells send a signal to the auditory nerve,

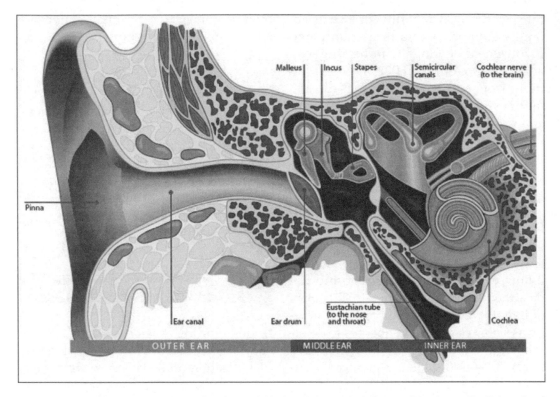

Figure 3–1. Anatomy of the ear. Courtesy of National Acoustic Laboratories: Australia. Taken from http://www.nal.gov.au/hearing-loss_tab_conductive.shtml

which then is transmitted to the auditory cortex in the brain. The central auditory system includes a pathway of input and signal transmission going up from the auditory nerve, through the brainstem, basal ganglia, and reaching the auditory cortex in the brain.

Understanding the anatomy in this pathway allows a framework for considering problems that can occur within each area. For example, the external ear can have issues with being blocked by cerumen or infection (e.g., external otitis media). Microtia (underdeveloped pinna) or atresia (narrowing) of the external auditory meatus are congenital conditions that also affect the external ear. The middle ear can have ear infections (acute or chronic

otitis media), persistent fluid (serous otitis media), or problems with the tympanic membrane such as retraction (often causing a popping sensation), perforation in the membrane, or cholesteatomas (benign tumor). The eustachian tube is the pathway from the middle ear to the back of the throat. Eustachian tube dysfunction can lead to difficulties with drainage of fluid out of the middle ear cavity. Otitis media (serous, acute, or chronic) are common childhood infections (Coker et al., 2010). The types of problems that can occur within the inner ear not only include sensorineural hearing loss but also infections (e.g., labyrinthitis) and malformations, such as enlarged vestibular aqueduct or Mondini deformity. If there are problems with the central auditory system such as an acoustic neuroma, injury to, or malformed auditory cortex, this can impact the brain's ability to process the auditory signals.

TYPES OF HEARING LOSS

There are many ways to characterize hearing loss when determining its type, degree, and configuration (Table 3–1). Classification can be based on whether the hearing loss is temporary or permanent, stable, fluctuating, or progressive, unilateral or bilateral, conductive, sensorineural, mixed hearing loss, or auditory neuropathy, and based on the pattern or configuration of the hearing loss (i.e., sloping, flat, "cookie bite," etc).

Children can have changes in their hearing over time. This would be described as fluctuating or progressive hearing loss. Some conditions put children at greater risk for progressive or fluctuating

Table 3–1. Types of Hearing Loss

Type	Conductive: Bone conduction thresholds are within normal limits; Air conduction thresholds are not within normal limits
	Sensorineural: Both bone conduction and air conduction thresholds are not within normal limits and are within 10 dB of each other
	Mixed hearing loss (conductive and sensorineural component): Both bone conduction and air conduction thresholds are not within normal limits and are greater than 10 dB from each other
	Auditory Neuropathy: Normal OAEs but abnormal ABR/AR
Stability	Temporary
	Fluctuating
	Permanent
	Progressive
	Stable
Side	Unilateral: hearing loss is present in only one ear
	Bilateral: hearing loss is present in both ears
Degree of Hearing Loss in Children	Normal: 0–15 dB HL
	Slight: 16–25 dB HL
	Mild: 26–40 dB HL
	Moderate: 41–55 dB HL
	Moderately Severe: 56 – 70 dB HL
	Severe: 71–90 dB HL
	Profound: 90+ dB HL
Configuration	Sloping/Precipitous Sloping
	Up-sloping/Rising
	U-shaped (Cookie Bite)
	Flat

Source: From Australian Hearing Hub website. Used with permission.

hearing loss (i.e., enlarged vestibular aqueduct syndrome or CMV infection during utero) and thus, require more frequent monitoring.

Children with conductive hearing loss have problems that occur in the outer or middle ear. When there are problems in the outer or middle ear, the ability for sound to be transmitted to the inner ear is impacted. Sensorineural hearing loss occurs due to problems in the inner ear, such as malfunctioning hair cells impacting the transmission of sound to the auditory nerve. Mixed hearing loss occurs when there are problems with both conductive and sensorineural hearing loss. For example, a child may have a mild sensorineural hearing loss as well as a problem in the middle or external ear that adds a barrier to sounds, thus impacts hearing levels further to a more severe level of hearing loss. Because both the nerve and middle/outer ear is affected, this type of hearing loss is described as mixed.

Auditory Neuropathy Spectrum Disorders (ANSD) are a less common group of disorders characterized by absent or severely abnormal auditory brainstem response (ABR) with normally functioning outer hair cells within the cochlea, as demonstrated by the presence of evoked otoacoustic emissions and/or cochlear microphonics (Nikolopoulos, 2014; Roush, Frymark, Venediktov, & Wang, 2011; Starr, Sininger, & Pratt, 2000). The signals are not transmitted properly through the auditory nerve and/or brain and the nerve fires dyssynchronously. To identify this type of hearing loss requires a specific testing protocol. There are risk factors for auditory neuropathy spectrum, such as high levels of bilirubin during infancy, but genetic etiologies can also occur. Auditory neuropathies can occur as part of broader peripheral neuropathies as well.

An absent auditory nerve can also present with an audiometric pattern of ANSD.

Vignette 3

The family is seeing their primary care provider for their 2-month well child checkup. Their primary care provider has appropriately received the child's screening results, ensured they were getting through the diagnostic process and now asks how things are going for their son. The family has completed the diagnostic evaluation, and their son was diagnosed with a mild bilateral sensorineural hearing loss. The family asks about all of the appointments that have been suggested by the audiologist and are feeling a little overwhelmed. They also indicated the state's Part C Early Intervention program has been trying to get in touch with them. They ask how to prioritize their next steps.

MEDICAL HOME AND TEAM MANAGEMENT

The medical home is a concept about how to provide care rather than describing a specific place where care is provided. It is concept to which medical providers aspire. Most providers who consider their practice as providing a medical home realize their care model can continue to improve even when already highly effective.

The concept of medical home has long been established for children and adults. In 2002, the American Academy of Pediatrics (AAP) published a policy statement guided by Medical Home Initiatives for Children with Special Needs Project Advisory Committee that further defined the desirable characteristics of a medical home with regards to children with special needs. **Medical home** and services need to be: *accessible, family-centered, continuous, comprehensive, coordinated, compassionate, and culturally effective* (Medical Home, 2002). The AAP further identified barriers such as geography, personnel constraints, practice patterns, and economic and social forces in the implementation of an effective medical home. All clinicians should advocate and support parents to establish a medical home.

Beyond the typical implementation of these constructs in delivering health care, these characteristics have specific applications for children and youth with hearing loss. Children with hearing loss have unique needs related to communication as well as in coordinating and partnering with the various disciplines that are often a part of management and intervention services.

In terms of accessibility, communication is one key factor for children with hearing loss. If children or parents use sign language, practices should have technology to handle video relay calls and interpreters during visits if needed to ensure that communication needs are specifically met. Relying on lip-reading or writing is not an appropriate form of communication within the medical setting. Furthermore, involving an interpreter early on in care allows children full access to their health information if the child is also signing. Families should not serve as the interpreter in the medical setting as their role is as parents/caregivers. It is challenging to listen and convey information to the provider while also meeting the communication needs of the child.

Having an interpreter within the medical visit may require a little more time during the visit. It is helpful to consider this need when scheduling appointments.

Accessibility to care can also be affected by financial constraints. For example, for children who use amplification, funding can be a substantial challenge due to variable insurance coverage for hearing aids. States across the United States have varying coverage for hearing aids, with insurance companies in many states not providing financial support for these needs. Frequency Modulation (FM) systems are rarely paid for through insurance means. Families may need to seek out charitable funding sources when no coverage is available. Some states allow coverage of amplification through Medicaid, State Children's Health Insurance Programs, and/or Title V State Programs for Children With Special Health Care Needs. Understanding funding sources can guide options for ensuring children receive appropriate and early amplification.

In providing **family-centered and culturally effective care**, clinicians should recognize that families of children with hearing loss should be provided information about communication modalities and technology needs to guide their decisions. Their decisions should be respected and supported by the clinical and educational team. As there are many avenues that are possible for educational and communication support, families may receive a great deal of information, some of which is conflicting. Sometimes decisions families make at one point in time may not be appropriate at another point of time. Supporting families when they decide to change intervention strategies empowers them to continue to make good decisions as their child grows and develops. (See Chapter 12.)

The continuity of care and coordinated care needs for children with hearing loss span many systems, including EHDI systems, Early Intervention (Part C) systems, educational systems, deaf educators, audiologists, speech-language pathologists, pediatric specialists (e.g., otolaryngologists, geneticists), technology vendors, interpreters, deaf mentors, family-to-family support, and psychosocial supports, to name a few. One role of the medical home is to ensure that families receive appropriate care and follow-up from birth and initial hearing screenings through identification and intervention. Ensuring that the physician's office has a tracking system for newborn hearing screening results as well as monitoring for late-onset hearing loss is important within the primary-care setting. Providing families with support and information at each step as well as helping families understand information and reports are essential in providing the optimal care for children with hearing loss. Linking families to support networks and family-to-family support should be an early aspect of the provision of care.

Comprehensive care entails a well-trained provider who is able to manage and facilitate all aspects of care following evidence-based guidelines. It is rare that a primary care provider/medical home can easily remain current on information related to hearing loss, in part due to the relatively infrequent occasion of having a child with hearing loss within a practice. The changes in technology and educational interventions and supports are also make it difficult to maintain a strong knowledge base. This makes it even more critically important to rely on a strong team of professionals, to refer to those who are active in the care of children with hearing loss, and to listen to families when they provide information or ask questions.

PEDIATRICIAN AND FAMILY MEDICINE PHYSICIANS

In general, there is a lack of medical training and knowledge in the area of hearing loss. Primary care providers can be uncertain about the most appropriate next steps in the care of a child with hearing loss (Moeller, White, & Shishler, 2006). Although there are other rare conditions for which providers seem to have a stronger knowledge base, this is often because of more substantial medical implications of these conditions. Children with hearing loss are often relatively healthy and most general practitioners (physicians) will only care for 6 to 10 such children within the duration of an individual provider's practice. This limits the provider's perceived need to stay up to date on medical and therapeutic interventions. Despite these limitations in knowledge, a key aspect to providing strong primary care is listening to families' needs and responding appropriately by coordinating the services children are receiving and referring to professionals with expertise for each concern. Scheduling visits for the family to review results from referrals or evaluations can ensure that families are receiving the quality of care they require. Advocating for interventions may be needed, particularly if therapies are needed but limited in insurance coverage plans.

There are some specific special medical considerations in children with hearing loss. Otitis media should be aggressively managed to avoid conductive hearing loss in addition to the child's baseline hearing loss. In children who have received or planned to receive a cochlear implant, a 23-valent pneumococcal vaccine should be administered after the second birthday. The purpose for this vaccine is to lower the risk associated with meningitis in children with implants (Reefhius et al., 2003; U.S. Food & Drug Administration, 2002).

Vignette 4

The family is seeing the pediatric otolaryngologist who has suggested a great deal of testing. They have many questions about all of the tests that are required and the reason for all of the tests. They are wondering if all of the evaluations are necessary and how they will impact next steps for their son.

MEDICAL WORKUP AND FOLLOW-UP

The medical workup of hearing loss starts with a thorough history and physical. The questions and physical examination should focus on possible causes of hearing loss. Many aspects of the medical history can identify risk factors for hearing loss (Table 3–2). A three-generation family history (pedigree) can identify a specific genetic pattern for hearing loss and/or provide clues for syndromes associated with hearing loss. Prenatal and perinatal history may identify the possibility of an infection or neonatal factors that cause hearing loss. Evaluating exposures to ototoxic medications is also important as well

as eliciting any history of head trauma, particularly fractures of the temporal bone, which may identify a potential cause of hearing loss. The JCIH has identified a number of risk factors for hearing loss. (See Table 3–2.) A full review of systems also can target underlying genetic conditions.

A physical examination should be comprehensive and target aspects that can guide further workup. Growth parameters (especially head circumference) may indicate concerns with brain growth from the impact of congenital infections, such as cytomegalovirus (CMV). Dysmorphic features can provide information to consider possible syndromes associated with hearing loss. It is also helpful to perform a full examination of the outer ear and tympanic membrane (including pneumatic otoscopy). Of course it is always important to also assess the eye and determine if there may be concerns related to vision that also need to be identified and addressed.

Commonly, children do not have specific risk factors or physical examination findings associated with known causes of hearing loss. Often medical workup focuses on genetic testing and imaging of the temporal bone and internal auditory canal. Some studies have considered tiered testing which takes a step-wise approach to identifying a cause of hearing loss (Preciado et al., 2004; Preciado et al., 2005; Table 3–3). Many blood and urine studies have been considered in the workup of hearing loss, but these studies tend to have a low yield. Specific laboratory investigation should be guided by clinical suspicion (Mafong, Shin, & Lalwani, 2002). Despite a low likelihood of Jervell and Lange-Nielsen syndrome, an electrocardiogram (ECG) is still considered

Table 3–2. Historical Indicators of Syndromes and JCIH Risk Factors for Hearing Loss

Historical Indicator	Symptoms and Signs	Possible Syndrome
Family History	Premature graying/white patches of skin, autosomal dominant pattern with variable penetrance	Waardenburg syndrome
	Kidney failure	Alport syndrome
	Sudden death (prolonged QT syndrome), fainting spells	Jervell and Lange-Nielsen syndrome
	Problems with night vision (retinitis pigmentosa), balance problems	Usher syndrome
	Thyroid problems	Pendred syndrome (associated with enlarged vestibular aqueduct)

Child Factors	Category	Causes of Hearing Loss
Prenatal Events	Infection	Congenital CMV, Toxoplasmosis, Rubella
Perinatal Events	Hypoxic birth	Low Apgars at 10–15 minutes
	Ototoxic medications	Gentamicin, Furosemide, etc.
	Prematurity/NICU stay	Mechanical ventilation, Extracorporal Membrane Oxygenation (ECMO) Persistent pulmonary hypertension
	Infection	Meningitis
Postnatal Events	Ototoxic medications	Gentamicin, Furosemide, etc.
	Jaundice	High bilirubin level
	Infections	Meningitis, measles, mumps
	Trauma	Temporal bone fracture

Source: JCIH, 2007.

Table 3–3. Selected Laboratory Tests in the Workup of Hearing Loss

Lab Test	Associated Syndromes or Etiology
ANA, ESR	Autoimmune disorders, systemic lupus, etc.
Rheumatoid factor	Autoimmune disorders, rheumatoid arthritis
CBC	Anemia, infections
Platelet count	Fechtner syndrome
Urinalysis, BUN, Creatinine	Alport syndrome
Serum glucose	Diabetes, Alstrom syndrome
Thyroid studies (TSH, free T4)	Pendred syndrome, congenital hypothyroidism
RPR, FTA-ABS	Syphilis
ECG	Jervell and Lange-Nielsen syndrome
Renal ultrasound	Branchio-Oto-Renal syndrome

Source: Bamiou et al., 2000; Mafong et al., 2002.

important in children with no identifiable cause of hearing loss due to the great danger in missing a fatal arrhythmia, such as prolonged QT (Association of Audiovestibular Physicians, 2008). Medical geneticists and pediatric otolaryngologists knowledgeable in hearing loss can assist in the evaluation of children with hearing loss. All children with hearing loss should be evaluated by an otolaryngologist, ophthalmologist, and geneticist (JCIH, 2007).

Otolaryngology

The pediatric otolaryngologist (ENT) often assists with the medical workup of hearing loss, performs medical clearance for hearing aid (HA) fitting, performs cochlear implant and other implantable device surgeries, and provides surgical management for persistent middle ear issues. They are often the providers who initiate the medical evaluation and work-up as described above (i.e., comprehensive history, physical exam, imaging, blood work, ECG).

Genetics

As half of children with sensorineural hearing loss have an underlying genetic etiology (Van Camp & Smith, 2014) geneticists have a crucial role in the evaluation of children with hearing loss. Geneticists work in collaboration with genetic counselors. They assist in investigating the underlying cause of syndromic and nonsyndromic hearing loss. While it is common for children to receive genetic testing for common genetic mutations, such as connexin 26, as part of hearing genetic testing panels, geneticists also have expertise in the recognition of dys-

morphic features that guides more refined genetic or molecular studies. Geneticists also guide a broader genetic evaluation in situations where intellectual disability co-occurs (Miller et al., 2010). The expertise from geneticists allows earlier recognition of possible coexisting conditions that require management or interventions. Even among children with risk factors related to prematurity, genetic causes of hearing loss can also be present and may have an impact on genetic counseling related to risk of hearing loss in siblings and the child's offspring (American College of Medical Genetics, 2002).

Ophthalmology

An ophthalmologist may identify conditions that require treatment but also provide possible clues towards specific etiologies of hearing loss. Due to the high rate of vision problems in children with hearing loss (Guy, Nicholson, Pannu, & Holden, 2003; Johnston et al., 2010; Nikolopoulos, Lioumi, Stamataki, & O'Donoghue, 2006; Sharma, Ruscetta, & Chi, 2009), referral for an ophthalmological evaluation is essential. Ophthalmologists identify and manage vision issues that can co-occur with hearing loss.

Vignette 5

Our family is seeing the genetic specialist as part of the workup of hearing loss. They have been talking to other families and doing an internet search. They indicate they understand that up to 40% of children with hearing loss have other issues. They ask about their son's risk for other issues.

DISORDERS ASSOCIATED WITH HEARING LOSS

The prior section on medical workup of hearing loss gives a starting place of understanding that comorbidities can occur in children with hearing loss. Etiology of hearing loss sometimes points to medical and developmental issues that can coexist in a child with hearing loss. It is important to recognize, however, that the etiology of hearing loss does not necessarily protect a child from other medical and developmental conditions. Even with a known genetic cause of hearing loss that may not be perceived as being associated with other problems, children can carry other genetic or environmental risks for medical or developmental problems. As such, children with hearing loss warrant the same type of medical care and anticipatory guidance as hearing children.

Table 3–4 describes some of the syndromes associated with hearing loss and associated problems that can occur. The reliance on a multidisciplinary approach for children with hearing loss is necessary for identifying and intervening for all of a child's needs. If a child has had a comprehensive medical evaluation by otolaryngologists, ophthalmologists, and geneticists with knowledge about conditions associated with pediatric hearing loss, syndromes and associated medical conditions may be identified. Children with developmental delays, concerns with vision or visual tracking, or those with medical complexities should receive comprehensive evaluations by providers to ensure all needs are being addressed (Bull & Committee on Genetics, 2011).

CONCLUSION

The medical workup and management of hearing loss is founded initially in understanding the type, degree, and configuration of hearing loss as this guides the subsequent workup and management. Aggressive monitoring and management of middle ear issues is critical as well as ensuring children receive appropriate evaluations from including otolaryngology, genetics, and ophthalmology. Genetic testing is a rapidly expanding and these changes can make it challenging to maintain the most up to date information for families.

The early identification and management of hearing loss requires a multisystems approach with good communication across providers, support for families in a manner that empowers them to follow through with next steps. Family-to-family support is an essential component of this journey. Supporting families through the medical evaluations allows families to understand their child's unique needs and to be proactive in providing appropriate medical care for their child.

Table 3–4. Common Syndromes and Causes of Hearing Loss and Associated Conditions

Syndromes	Distinctive Aspects of Hearing Loss	Possible Associated Conditions
Alport syndrome	Late-onset SNHL	Kidney problems
Down syndrome	Conductive, SNHL, or mixed	Vision, cardiac, gastrointestinal, thyroid, developmental issues
CHARGE syndrome	Structural abnormality of inner ear and vestibular anatomy, outer ear shape atypical	Multiple systems can be involved, vision (coloboma), congenital heart disorders, cleft lip/palate, kidney problems, difficulties with growth
Goldenhar syndrome	Conductive or SNHL, ear anomalies	Vision, brain, spine, heart, kidney anomalies
Jervell and Lange-Nielsen syndrome	Severe bilateral SNHL	Heart arrhythmia (prolonged QT) associated with sudden death
Pendred syndrome	Enlarged vestibular aqueduct, can have progressive SNHL	Thyroid problems
Stickler syndrome	SNHL, conductive, or mixed, usually milder hearing loss	High myopia, risk for retinal detachment, glaucoma, bone and joint problems,
Treacher Collins	Conductive or SNHL, ear anomalies	Vision, congenital heart disorders, narrow airway, cleft palate
Usher syndrome (type I, II, III)	Degree of SNHL and progression depends on type	Progressive vision loss due to retinitis pigmentosa, type I balance issues
Waardenburg syndrome	SNHL or no hearing loss	Vision issues, patches of white skin, early graying, one subtype with Hirschprung's disease
Infectious Causes	**Distinctive Aspects of Hearing Loss**	**Possible Associated Conditions**
Congenital Symptomatic CMV	SNHL, at risk for progressive hearing loss	Calcifications of the brain, microcephaly, seizures, developmental delays
Bacterial meningitis	SNHL	Can have broader developmental problems if also associated with encephalitis or abscess formation

Note. SNHL = sensorineural hearing loss.

REFERENCES

American College of Medical Genetics. (2002). Genetics evaluation guidelines for the etiologic diagnosis of congenital hearing loss. Genetic evaluation of congenital hearing loss expert panel. ACMG statement. *Genetics in Medicine, 4,* 162–171.

Association of Audiovestibular Physicians. (2008). *Guidelines for investigating infants with congenital hearing loss identified through newborn hearing screening.* Retrieved from http://www.bapa .uk.com/userfiles/Congenital%20Hearing %20Loss%20Investigation%20in%20the%20 Newborn%20BAAP%20BAPA%20Guideline %202008(1).pdf

Bamiou, D. E., MacArdle, B., Bitner-Glindzicz, M., & Sirimanna, T. (2000). Aetiological investigations of hearing loss in childhood: A review. *Clinical Otolaryngology and Allied Sciences, 25,* 98–106.

Bull, M. J., & Committee on Genetics. (2011). American Academy of Pediatrics Clinical Report: Health supervision for children with Down syndrome. *Pediatrics, 128*(2), 393–406.

Centers for Disease Control and Prevention (CDC). (2013). *Summary of 2011 national CDC EHDI data.* Retrieved from http://www.cdc. gov/ncbddd/hearingloss/2011-data/2011_ ehdi_hsfs_summary_a.pdf

Centers for Disease Control and Prevention (CDC). (2014). *Preliminary summary of 2012 national CDC EHDI data.* Retrieved from http:// www.cdc.gov/ncbddd/hearingloss/2012- data/2012_ehdi_hsfs_summary_b.pdf

Coker, T. R., Chan, L. S., Newberry, S. J., Limbos M. A., Suttorp, M. J., Shekelle, P. G., & Takata, G. S. (2010). Diagnosis, microbial epidemiology, and antibiotic treatment of acute otitis media in children: A systematic review. *Journal of the American Medical Association, 304*(19), 2161–2169.

Fitzpatrick, E. M., Whittingham, J., & Duriuex-Smith, A. (2014). Mild bilateral and unilateral hearing loss in childhood: A 20-year view of hearing characteristics, and audiologic practices before and after newborn hearing screening. *Ear and Hearing, 35*(1), 10–18.

Guy, R., Nicholson, J., Pannu, S. S., & Holden, R. (2003). A clinical evaluation of ophthalmic assessment in children with sensorineural deafness. *Child Care and Health Development, 29*(5), 377–384.

Johnston, D. R., Curry, J. M., Newborough, B., Morlet, T., Bartoshesky, L., Lehman, S., . . . O'Reilly, R. C. (2010). Ophthalmologic disorders in children with syndromic and nonsyndromic hearing loss. *Archives of Otolaryngology-Head & Neck Surgery, 136*(3), 277–280.

Joint Committee on Infant Hearing (JCIH). (2007). JCIH year 2007 position statement: Principles and guidelines for early hearing detection and intervention programs. *Pediatrics, 120,* 898–921.

Joint Committee on Infant Hearing (JCIH). (2013). JCIH: Supplement to the JCIH 2007 position statement: Principles and guidelines for early intervention after confirmation that a child is deaf or hard of hearing. *Pediatrics, 131*(4), e1324–e1349.

Kennedy, C. R., McCann, D. C., Campbell, M. J, Law, C. M., Mullee, M., Petrou, S., . . . Stevenson, J. (2006). Language ability after early detection of permanent childhood hearing impairment. *New England Journal of Medicine, 354*(20), 2131–2141.

Mafong, D. D., Shin, E. J., & Lalwani, A. K. (2002). Use of laboratory evaluation and radiologic imaging in the diagnostic evaluation of children with sensorineural hearing loss. *Laryngoscope, 112,* 1–7.

Medical Home Initiatives for Children With Special Needs Project Advisory Committee, & American Academy of Pediatrics. (2002). The Medical Home. *Pediatrics, 110*(1 Pt. 1), 184–186.

Meinzen-Derr, J., Wiley, S, & Choo, D. I. (2011). Impact of early intervention on expressive and receptive language development among young children with permanent hearing loss. *American Annals of the Deaf, 155*(5), 580–591.

Miller, D. T., Adam, M. P., Aradhya, S., Biesecker, L. G., Brothman, A. R., Carter, N., . . . Ledbetter, D. H. (2010). Consensus statement: Chromosomal microarray is a first-tier clinical diagnostic test for individuals with developmental disabilities or congenital anomalies. *American Journal of Human Genetics, 86*(5), 749–764.

Moeller, M. P. (2000). Early intervention and language development in children who are deaf and hard of hearing. *Pediatrics, 106*(3), e43–e51. doi:10.1542/peds.106.3.e43

Moeller, M. P., White, K. R., & Shisler, L. (2006). Primary care physicians' knowledge, attitudes, and practices related to newborn hearing screening. *Pediatrics, 118*(4), 1357–1370.

Nikolopoulos, T. P. (2014). Auditory dyssynchrony or auditory neuropathy: Understanding the pathophysiology and exploring methods of treatment. *International Journal of Pediatric Otorhinolaryngology, 78*(2), 171–173.

Nikolopoulos, T. P., Lioumi, D., Stamataki, S., & O'Donoghue, G. M. (2006). Evidence-based overview of ophthalmic disorders in deaf children: A literature update. *Otology & Neurotology, 27*(2 Suppl. 1), S1–24, discussion S0.

Pimperton, H., & Kennedy, C. R. (2012). The impact of early identification of permanent childhood hearing impairment on speech and language outcomes. *Archives of Diseases in Children, 97*(7), 648–653.

Preciado, D. A., Lawson, L., Madden, C., Myer, D., Ngo, C., Bradshaw, J. K., . . . Greinwald, J. H. (2005). Improved diagnostic effectiveness with a sequential diagnostic paradigm in idiopathic pediatric sensorineural hearing loss. *Otology & Neurotology, 26*(4), 610–615.

Preciado, D. A., Lim, L. H., Cohen, A. P., Madden, C., Myer, D., Ngo, C., . . . Greinwald, J. H. (2004). A diagnostic paradigm for childhood idiopathic sensorineural hearing loss. *Otolaryngology-Head & Neck Surgery, 131*(6), 804–809.

Reefhuis, J., Honein, M. A., Whitney, C. G., Chamany, S., Mann, E. A., Biernath, K., . . . Boyle, C. (2003). Risk of bacterial meningitis in children with cochlear implants, USA 1997–2002. *New England Journal of Medicine, 349*, 435–445.

Roush, P., Frymark, T., Venediktov, R., & Wang, B. (2011). Audiologic management of auditory neuropathy spectrum disorder in children: A systematic review of the literature. *American Journal of Audiology, 20*(2), 159–170.

Sharma, A., Ruscetta, M. N., & Chi, D. H. (2009). Ophthalmologic findings in children with sensorineural hearing loss. *Archives of Otolaryngology-Head & Neck Surgery, 135*, 119–123.

Sininger, Y. S., Martinez, A., Eisenberg, L., Christensen, E., Grimes, A., & Hu, J. (2009). Newborn hearing screening speeds diagnosis and access to intervention by 20–25 months. *Journal of American Academy of Audiology, 20*(1), 49–57.

Starr, A., Sininger, Y. S., & Pratt, H. (2000). The varieties of auditory neuropathy. *Journal of Basic Clinical Physiology and Pharmacology, 11*(3), 215–230.

U.S. Food and Drug Administration. (2002). *FDA public health web notification: Risk of bacterial meningitis in children with cochlear implants.* Retrieved from http://www.fda.gov/Medical Devices/Safety/AlertsandNotices/Public HealthNotifications/ucm064526.htm

Uus, K., & Bamford, J. (2006). Effectiveness of population-based newborn hearing screening in England: Ages of interventions and profile of cases. *Pediatrics, 117*(5), e887–893.

Van Camp, G., & Smith, R. J. H. (2014). *Hereditary hearing loss homepage.* Retrieved from http://hereditaryhearingloss.org

Vehaert, N., Willems, M., Van Kerschaver, E., & Desloovere, C. (2008) Impact of early hearing screening and treatment on language development and education level: Evaluation of 6 years of universal newborn hearing screening (ALGO) in Flanders, Belgium. *International Journal of Pediatric Otorhinolaryngology, 72*(5), 599–608.

Yoshinaga-Itano, C., Sedey, A. L., Coulter, D. K., & Mehl, A. L. (1998). Language of early- and later-identified children with hearing loss. *Pediatrics, 102*(5), 1161–1171.

Young, N. M., Reilly, B. K., & Burke, L. (2011). Limitations of universal newborn hearing screening in early identification of pediatric cochlear implant candidates. *Archives of Otolaryngology-Head & Neck Surgery, 137*(3), 230–234.

CHAPTER 4

Auditory Assessments

Allan O. Diefendorf, Donna Fisher Smiley, and Tamala S. Bradham

KEY POINTS

- Due to transformational changes in health care today, audiology service models are changing. As health care transitions from fee-based services to value based services, audiologic protocols must be efficient, effective, and safe. Practicing audiologists must deliver *"the right care, at the right time, for the right patient."*
- Implementing a "value added practice management program" to achieve optimal outcomes for children with hearing loss and their families, audiologists must design their practice around why the patient is being seen for services.
- By identifying and selecting appropriate measures used to assess auditory skills and measure developmental milestones, the audiologists will be able to initiate optimal interventions and amplification device selection.
- In value-added practice, audiologists will no longer be afforded the luxury of having a child return for annual audiological testing without reason or data to support such follow-up.

Understanding discharge strategies and continuous care management is essential to justify the medical necessity of audiological care.

INTRODUCTION

Hearing is essential for speech, language, and literacy development. With early identification and intervention of hearing loss, the negative consequences that are often associated with hearing loss on a child's development of spoken communication can be minimized (Sininger, Grimes, & Christensen, 2010; Yoshinaga-Itano, Baca, & Sedey, 2010). It was not too long ago that families often did not learn that their child had a hearing loss until the child was 2½ or 3 years of age (Harrison, Roush, & Wallace, 2003). However, with the refinement of advancing technologies to evaluate the subtleties of auditory function from the outer ear to the auditory cortex, audiologists can diagnose hearing loss from mild to profound within days of an infant's birth. Moreover, throughout the early developmental period of an infant and toddler, audiologists can adapt their assessment plans to monitor these infants and young children with hearing loss for suspected progression as well as re-evaluate infants and young children at risk for delayed onset of hearing loss.

Today's practicing audiologists' service delivery model is drastically different than it was even ten years ago. Tomorrow's practicing audiologists' service delivery model, hopefully, will be very different than today. Why these changes in practices? In 2011, 97.9% of all infants were screened prior to discharge (CDC, 2013) versus 65.4% in 2001 (Curry & Gaffney, 2010). Two to three of every 1,000 children born in the United States will present with hearing loss that is significant enough to impact spoken language development (Finitzo, Albright, & O'Neal, 1998). This shift alone is significant, because audiologists are providing care to much younger children, a 1-month-old versus a 3-year-old. Technologies, hearing science research, public policies, and healthcare reform also play important roles in the changes in what and how audiologists deliver services. Audiologists are combining physiologic and behavioral assessment tools to facilitate audiologic assessments that are age-appropriate, evidence-based, reliable, efficient, and cost-effective. Parents, third-party payers, and healthcare policy makers demand this level of service provision during a time when all healthcare services are being scrutinized by mandatory reported outcomes for all aspects of a patient's care.

The purpose of this chapter is to provide an overview of the measures used by audiologists to assess the auditory system, best practices on selecting appropriate measures based on episodes of care, and monitoring auditory function after diagnosis. For children who are developing listening skills and spoken language, the auditory assessment provides essen-

tial information for establishing an initial care plan for implementation (American Speech-Language-Hearing Association [ASHA], 2006).

QUALITY CARE VALUE–ADDED PRACTICE IN PEDIATRIC AUDIOLOGY

Due to changes in health care, audiology service models are changing. Healthcare reimbursement models are moving steadily towards payment for outcomes versus payment for procedures. In the past, practicing audiologists have been taught to apply the cross-check principles due to lower sensitivity and specificity of the tests administered. This approach also was rewarded under a payment for procedures reimbursement climate. Today, however, health care is transitioning from fee-based services to value-based services. This emerging philosophy of payment for outcomes will eventually impact the diagnostic practice of audiology. Third-party payers may only reimburse a single amount for completion of an **episode of care**. Using the diagnostic process to identify hearing loss in children to illustrate the episode of care reimbursement model, audiologists will be reimbursed one fee for their services regardless of the number of procedures and the number of sessions required for acquiring information necessary to make a specific diagnosis. Moreover, errors in diagnosis may result in total or partial forfeiture of reimbursement revenue.

To assist the audiologist in service delivery model changes, the Institute of Medicine (IOM) provides six aims for improvement that affect outcomes (IOM, 2001). As mentioned in Chapter 1, these six aims should be considered when designing innovative care in this new era of health care (Table 4–1).

By incorporating these six aims, audiologists will be able to facilitate better access to care and initiate plans of care that ameliorate the consequences of late-diagnosed hearing loss.

Audiologic protocols must be efficient, effective, and safe as audiologists incorporate changes essential for sustainable professional practice. Now, practicing audiologists must deliver *the right care, at* *the right time, for the right patient*. Based on case history and presenting complaints, audiologists need to determine what test(s) will address the reason(s) for the patient's visit. Depending on the outcomes of the assessment, the payment for services will follow. By providing value-based services and by measuring outcomes through systems such as the Physician Quality Reporting System (PQRS), audiologists should be well positioned to meet the patient's needs and remain viable.

Table 4–1. Questions to Consider for an Audiology Program in Meeting the IOM Quality Outcome Aims

- *Safe*
  - Do you clean your sound room after each patient encounter?
  - Do you dispose of your probes and tips in a manner that is not retrievable by a curious explorer?
- *Effective*
  - Have you visited the ASHA's Evidence Maps at http://www.ncepmaps.org/?
  - Do you review your journals, stay up-to-date on continuing education on a regular basis?
  - Can you justify why the tests administered were necessary?
  - Do you actively collaborate and communication with your colleagues in the field and in the community to exchange information and coordination of care?
- *Patient-centered*
  - How do you practice patient-centered care?
  - Have you taken a self-assessment inventory such as the Patient- and Family-Centered Care: A Hospital Self-Assessment Inventory (http://www.ipfcc.org/tools/downloads-tools.html)?
  - Did you anticipate your patient's need rather than simply reacting?
- *Timely*
  - Are you meeting the 1-3-6 JCIH benchmarks?
  - Is your audiology practice responsive at all times?
  - Do you have systems in place to be responsive to your patient needs besides face-to-face such as telephone and internet?
- *Efficient*
  - When was the last time you had a Plan-Do-Study-Act (PDSA)?
  - Do you have a current PDSA targeting efficiency and quality care?
  - Do you minimize your patient wait time?
- *Equitable*
  - Does your mission and practice support equitable care?
  - Is your practice transparent in that you make information available to your patients and their families that allows them to make informed decisions when selecting treatment options?

MEASUREMENTS USED IN AUDITORY ASSESSMENTS

Case History

Before administering any auditory assessments, the audiologist should obtain a case history. This can be accomplished in multiple ways such as using an interview style, mailing a case history form for parents/caregivers/relatives to bring with them, asking them to complete a case history in the waiting room prior to the appointment, reviewing medical records, and/or communicating with the referral source. It is important to establish from both the referral source as well as the family why they were referred for an audiological evaluation. Based on the information obtained from the case history and from talking with the family, the audiologist will be able to determine which procedures should be administered in the time allowed. At this point, the audiologist (or any service provider) should be thinking *the right care, at the right time, for the right patient.* For some practices, the audiologist may have the scheduler ask a few specific questions to determine how best to schedule the patient to ensure appropriate time is allowed for the evaluation.

Visual Inspection of the Outer Ear and Otoscopy

Regardless of the age of the child, visual inspection of the outer ear, ear canal, and tympanic membrane is standard practice when evaluating the hearing of children. Visual inspection of the outer ear is typically performed by simply looking at the outer ear and noting any abnormalities such as deformity of the pinna, unusual shape or position of the pinna, or preauricular skin tags or ear pits in front of the ear. In some cases, but certainly not all, these visual cues could be outer signs of other auditory system abnormalities and subsequent hearing involvement. For example, Roth et al. (2008) studied the prevalence of hearing loss in a large cohort of infants with preauricular skin tags or ear pits in comparison to newborns without these outer ear abnormalities. Overall, they found a significantly higher prevalence of permanent hearing loss in the infants with preauricular skin tags or ear pits (8 of 1000) when compared to the infants without tags or pits (1.5 of 1000).

Otoscopy is used to visually inspect the ear canal and the tympanic membrane. Otoscopes are equipped with a light source as well as a low power magnifying lens. Otoscopes are available in wall-mounted and portable versions and some otoscopes are connected to a video source which allows the individual and/or family members to see the ear canal and tympanic membrane. Visual inspection with an otoscope prior to a hearing evaluation in a child serves several purposes for the audiologist, including allowing for the visualization of:

1. Obstructions, such as earwax or foreign objects that may be in the ear canal;
2. Anatomical abnormalities in the ear canal such as stenosis (unusual narrowing of the canal), cysts, lesions, infection, or collapsing ear canals; and
3. The health of the tympanic membrane including the presence of a perforation, pressure equalization tubes, or retraction of the membrane.

Otoscopy findings assist the audiologist in ruling out any contraindications for placing a probe tip or inserting an earphone into the canal of the child for audiological testing. Otoscopic findings also may prompt a referral for medical treatment, regardless of the outcome of the hearing evaluation. An example would be when the child has excessive **cerumen** or a foreign object in the ear canal. Cerumen may not be completely occluding the ear canal so as to affect the hearing sensitivity of the child; however, over time hearing could be affected with continued buildup of cerumen. Therefore, the audiologist may either choose to remove the cerumen or make a referral to have it extracted by a medical provider.

Visual inspection of the outer ear does not usually require the use of magnification provided by an otoscope. This visual inspection can be accomplished before the audiologist begins his or her otoscopic exam of the ear canal and tympanic membrane.

Pediatric patients vary in their acceptance of the otoscopic exam. Some children will be resistant to the procedure and the audiologist will need to try to make the process as child-friendly as possible. In many cases, a child's reaction to otoscopy guides the audiologist in knowing what to do next. If a child is resistant to otoscopy, the audiologist may choose to do basic audiometry procedures next (e.g., sound field testing or play audiometry) and come back to tympanometry or otoacoustic emissions later after the child has had a chance to acclimate to the testing environment.

Auditory Brainstem Response (ABR) and Auditory Steady–State Response (ASSR)

Achieving an audiologic diagnosis by 3 months of age requires adherence to the six dimensions framing quality care addressed earlier. Value-based service necessitates detailed diagnostic assessment requiring frequency-specific thresholds and identification of the type of hearing loss, including neural conduction deficits, within weeks of referral. These outcomes are essential to inform decisions regarding medical follow-up, audiologic planning, and early intervention commensurate with the 1–3–6 EHDI benchmarks (screening completed by 1 month; audiologic assessment by 3 months; intervention by 6 months). Uncertainty with regard to hearing loss type leads to large delays in medical treatment and audiologic intervention (Gravel, 2002).

Auditory evoked potentials (AEPs) with high correlation to frequency-specific behavioral thresholds are essential to facilitate confirmation and characterization of hearing loss (of a mild degree or worse) by age 3 months (JCIH, 2007). Moreover, measurements must include bone conduction thresholds to frequency-specific stimuli to distinguish between sensorineural, conductive, and mixed hearing losses, in turn facilitating early referral for medical and/or audiologic intervention.

The ABR to air and bone conducted (A/C and B/C respectively) brief tones has had a long history of successful clinical use. In comparison, the ASSR has a more limited history, but evidence continues to grow suggesting the ASSR has an emerging record of successful clinical use for infant threshold measurement for both A/C and B/C as well. Infant data relative to ASSR B/C are still evolving (Stapells, 2011); as such clinicians can balance ABR B/C when assessing cochlear reserve with ASSR B/C for confirming normal cochlear function when this strategy facilitates quality care in infant assessment protocols.

An important point to establish is that physiological thresholds rarely equal those measured behaviorally; after all, the procedures and measurements are fundamentally different. If a physiological method, however, is to predict auditory status successfully across all age groups (with dynamic developmental considerations especially in infants), it is essential that appropriate correction factors are applied to the physiological thresholds to estimate the behavioral thresholds. As such, both physiologic measures are particularly well-suited for the purposes of hearing loss estimation for the following reasons: (1) tone-evoked ABRs and ASSRs accurately approximate behavioral pure tone thresholds; (2) the responses do not habituate and are stable over time and therefore suitable for acquiring the multiple responses necessary for frequency-specific hearing level estimation; and (3) the responses are unaltered by sleep or sedation and thus useful for the many infants and children who are unable to fully cooperate during a recording session.

The ABR response in infants occurs within a time-window of 25 ms, which places the anatomic origin of the response at the brainstem level. Additionally, the recommended stimulus to elicit an ABR threshold is a frequency-specific tone-burst whose acoustic characteristics are designed to maximize frequency specificity for both air and bone conducted signals. Such brief tones demonstrate reasonable frequency specificity (Oates & Stapells, 1997; Purdy & Abbas, 2002), and provide good estimates of the audiogram. While not recommended for threshold assessment, a click-evoked ABR is recommended to provide important information regarding neural integrity.

Like the ABR, the ASSR is obtained by presenting periodic signals and recording the synchronous neuro-electrical activity from the brain. The stimulus used to elicit the ASSR is a continuous sinusoidally amplitude-modulated (AM) tonal stimulus and, thus, differs from the series of tone bursts used to evoke the ABR. Yet, a continuous sinusoidal AM stimulus is very frequency-specific, thus meeting the necessity of assessing frequency-specific threshold responses.

Knowing the modulation frequency of the signal allows one to predict with certainty the modulation frequency of the response. The amplitude and phase of the response at the rate of stimulation, as well as measures of response noise, are measured entirely objectively and automatically by a computer. The use of objective measures for the ASSR has been emphasized as an "advantage" of the ASSR over the ABR. Response detection of the ABR waveform is usually carried out using subjective criteria that likely vary across time and examiner. This advantage, however, is minimized when ABR interpretation is conducted by audiologists who specialize in pediatric assessment and applies the same rules for interpretation across all ABRs.

Another feature of modulated signals is that more than one carrier frequency can be presented at the same time. Modulating each carrier with a slightly different frequency produces an ASSR that contains carrier-specific modulation components. Through analysis of the response on the basis of the individual components, the simultaneous measurement of hearing thresholds at several test frequencies is possible. First demonstrated by Lins and Picton (1995), this multiple-stimulus ASSR technique has subsequently been developed to allow simultaneous assessment of responses from both ears and four carrier frequencies (i.e., eight different modulation rates). Adopting this strategy may speed up the acquisition process considerably compared to the standard ABR protocol where only one ear and one frequency can be tested at the same time.

Moderate Sedation

The ABR and ASSR are unaltered by sedation and/or sleep. This is an advantage when recording these physiologic responses from infants and children who are unable to fully cooperate or remain quiet during assessment protocols. As such, sedation may be necessary to optimize assessment outcomes. In turn, safety, efficiency, effectiveness, and patient-centered elements of quality care must be carefully implemented to facilitate favorable clinical outcomes and ensure patient safety, while meeting family expectations.

The Joint Commission (TJC), formerly known as the Joint Commission on the Accreditation of Healthcare Organizations (JCAHO), calls for pre-anesthesia assessment, monitoring under sedation, and discharge from post-anesthesia recovery by a licensed healthcare practitioner. The current terminology of the American Society of Anesthesiologists (2002) has replaced the term conscious sedation with the term moderate sedation.

Otoacoustic Emissions (OAEs)

Low-intensity sound energies generated by the cochlea and measurable within the ear canal are termed otoacoustic emissions (OAEs) and were first demonstrated by Kemp in 1978. Considerable research has been conducted on OAEs since the time of their first description, and they now assume an essential role in the pediatric audiology test battery.

The cochlear origin of OAE generation is well accepted. OAEs arise because mammalian auditory systems have evolved a special mechanism to enhance hearing sensitivity and frequency responsiveness. The mechanism is known as the cochlear amplifier and it depends on the specialized type of cells found in the inner ear and identified as outer hair cells. Outer hair cells react mechanically to stimulation. They change length rapidly, releasing their own vibration. OAEs arise because some of the energy generated by outer hair cells escapes back into the ear canal. OAEs are not in and of themselves necessary for hearing, nor are they a mechanism of hearing; rather, OAEs reflect the status of structures that are necessary for hearing.

OAEs expand the pediatric audiology test battery by providing a physiologic means of assessing preneural auditory function. Knowledge of the physiology underlying the generation of OAEs makes them a powerful tool in the diagnostic test battery. Because they are indicative of mechanical, preneural activity, audiologists have an idea whether there is a sensory component to a more commonly described sensorineural hearing loss. Used in conjunction with other AEPs (e.g., ABR; ASSR), OAEs are not only useful in the differential diagnosis of cochlear hearing loss but also in the identification of children with neurological dysfunction. Additionally, with the pediatric population, OAEs offer the clinician the opportunity to obtain ear specific data since behavioral audiometric measures obtained in sound field testing are not able to delineate individual ear information.

Evoked otoacoustic emissions can be elicited by various signals. Transient signals are effective in generating transient evoked OAEs (TEOAEs). Although the click stimulus is a broadband stimulus that is not frequency specific, the response is analyzed in the frequency domain, thus providing information across frequencies from 500 to 5000 Hz.

Emissions also can be recorded as acoustic distortion products (DPOAEs) which originate in the cochlea as a result of interference (distortion) between two simultaneously present frequencies (f1 and f2). DPOAEs can be elicited at any frequency throughout the range of human hearing. Whether TEOAEs or DPOAEs are used, these data provide clinicians the information needed to make an informed clinical decision regarding cochlear function and hearing status.

Also of interest, OAE responses are affected by even slight changes in the middle ear. Although the cochlea produces OAEs, the evoking stimulus must pass through the external and middle ears to the cochlea to evoke the OAEs. The OAEs subsequently travel back through the middle ear into the ear canal, so minor changes can alter their levels.

OAEs have the clinical capability to indicate normal cochlear function when it exists. For pediatric audiology, this is particularly helpful when used in conjunction with other hearing assessment tools, such as the ABR/ASSR and tests of middle ear function (tympanometry). For example, in children with neurologic involvement, an absent brainstem response can be the result of either severe cochlear involvement or lack of neural synchrony at the level of the brainstem. A finding of normal OAEs and normal middle ear function indicates normal peripheral (i.e., middle ear and cochlea) functioning, thus isolating the disorder to the brainstem auditory pathway. This finding illustrates an increasingly common audiologic challenge. Normal OAEs in combination with

abnormal brainstem function represents the hallmark signs in infants and children of some form of auditory nerve pathology, brainstem neuropathy, or brainstem conduction defect.

Behavioral Audiometry

A comprehensive, behavioral audiological evaluation includes pure tone air conduction, pure tone bone conduction, and speech audiometry measures and is considered the gold standard of audiological practice. The information from the audiological evaluation provides the audiologist and others with a picture of the child's hearing abilities.

As was outlined in Chapter 3, the human auditory system is composed of four main sections: the outer ear (pinna and ear canal), the middle ear (tympanic membrane and ossicular chain), the inner ear (the auditory portion or cochlea and the vestibular portion) and the auditory nerve and central auditory pathways. The outer ear collects and amplifies sound while the middle ear changes sound waves into vibrations. The inner ear transduces sound vibrations into neural signals which travel via the auditory nerve to the brain for processing. A deficit or problem in any of these areas may result in a hearing loss.

Behavioral audiometry is accomplished by assessing two pathways of hearing. The air conduction pathway involves the entire auditory system (Figure 4–1). Sound waves travel through the air, are picked up by the outer ear and eventually reach the auditory cortex in the brain. The bone conduction pathway is assessed by vibrating the skull to stimulate the inner ear directly. Bone conduction bypasses the outer and middle ear

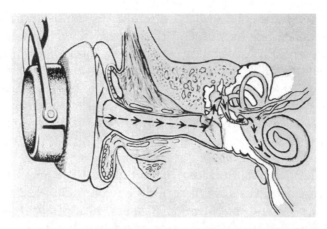

Figure 4–1. Air conduction pathway of the auditory system. Courtesy of Allan Diefendorf.

systems and tests the inner ear (cochlea), auditory nerve and central auditory pathways (Figure 4–2). Air and bone conduction pathways can be used in both pure tone and speech audiometry measures.

Pure Tone Audiometry

Pure tone audiometry is a subjective behavioral test of hearing sensitivity. The overall goal of pure tone audiometry is to determine the child's ear specific hearing thresholds (i.e., right and left separately) at different frequencies.

Pure tone signals are generated by an audiometer at specific frequencies (e.g., 1000 Hz) and with variable intensity (e.g., 25 dB HL). Although the human ear can detect frequency information from 20 to 20,000 Hz, hearing sensitivity is measured across several speech frequencies (250 through 8000 Hz) and intensity is measured using a dB scale ranging from –10 to 115 dB HL in 5 dB increments.

An audiometric (or hearing) threshold is the softest intensity at which the child can perceive a given sound. For example, if the child's response in the left

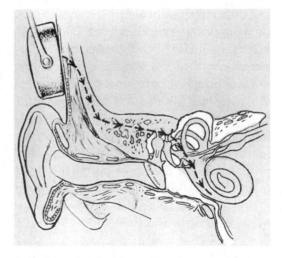

Figure 4–2. Bone conduction pathway of the auditory system. Courtesy of Allan Diefendorf.

ear to 1000 Hz is reported at 10 dB HL, then 10 dB HL is the softest intensity at which the child can perceive the 1000 Hz pure tone. In very young children, the pediatric audiologist does not expect to obtain an exact audiometric threshold. Instead, very young children will provide a response to auditory input at a minimum response level (MRL; Matkin, 1977). As the infant's auditory system matures, the child's MRL will move closer to his or her true audiometric threshold. In typically developing infants, it is expected that at 3 months of age the MRLs will be 15 to 30 dB higher than those of adults and at 6 to 12 months of age, MRLs will be 10 to 15 dB higher especially in the lower frequencies (Olsho, Koch, Carter, Halpin, & Spetner, 1988).

Pure tone audiometry allows the audiologist to measure hearing sensitivity and to report degree, type, and configuration of any hearing loss that may be present. Air conducted pure tone signals travel through the entire auditory system and give the audiologist information about the degree and configuration of the hearing loss. Air conducted pure tones can be presented to the child through one of several transducers: headphones, insert earphones, or through a sound field speaker. Bone conducted pure tone signals bypass the outer and middle portions of the auditory system via a bone conduction oscillator or vibrator. This bone conduction oscillator is placed either on the mastoid process behind the ear or on the forehead of the child. Bone conduction pure tone thresholds are compared to air conduction thresholds and help the audiologist determine the *type* of hearing loss. (See Chapter 3 for an overview of degree and types of hearing losses.)

Techniques for obtaining pure tone thresholds (air and bone conduction) via behavioral assessment on children fall into three categories: visual reinforcement audiometry, conditioned play audiometry, and conventional audiometry. The technique used will depend on several factors, including age and developmental status.

Visual reinforcement audiometry (VRA) uses the concept of conditioning to elicit the desired response. The conditioning paradigm involves presenting a stimulus (e.g., pure tone signal), getting the desired response (e.g., head turn to the sound source), rewarding or reinforcing the response (e.g., animated toy is activated or movie appears in monitors next to speakers) and repeating. VRA and conditioned orientation reflex (COR) audiometry are types of reinforcement audiometry and differ slightly in their techniques. VRA and COR audiometry may be conducted through sound field speakers, headphones, insert earphones or a bone conduction oscillator. In a typically developing child, the audiologist will use reinforcement audiometry techniques with children between the ages of 6 months and 2½ to 3 years. Importantly, visual reinforcement audiometry techniques are often necessary and successful in infants and toddlers or children who are developmentally delayed or who have motoric limitations.

Conditioned play audiometry (CPA) techniques are appropriate for children between the ages of 3 and 5 years. The use of a play task (e.g., throwing a block in a bucket) while attempting to obtain hearing thresholds on children is somewhat of a mix between reinforcement audiometry and conventional audiometry. While play audiometry may appear to rely solely on a child's ability to understand what the audiologist is asking him or her to do (i.e., put the toy car in the garage WHEN you hear the sound), it also continues to use the principles of conditioning and reinforcement. This is most evident in younger children and even in children who speak a different language than the audiologist. If the audiologist presents the pure tone stimulus at an intensity that is above the anticipated threshold and assists the child in the motor task that is being used (e.g., putting the peg on the board) several times, this is likely to condition the child to make the response when he or she hears the pure tone stimulus in the future. As children get older, they will understand the idea of performing the task in response to hearing the auditory stimulus. The use of play audiometry does require a specialized skill set and is more involved than the scope of this chapter allows especially in threshold determination. Play audiometry techniques may be used in children older than 5 who are developmentally delayed or who need the reinforcement of this technique to stay engaged in the task of the pure tone hearing test.

Conventional audiometry is used in older children and requires that the child raise his or her hand, provide a verbal response (e.g., "yes"), or presses a button (e.g., audio game–zap the sound) when he or she hears the pure tone stimulus. School-aged children are usually able to participate in pure tone testing using conventional audiometry techniques.

Regardless of the technique employed in pure tone testing, thresholds are obtained and plotted on an audiogram which provides a picture of a child's hearing sensitivity. Age-specific audiometric profiles are provided later in the chapter as well as a dissection of the audiogram to assist the reader in further understanding the results of the audiological evaluation.

Speech Audiometry

Although the pure tone audiogram is a prominent piece of information in the audiological evaluation, alone, it does not describe the full effects of hearing loss on a person's ability to perceive sound, especially speech. Speech audiometry measures provide information about a child's degree of hearing loss for speech stimuli and their ability to recognize and differentiate speech sounds in words, phrases, and sentences. In addition, speech audiometry techniques are used to assess a child's ability to understand speech in the presence of background noise. In most cases, when hearing sensitivity is measured to be normal for pure tone stimuli, speech audiometry results also will be normal. In the presence of hearing loss, however, speech audiometry results may vary from person to person—even if the pure tone audiograms look the same.

The primary speech audiometry measures used with children include determining the threshold for speech stimuli and evaluating the child's ability to recognize speech at different levels of audibility (soft speech, average speech and loud speech) relative to the pure tone thresholds. Speech audiometry measures can be administered via air conduction transducers or bone conduction transducers. Age and the developmental level (including the child's level of language development) will determine what speech audiometry measures may be used as well as how much information can be obtained.

Speech Threshold Measures. A speech detection threshold (SDT) or speech awareness threshold (SAT) is the lowest intensity level at which a child can detect or show awareness for speech. These measures are used with infants and young children who can demonstrate awareness of speech but who cannot demonstrate that they understood the speech. For example, an 11-month-old child may look up from a toy when someone talks to him but he cannot repeat what the person said.

Speech reception thresholds (SRT) can be obtained when a child can point to a picture of the word that he or she heard or can repeat the word back to the audiologist. Audiologists typically use spondaic words (two-syllable words with equal stress on each syllable; hotdog, baseball, toothbrush) as the stimulus for SRTs. As children begin to be able to demonstrate some understanding of speech, pediatric audiologists will use a modified SRT procedure and estimate threshold for speech by requesting that a child follow a direction: point to your nose, point to your ear; where is momma?; where is your daddy?

For pediatric hearing assessments, speech threshold measures are often used early in the evaluation because children may be more comfortable responding to speech. The audiologist can then use the speech threshold data to inform his or her pure tone testing. Speech thresholds should match (within 5 dB) the pure tone average of 500, 1000, and 2000 Hz. For example, if the audiologist obtains an SRT on a 5-year-old at 10 dB HL, then as the audiologist begins his pure tone testing on this child, he can estimate that pure tone thresholds in the 500, 1000 and 2000 Hz range should be around 10 dB HL. Pure tone testing will start at intensity levels above the threshold (e.g., 30–50 dB HL). If the child is not responding at this suprathreshold level, then the audiologist may need to reinstruct the child or retrain the child for the task. Speech threshold measures serve as a cross-check for pure tone data. (See "dissection of the audiogram" in this chapter for more information on the utility of these data to non-audiologists.)

Speech Recognition/Perception. Pure tone testing data, as well as speech threshold data, provide information about *audibility*. Is the sound or speech heard? However, the chief complaint of many individuals with hearing loss is that they can hear speech, but they can't understand it; it isn't intelligible. Speech needs to be both audible and intelligible to the person with hearing loss. Speech recognition and per-

ception testing allows the audiologist to measure the intelligibility of speech for a child in different listening conditions (e.g., quiet, noisy, soft speech, average speech). Speech recognition testing can be performed using words and sentences. These stimuli can be presented at different intensity levels relative to the child's pure tone and speech thresholds. In addition, these stimuli can be presented in quiet or in the presence of background noise.

Decisions by the audiologist on what speech recognition testing needs to be performed should be based on the primary reason for the visit. For children with documented hearing loss, it will not be possible to measure speech recognition in every condition at every visit. The choice of what materials to use (words or sentences) and under what conditions to present the speech recognition tasks will vary from child to child. It is important, however, to include this component in the audiological evaluation.

Speech audiometry results are often useful to parents, school personnel, and other individuals besides the audiologist. These results may assist teachers and parents in making modifications for a child who may need additional supports for information that is presented auditorially. The speech-language pathologist may find speech audiometry data helpful in planning for therapy. The combination of the pure tone and speech audiometry data should provide a thorough picture of a child's hearing and listening abilities.

Equipment Needed to Test Children for Pure Tone and Speech Audiometry

The audiologist who sees pediatric patients will often have an office setup that looks different from the audiologist who primarily sees adults. Child-friendly practices often have toys that children can play with in the waiting area as well as toys that can be used for play audiometry as well as "distractors" (e.g., small books with bright pictures) for use in visual reinforcement audiometry.

It may take two people to test young children, especially when behavioral audiometry is being used. An audiologist will need to be at the audiometer in the control room of the sound suite. A second person may be needed to sit in front of the child and keep him or her on task during testing. It is critical that this second person be trained in his or her duties (what to do, what NOT to do) as this task is as important as that of the audiologist behind the audiometer. The second person should wear attenuators or headphones with masking noise to minimize their ability to hear the presented stimuli, so as to not cue the child.

Additional equipment and materials will also be found in the office of an audiologist who sees pediatric patients. A larger sound booth may be used because of the need for sound field speakers, along with equipment that allows for visual reinforcement (i.e., animated and lighted toys in boxes behind dark plexiglass or movie on the monitor). Another consideration in the size of the sound booth is that with children, parents should be allowed to accompany the child for testing. This often requires more seating space in the sound room.

A small, portable audiometer may be needed on the patient side of the sound booth for children who can participate in ear-specific pure tone audiometer, but who need "side by side" attention from the audiologist to understand the task and to stay focused and engaged. At a minimum, this audiometer should provide air- and bone conduction testing capabilities along with masking.

Testing materials, in addition to toys, should include picture cards for speech threshold testing. Assessments for speech recognition testing that include pictures (such as the Word Intelligibility by Picture Identification test; Ross & Lerman, 1971) should be available for children who cannot perform traditional measures. For example, a child who has poor speech production/articulation may be able to pick out a picture of the word he or she heard (from a choice of six), but if asked to repeat that word, it would not be clear enough for the audiologist to know which of those words the child said.

Last, the audiologist who sees pediatric patients will want to have written materials and resources appropriate for a parent of a child with hearing loss. Materials relative to normal speech and language milestones as well as information on pediatric hearing technology will help the family understand what the child is experiencing. Resources about speech-language-listening therapy, financial assistance for technology, early intervention services, and family support opportunities will be of interest to families, facilitate future informed decision making, and strengthen professional relationships.

Immittance

Acoustic immittance in the pediatric population contributes important information by verifying the functional status of the conductive auditory system. Immittance is a measurement of energy or air pressure flow, which involves the ear canal, tympanic membrane, ossicular chain, tensor tympani, stapedius muscle, cochlea, and cranial nerves VII and VIII. Mass, mobility, and resistance of the outer and middle ear systems affect this test. Immittance testing includes, but is not limited to, tympanometry and acoustic reflexes. Tympanometry is the measure of acoustic admittance of the middle ear system. Acoustic reflexes measure the integrity of the acoustic reflex pathway ipsilaterally and contralaterally.

One reason why immittance testing is important is that otitis media is one of the most common causes of hearing loss in children. Between 50% and 85% of children under the age of 3 years experience at least one episode of acute otitis media (Klein, 1989). Otitis media with effusion can affect as many as 80% of children with approximately 2.2 million cases of otitis media identified annually in the United States of America (van Zon, van der Heijden, van Dongen, Burton, & Schilder, 2012).

Children under the age of 7 years are more prone to otitis media due to an anatomical predisposition. The eustachian tube is horizontal and shorter, allowing potential pathogens to enter the middle ear cavity with minimal resistance. As the child matures, the eustachian tube becomes vertical and longer, making it more difficult for pathogens to enter the middle ear cavity after age 7 years. There are two commonly used tests for identifying middle ear dysfunctions: pneumatic otoscopy and tympanometry testing (AAFP; AAOHNS, 2004).

Pneumatic otoscopy and tympanometry both assess the mobility of the tympanic membrane by varying ear canal pressure. A physician commonly uses pneumatic otoscopy to visualize the tympanic membrane while varying pressure. With tympanometry, as the pressure is varied, a probe measures the mobility of the tympanic membrane by means of sound reflection (Table 4–2). This diagnostic tool is commonly used by audiologists, nurses, and family medical practices.

Tympanometry obtains four measurements: equivalent ear canal volume, peak pressure point, tympanic width, and static acoustic compliance (Table 4–3). Together, these measurements are depicted on a graph for interpretation and provide information on the status of the middle ear function.

With children under the age of approximately 6 months, interpretation of tympanograms is compromised when a conventional low-frequency (220- or 226-Hz) probe tone is used. As such, a higher probe-tone frequency (e.g., 1000 Hz) is recommended for identifying middle ear

Table 4–2. Otoscopy, Tympanometry, and Acoustic Reflex Testing Suggestions

Call the otoscope a flashlight
Help the child look in the parent's ear
For tympanometry, say to the child, "Did you know your ear can draw a picture? Will your ear draw a flat road or a mountain?"
Have the child feel the tip of the probe
Test the parent's ear first
Have the child watch a video during the testing

Table 4–3. Norms for Individuals With Normal Anatomy

Ear Canal Volume
Adults: 0.9–2.0 cc
Pediatrics (2.8–5.8 years): 0.3–0.9 cc
Peak Compliance
Adults: 0.3–1.7 cc
Pediatrics (2.8–5.8 years): 0.2–1.0 cc
Normal Pressure
Adults: −150/+50
Pediatrics (2.8–5.8 years): −150/+50

Source: Margolis and Heller, 1987; Wiley et al., 1996.

disorders in infants less than 6 months of age (JCIH, 2007). While the test only takes a couple of minutes to perform for both ears, it should only be performed when the case history or patient symptoms indicates the necessity of this procedure.

If abnormal results are obtained, a referral to a primary care provider or an otolaryngologist is warranted. At this point, the audiologist will need to determine if testing should continue based on the case history, presenting complaints, and the abnormal tympanometry. See Figure 4–3 for examples on decision matrix.

The other primary immittance measurement performed on children is called

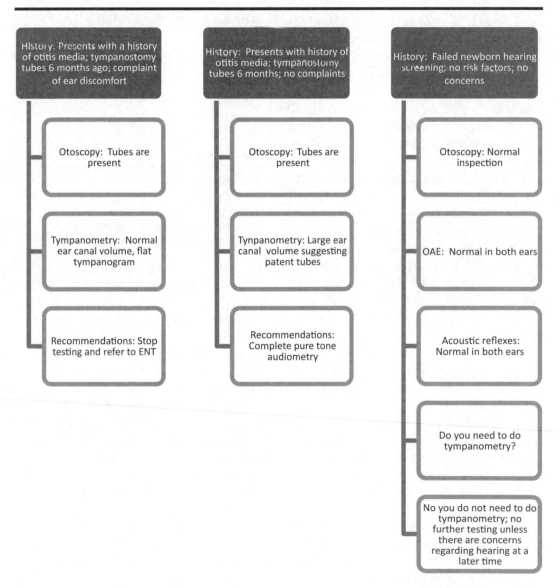

Figure 4–3. Hearing evaluation decision matrix.

acoustic reflexes. The acoustic reflex provides supplemental information relevant to the functional status of the middle ear, cochlea, and lower brainstem pathway. The measurement is a response to the contraction of middle ear muscles/tendons to a sound stimulation. Although only one ear is measured at a time, the contraction of the middle ear muscles and tendons occur in both ears at the same time.

In the middle ear, the tensor tympani muscle is connected to the malleus and is innervated by the trigeminal (V) nerve. The stapedius muscle is connected to the stapes and is innervated by the facial (VII) nerve. These middle ear muscles contract when sounds exceed 70 dB HL. At this point, the middle ear system stiffens and compliance decreases. There are four combinations measured for this test: ipsilateral right (probe and stimulus right ear), contralateral right (probe left ear, stimulus right ear), ipsilateral left (probe and stimulus left ear), and contralateral left (probe right ear, stimulus left ear). The measurements recorded are always in response to the stimulus presented, regardless of which ear the probe measurement is occurring. Frequencies tested include 500, 1000, and 2000 Hz (Table 4–4). A threshold is recorded to the minimum stimulus-intensity level that activates the acoustic reflex response of a 0.2 deflection.

A word of caution: immittance testing should not be completed when contraindications exist such as middle ear surgery within 6 months or patient reports of extreme discomfort. Together, these measures are fundamental components of the pediatric audiology test battery but only should be performed when indicated by the referral source, patient's case history, or patient complaints or findings at the time of examination.

Table 4–4. Acoustic Reflex Normative Values

Hearing thresholds 0–25 dB HL
500 Hz: <95
1000 Hz: <95
2000 Hz: <95
Hearing thresholds 30–45 dB HL
500 Hz: <95
1000 Hz: <95
2000 Hz: <105
Hearing thresholds 50–65 dB HL
500 Hz: <110
1000 Hz: <110
2000 Hz: <115
Hearing thresholds 30–45 dB HL
500 Hz: >115
1000 Hz: >115
2000 Hz: >115

Source: Gelfand, 1990.

Auditory Skills Assessments

Measuring hearing sensitivity as reported in the audiogram is an important component in developing the child's audiologic profile, but it doesn't tell the whole story. Once degree, type, and stability of the hearing loss are established, the next step is to determine *how* the child is using his or her hearing (with or without his or her technology) in everyday situations. Completing auditory skills assessments during the audiological evaluation provides the audiologist important information to help direct management of child's hearing care and also provide opportunities to determine effectiveness of treatment.

The use of criterion-referenced tests and functional outcome measures early in an episode of care establishes the baseline status of the child, providing a means to quantify change in functioning levels as the child grows. Functional outcome measures, along with other measures used throughout the episode of care, as part of periodic re-evaluation, provide information about whether predicted outcomes are being realized. When the child is discharged from interventional services and/or the end of the episode of care, the audiologist will still need to continue to monitor outcomes to ensure that there are no changes in hearing status.

Using functional outcomes measures provides a common language with which to evaluate the success of auditory interventions. Measuring outcomes of listening, talking, comprehending, and literacy among children with the same diagnosis is the foundation for determining which intervention approaches optimize best clinical practice. Furthermore, some healthcare reimbursement models, like Medicare, are now tying reimbursement with claim-based outcome reporting (CBOR) for therapy and PQRS. Audiologists and speech-language pathologists registered with Centers for Medicare and Medicaid Services (CMS) are required to report at least one claim for one beneficiary that includes one of the approved PQRS codes or face a reduction of 1.5% in all 2015 claims and 2% reduction in 2016 (CMS, 2014).

There is a variety of criterion measures available for assessing functional outcomes. These measures allow audiologists to assess a child's performance over time. Since many factors can impact a child's development of listening and spoken language, using functional outcomes will help audiologists determine what potential intrinsic and extrinsic factors are contributing to the child's performance.

Intrinsic factors include overall cognition, learning style, processing abilities, and/or the presence of other developmental disabilities. Extrinsic factors are related to family support and follow-through, appropriately fit technology and management, type of intervention provided, and/or services provided by a highly qualified provider (Perigoe & Paterson, 2015). Depending on what skills need to be assessed will guide the examiner as to which test(s) to administer.

Functional outcome measures can be categorized into questionnaires (Table 4–5), closed set auditory assessment, open-set auditory assessment, and comprehensive assessment (Perigoe & Paterson, 2015). Some questionnaires are interview style whereas others are forms that the parents, teachers, and/or the children themselves complete. Closed- and open-set auditory assessments are typically completed in the sound room by the audiologist as described above. Comprehensive assessments may use a battery of tests or measures and assess a variety of auditory skills.

Regardless of the instrument used, a review of content reliability is essential to verify that it is measuring what you intend to assess.

Functional outcomes seem to have become the "gold standard" (Mendel, 2009). How hearing loss impacts a child cannot be simulated in the office. The use of functional assessments, however, provides the examiner information about how a child is benefitting from the use of hearing technology. As health care continues to evolve, specifically new payment models like **Bundled Payments for Care Improvement (BPCI)**, audiologists will enter into reimbursement models that are based on episodes of care and on how the patient is functioning (CMS, 2014). These models will require more coordinated care, which ultimately will lead to higher quality and lower cost. Auditory assessment tools that measure functional skills will be critical in this new model.

Table 4–5. List of Commonly Used Questionnaires and Functional Outcomes Measures

Name of Measure	Age Range	Descriptions	Reference(s)
Questionnaires			
ASHA's National Outcome Measures (NOMS)	Preschool age	Seven-point scales to assess functional change in communication abilities over time. Six functional communication measures (FCM) are available for prekindergarten: Articulation, cognitive orientation, pragmatics, spoken language comprehension, spoken language production, and swallowing.	ASHA (2011)
Auditory Skills Checklist (ASC)	No age limits reported	Thirty-five item checklist administered via parent interview in three-month intervals to assess auditory skill development.	Meinzen-Derr, Wiley, Creighton, & Choo (2007)
Children's Auditory Performance Scale (CHAPS)	7+ years	A scaled questionnaire that quantifies observed behaviors in the classroom and compares them to children without hearing difficulties.	Smoski, Brunt, & Tannahill (1992)
Children's Home Inventory for Listening Difficulties (CHILD)	7–12 years	Child and parent questionnaires which rate how well the child understood speech in 15 different situations.	Anderson & Smaldino (2000)
Children's Observation Worksheet (COW)	4–12 years	Worksheets can be completed by the teacher, parent, and/or the child who are asked to specify five situations where improved hearing is desired.	Williams (2003)
Early Listening Function (ELF)	5 months–3 years	Observation worksheet for the audiologist and/or parent to record the child's responses to auditory stimuli in 12 listening situations.	Anderson (2002)
Functional Auditory Performance Indicators (FAPI)	No age limits reported	Examines seven categories of auditory development: sound awareness, sound as meaningful, auditory feedback, localizing sound source, auditory discrimination, short-term auditory memory, and linguistic auditory processing.	Stredler-Brown & Johnson (2001)
Functioning After Pediatric Cochlear Implantation (FAPCI)	2–5 years	Parent questionnaire to evaluate the child's real-world verbal communication performance.	Lin, Ceh, Bervinchak, Riley, Miech, & Niparko (2007)
Meaningful Auditory Integration Skills (MAIS)	3–4 years	Ten-item parental interview that evaluates how the child uses sound in everyday situations (hearing technology attachment, alerting to sound, and attaching meaning to sound).	Robbins, Renshaw, & Berry (1991)
Infant-Toddler Meaningful Auditory Integration Skills (IT-MAIS)	Birth–3 years	Ten-item parental interview that evaluates how the child uses sound in everyday situations (vocal behavior, hearing technology attachment, alerting to sound, and attaching meaning to sound).	Zimmerman-Phillips, Robbins, & Osberger (2000)

Table 4–5. *continued*

Name of Measure	Age Range	Descriptions	Reference(s)
Listening Inventory for Education (LIFE)	6 years and up	Two questionnaires: the child version has 15 items and the teacher version has 16 items. LIFE identifies challenging classroom situations.	Anderson & Smaldino (1996)
LittlEARS Auditory Questionnaire	Birth–2 years	Available in 16 languages, this 35-item parent questionnaire provides information about auditory development and early speech production development.	Tsiakpini et al. (2004); Coninx et al. (2009)
Parent's Evaluation of Aural/Oral Performance of Children (PEACH)	3–6 years	Fifteen item parent interview targeting everyday listening situations (use, quiet, noise, telephone, and environment).	Ching & Hill (2005)
Pragmatic Language Observation Scales (PLOS)	8 years–17 years, 11 months	Thirty-item norm-referenced teachers' 5-point rating scale that can be used to assess students' daily classroom spoken language behaviors.	Newcomer & Hammill (2009)
Preschool Screening Instrument For Targeting Educational Risk (Preschool SIFTER)	3–6 years	Fifteen-item teacher questionnaire that identifies children at risk for educational failure (academics, attention, communication, participation, and behavior).	Anderson & Matkin (1996)
Secondary Screening Instrument For Targeting Educational Risk (Secondary SIFTER)	Children enrolled in 6th through 12th grade.	Fifteen-item teacher questionnaire that identifies children at risk for educational failure (academics, attention, communication, participation, and behavior).	Anderson (2004)
Screening Instrument For Targeting Educational Risk (SIFTER)	Grades 1st through 5th grade	Fifteen-item teacher questionnaire that identifies children at risk for educational failure (academics, attention, communication, participation, and behavior.	Anderson (1989)
Listening Inventory For Education–Revised (LIFE-R)	No age limits reported	Pretest and post-test format that provides documentation of the effectiveness of intervention used to improve the classroom listening environment. Student and teacher versions are available in three languages.	Anderson, Smaldino, & Spangler (2011)
Teachers' Evaluation of Aural/Oral Performance of Children (TEACH)	Preschool to 7 years	Thirteen-question teacher interview targeting the child's everyday environment. Includes scoring for five subscales: use, quiet, noise, telephone, and environment.	Ching, Hill, & Psarros (2000)

Closed–Set Auditory Assessments

Name of Measure	Age Range	Descriptions	Reference(s)
Early Speech Perception Test (ESP)	6+ years	Thirty-six words in three subtests that provide information about the child's speech discrimination skill development.	Moog & Geers (1990)
Learning to Listen Sounds	Birth+	Onomatopoeic sounds that are associated with toys commonly used by babies and very young children.	Estrabrooks (1994)

continues

Table 4–5. *continued*

Name of Measure	Age Range	Descriptions	Reference(s)
Ling Six-Sound Test	Birth+	Six sounds that represent low-, mid-, and high-frequency aspects of speech.	Ling & Ling (1978)
Low-Verbal Early Speech Perception Test	2–6 years	Using stimuli that vary in pattern, the child is instructed to identify the word out of four items. This measure estimates speech perception abilities.	Moog & Geers (1990)
Mr. Potato Head Test	2 years+	Ten sentences using pieces from Mr. Potato Head are presented to the child for the child to perform the task (e.g., "Find his black hat").	Robbins (1993)
Northwestern University—Children's Perception of Speech (NU-CHIPS)	2.5 years+	Picture pointing word recognition test.	Elliot & Katz (1980)
Word Intelligibility by Picture Identification (WIPI)	4+ years	Picture pointing word recognition test.	Ross & Lerman (1971)

Open-Set Auditory Assessments

Name of Measure	Age Range	Descriptions	Reference(s)
Multi-syllabic Lexical Neighborhood Test (MLNT)	5 years+	Multi-syllabic word recognition test.	Kirk, Pisoni, & Osberger (1995)
Lexical Neighborhood Test (LNT)	5 years+	Twenty-five monosyllabic word recognition test.	Kirk, Pisoni, & Osberger (1995)
Phonetically Balanced Kindergarten Test (PBK-50)	6 years+	Monosyllabic word recognition test.	Haskins (1949)
Hearing in Noise Test for Children (HINT-C)	6–12 years	Sentence recognition test in background noise.	Nilsson, Soli, & Gelnett (1996)
Bamford-Kowal-Bench Sentence In Noise Test (BKB-SIN)	5+ years	Uses sentences in the presence of four talker speech babble to estimate the signal-to-noise ratio (SNR) loss.	Etymotic Research (2005)

Comprehensive Auditory Assessments

Name of Measure	Age Range	Descriptions	Reference(s)
Auditory Perception Test for the Hearing Impaired (APT-HI)	3 years+	Criterion-based test that provides an accurate determination of children's discrete auditory perception abilities by profiling in 16 different skill areas.	Allen (2008)
Cottage Acquisition Scales for Listening, Language, and Speech (CASLLS)	3 years & older (due to small parts that accompany the test)	Using language sampling, the CASLLS provides listening, language, speech, and cognitive milestones in five states of development: preverbal, presentence, simple sentences, complex sentences, and sounds and speech.	Wilkes (2001)

Table 4–5. *continued*

Name of Measure	Age Range	Descriptions	Reference(s)
Evaluation of Auditory Responses to Speech (EARS)	3–12 years	Available in 21 languages, EARS contains 5 closed-set tests, 2 open-set tests, and 2 questionnaires that provide information about detection, discrimination, identification, recognition, and comprehension.	Allum, Greisinger, Staubhaar, & Carpenter (2000)
Teacher Assessment of Spoken Language (TASL)	6 months+	Teacher rating form that evaluates the sentence structure of the child.	Moog & Biedenstein (1998)
TeenEARS	13–19 years	Available in two languages, TeenEARS contains 3 rating scales, 4 open-set tests, and 1 questionnaire that provide information regarding primary and secondary benefits of cochlear implantation.	Anderson, Philips, Robert, Jamieson, Costa, & Cross (2004)

SELECTING THE MEASURES

To facilitate a timely transition in the intervention stage, the diagnostic process must be outcome-driven and efficient. As stated above, the audiologist will be thinking about providing the right care, at the right time, for that child and his or her family. The age of the child as well as the case history will guide the audiologist in determining how to proceed.

Infant Audiometric Profile

Because test time may be limited, decisions about stimulus mode (air conduction [A/C] and bone conduction [B/C]) and frequency order must be made after each successive step in the assessment protocol. Effective clinical decision making at diagnostic appointments requires an approach to assessment that has both qualitative and quantitative outcomes. This approach facilitates diagnostic outcomes that are crucial for initiating fam-ily counseling, substantiating appropriate recommendations, and making a difference in subsequent management planning, yet are complicated by restricted test time.

An effective clinical approach is structured to seek answers to the following questions:

1. Can diagnostic testing be carried out in natural sleep or will moderate sedation be required?
2. What information will the family find useful for allaying/confirming their initial concerns?
3. What information will facilitate family counseling?
4. What information will guide medical referrals and facilitate medical management?,
5. What information will facilitate coordinated care, including audiologic intervention? (ASHA, 2006)

Obviously, clinical decision making during an evaluation is, by necessity, ongoing, patient-centered, and family-focused. Audiologists recognize the uniqueness of the pediatric population, pediatric assessment, and the vast differences between protocols uniquely aligned for infants and more conventional protocols recommended for adults. As such, the diagnostic protocol with infants requires the following qualitative and quantitative decisions:

1. What is the most efficient A/C sequence to distinguish normal hearing from hearing loss?
2. How soon is switching to B/C considered to distinguish between conductive hearing loss and sensorineural hearing loss?
3. What are the essential frequencies to assess that enhance efficiency without sacrificing accuracy?
4. What is the preferred order of obtaining frequency information?
5. What stimulus levels will provide the most information in the least amount of time in order to maximize safety (sedation-related) and maximize efficiency (obtaining both qualitative and quantitative information while the infant is in an optimal physical state)?

Infants from the well-baby nursery who were referred by screening ABR should not be evaluated initially as outpatients by OAEs and "passed," because such infants are presumed to be at risk for a subsequent diagnosis of auditory neuropathy/dysynchrony. Additionally, comprehensive outpatient assessment should be performed on both ears even if only one ear failed the hospital-based screening.

Most infants referred for diagnostic follow-up from hospital screening programs have normal hearing. As such, use of AEPs presented at low-intensity stimulus levels can address the initial concern about the presence of hearing loss. Start-ing at a low intensity will quickly obtain clinical results qualifying normal hearing bilaterally. Results for 2000 Hz are recommended, first in one ear and then the other. This strategy is based on the belief that knowing the qualitative status of both ears by A/C will, at a minimum, provide information to a family that helps inform their initial concerns. The order of frequency-specific information will certainly be influenced by the child's medical history and the family's primary concern.

When A/C testing suggests elevated responses, B/C testing should be considered sooner rather than later. Depending entirely on the infant's activity state and the outcome of the initial A/C data, immediate clinical decisions should be made to determine whether additional A/C information is desirable, or if B/C information will best facilitate the diagnostic process. The choice of stimulus mode and frequency preferences should be based on establishing quantitative results that expand information essential for content counseling, impacting medical management as necessary, and facilitating early intervention, particularly the selection and fitting of amplification systems.

OAEs also are useful in the diagnostic process to determine the presence or absence of auditory neuropathy/dysynchrony. Additionally, OAEs have an expanding role in on-going surveillance, particularly in the areas of monitoring for ototoxicity, noise exposure, and progressive hearing loss.

Toddler/Preschooler Audiometric Profile

At this point in the child's life, it is important to obtain the case history to determine the procedures that are needed.

Example 1

If the concern is that the child has passed newborn hearing screening and has no risk factors but is not talking yet, then the audiologist needs to administer a test battery that will rule out hearing loss as a primary concern for the delay in developing spoken language. For this scenario, the audiologist should consider starting with otoscopy and OAEs. If those are normal, the audiologist should administer a functional assessment. If there are no further concerns, the assessment may be complete. If, however, there are abnormal test findings or concerns raised during the functional assessment, then the administration of tympanometry and/or ear-specific air conduction testing is warranted.

Example 2

If the parent does have concerns regarding hearing, then a more comprehensive assessment should be considered. It is important to explore what concerns the family has about hearing. If the toddler has a positive history for otitis media, the test battery should start with otoscopy and OAEs. If those are normal, the audiologist should obtain ear specific speech-reception thresholds and air conduction thresholds for 2000, 500, 4000, and then 1000 Hz if possible to rule out minimal hearing loss. If the OAEs were abnormal, the audiologist should perform tympanometry. For abnormal tympanometric results, testing should stop at this point unless there is something else presented in the history that warrants moving on to air conduction and bone conduction testing. For normal tympanometric results, the audiologist should obtain acoustic reflexes and move on to ear spe-

cific speech-reception thresholds and air conduction thresholds for 2000, 500, 4000, and then 1000 Hz to determine the degree of hearing loss. The audiologist should administer bone conduction if a hearing loss is present for 500 and 2000 Hz and fill in with 4000 and 1000 Hz if time permits. Finally, the audiologist should administer a functional assessment before the family leaves to determine the impact of the hearing loss in a variety of listening conditions.

It is important to move to ear specific testing as soon as possible instead of performing sound field testing first. The audiologist can always drop back to sound field testing if the child refuses insertion of earphones or earphones.

Example 3

If the concern is that the child has passed newborn hearing screening but has risk factors for hearing loss, the audiologist can administer a test battery that confirms normal hearing. For this scenario, the audiologist should administer a functional assessment first. If there are no concerns, then the audiologist should obtain ear specific air conduction thresholds for 2000, 500, 4000, and 1000 Hz. If these results are normal, the assessment may be complete. In this scenario, it is assumed that the child has already had an electrophysiological test completed that included screening ABR/ASSR/ABR and OAEs. There is no reason to repeat these tests unless something in the history warrants repeating these measures. If only OAEs were performed for the newborn hearing screening, it is prudent for the audiologist to complete either an electrophysiological measure or acoustic reflexes to confirm the absence of ANSD.

School–Age Audiometric Profile

School-age children will be referred to an audiologist for many reasons. The audiologist should consider the reason for referral as he or she makes clinical decisions about what tests are appropriate to administer.

Example 1

A kindergarten student is referred for a hearing evaluation because he did not pass a hearing screening at school. The case history provided by the parent and the audiologist's initial observation of the child reveal that he has some articulation errors including difficulties with sounds such s, sh and f. The case history also indicates that the child passed his newborn hearing screening and that he has been in day care since age 3.

In this example, the audiologist starts with otoscopy and tympanometry to determine outer or middle ear involvement. Next the audiologist obtains ear specific SRTs and moves on to pure tone air conduction. The child's pure tone audiometry reveals a mild to moderate bilateral, high-frequency hearing loss (4000–8000 Hz). Bone conduction testing is performed and thresholds match air conduction. Speech recognition testing is performed at a level of 40 dB SL (which is 40 dB above the SRT) for words in quiet. In addition, the audiologist wants to obtain information about how well the child understands speech in the presence of background noise. Therefore, the audiologist administers another word list but uses some background noise at a level 5 dB below the level of the speech (+5 dB signal to noise ration or SNR).

The child is referred for a comprehensive medical evaluation. (See Chapter 3.) The pros and cons of amplification (i.e., hearing aids) on this high-frequency hearing loss are discussed with the family. At this time, they decide not to pursue the use of hearing aids. The audiologist, however, provides the family with suggestions for accommodations related to classroom and home listening environments. (See Chapter 9.) The audiologist further explains that if the child is having difficulty in the classroom listening to or hearing the teacher, the parent should discuss this with the school-based audiologist. The use of a classroom sound distribution system may need to be considered or a personal FM/DM system to improve the signal to noise ratio for the child in the classroom. The child is scheduled to return to see the audiologist in 3 months to confirm the hearing loss and to check for stability of hearing thresholds. The parents are counseled that if any changes are noted before that time, they should schedule an appointment sooner.

Example 2

Olivia is a 10-year-old with bilateral severe sensorineural hearing loss. Her hearing loss was identified at birth and she was fitted with hearing aids at 8 weeks of age. Hearing thresholds have remained stable since she was initially diagnosed. At Oliva's annual evaluation with her managing audiologist, Olivia and her family reported no concerns. The audiologist obtained ear impressions for new earmolds, and checked her hearing aids to ensure that appropriate amplification is being provided. The audiologist also verified that her pure tone thresholds were stable since her hearing loss is caused by enlarged vestibular aqueduct syndrome (which is known to be progressive). As her pure tone thresholds were stable, the audiologist completed the session.

Dissection of the Audiogram

Many professionals outside of the profession of audiology need to be able to understand and use hearing evaluation data. It is critical that the audiologist provide interpretation of the audiological information so that other professionals and parents are not left to guess what information has been provided. However, even with the audiometric interpretation, parents and other recipients may have to apply the information to their particular setting or need. Here are some tips on dissecting the audiological information:

1. Look for a description of the audiogram. This usually will involve details related to the degree, type, and configuration of hearing loss for each ear. Examples include:
   - Mild to moderate sensorineural hearing loss in the right ear OR
   - Moderate rising to mild conductive hearing loss in the left ear OR
   - Slight to severe sensorineural hearing loss in both ears
   This information will correspond to the marks on the audiogram (i.e., the graph that is a picture of the hearing thresholds).
2. Look for information related to tympanometry. Tympanograms are not a measure of hearing sensitivity. However, they are important in understanding middle ear system function and how it is affecting the child's overall hearing ability. If a child has abnormal middle ear function, he may be experiencing hearing loss that could impact his performance in the classroom. Even children with permanent childhood hearing loss can experience ear infections (or fluid in the middle ear) that cause their hearing thresholds to be even more elevated.
3. Examine the interpretations of the speech audiometry measures. In many cases, the audiologist will not interpret or discuss the speech threshold measures unless they do not match the audiometric hearing thresholds. Speech threshold measures are a cross-check in most cases and provide reliability data for the hearing thresholds. However, speech perception/recognition test data may be of interest to non-audiologists. The speech-language pathologist or teacher of the deaf or hard of hearing may find it helpful to know that when speech is intense (or loud) enough, the child has good (or poor) speech recognition ability for single words in quiet. The classroom teacher may find it helpful to know that in the presence of background noise the child has fair speech perception for sentences.

Audiologists who see pediatric patients of any age are strongly encouraged to provide a written explanation of the audiometric data in language that is usable by non-audiologists. The impact of hearing loss for children is far reaching and therefore, many individuals outside of the audiology clinic need to be able to use this information to make decisions about classroom accommodations, therapy goals, and expectations as well as health-related implications.

Olivia and her family are instructed to return in one year to check earmolds, hearings aids, and monitor pure tone thresholds. The family is advised to return sooner if there are issues with the hearing aids, changes in her hearing sensitivity, or notice difficulties hearing her teachers in school (see Chapter 9).

If Olivia or her parents have specific complaints regarding her ability to understand speech in certain situations, the audiologist should check pure tone thresholds and administer speech recognition testing. In this case, the audiologist uses sentence stimuli and administers the words in quiet and in noise. If the results of the testing indicate that in higher levels of background noise Olivia's ability to recognize speech is compromised, the audiologist would initiate a counseling conversation with Olivia and her family about strategies that can be used when trying to listen or communicate in noisy situations.

DISCHARGE VERSUS CONTINUOUS CARE

Determining when to discharge a patient from audiological management seems like it would be a very simple concept. A child passes the newborn hearing screening, end of story. Right? Or a child presents with hearing loss, thus they should continue to be monitored by the audiologist. The question though is how often?

Surveillance in Children Who Pass the Newborn Hearing Screening

Concern for hearing loss must not stop at birth. It must be recognized that limiting hearing screening to the neonatal period will result in excluding a number of children with hearing loss from the benefits of early detection. Most newborns and infants will pass initial hearing screening yet some will require periodic monitoring of hearing to detect delayed-onset hearing loss. Information on developmental milestones for hearing and communication should be provided to all parents upon discharge from a hospital and/or at the time of well-baby checkups. Increased parent awareness is an inexpensive approach to increase the likelihood of detecting an infant with hearing loss who had initially passed the newborn hearing screening.

Figure 4–4 illustrates four routine outcomes from universal newborn hearing screening and delineates the subsequent follow-up that should be implemented. As noted, on-going surveillance in the child's Medical Home and continued monitoring using risk indicators is recommended for all children. The Medical Home is part of the health-delivery system responsible for assuring that a child has follow-up screening and audiologic assessment scheduled. Moreover, the child's medical home insures that families and children attend appointments, and that they enter the early intervention system and healthcare intervention system in a timely manner. The physician also has the opportunity to articulate to parents the importance of follow-up and to actively demonstrate the importance through sustained monitoring as is indicated in the American Academy of Pediatrics periodicity schedule (Hagan, Shaw, & Duncan, 2008).

The JCIH (2007) identified 11 risk indicators (Table 4–6) associated with either congenital or delayed-onset hearing loss. These indicators guide continuing surveillance of all infants for delayed-onset hearing loss.

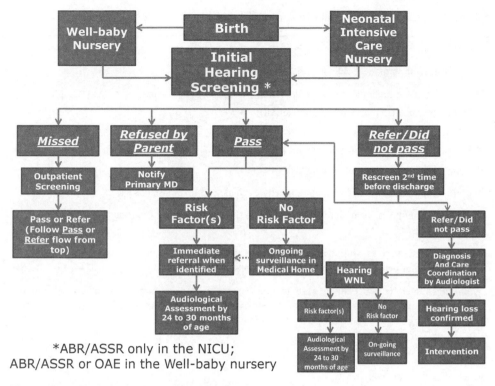

**ABR/ASSR only in the NICU;
ABR/ASSR or OAE in the Well-baby nursery*

Figure 4–4. Roadmap for initial hearing screening.

Transitioning Audiologic Surveillance Between EHDI Programs and School-Based Programs

Continued surveillance for hearing impairment that may interfere with communication, literacy, social and emotional development, and academic performance should continue for preschool children. There are, however, no systematic screening programs in most communities for children between birth and kindergarten. Unlike the newborn and school-age populations when nearly all children are accessible in hospitals and schools, preschoolers are generally not available in large, organized groups that lend themselves to universal detection of hearing loss. As such, an interdisciplinary, collaborative effort is particularly important for this age group.

Physicians who make up the child's medical home, audiologists who provide the initial care-coordination of hearing health care, speech-language pathologists and educators of children with hearing loss who provide early intervention services, and other professionals who specialize in children's healthy development should be at the core in planning and implementing hearing screening opportunities to maximize the likelihood of prompt referral of children suspected of hearing loss.

For this age group (3–5 years), screening for hearing impairment is a pass-refer procedure to identify individuals who require further audiologic evaluation or other assessments. Hearing impairment is defined as permanent, bilateral or unilateral, sensory-neural and/or conductive hearing loss greater than 20 dB HL in the

Table 4–6. Joint Committee on Infant Hearing (JCIH) 2007 High-Risk Indicators

1. Caregiver concern regarding hearing, speech, language, or developmental delay

2. Family history of permanent childhood hearing loss

3. Neonatal intensive care of more than 5 days or any of the following regardless of length of stay:
   - Extracorporeal membrane oxygenation (ECMO)
   - Assisted ventilation
   - Exposure to ototoxic medications (gentimycin and tobramycin) or loop diuretics
   - Hyperbilirubinemia requiring exchange transfusion

4. In utero infections, such as CMV, herpes, rubella, syphilis, and toxoplasmosis

5. Craniofacial anomalies, including those that involve the pinna, ear canal, ear tags, ear pits, and temporal bone anomalies

6. Physical findings, such as white forelock, that are associated with a syndrome known to include a sensory-neural or permanent conductive hearing loss

7. Syndromes associated with hearing loss or progressive or late-onset hearing loss, such as neurofibromatosis, osteopetrosis, and Usher syndrome; other frequently identified syndromes include:
   - Waardenburg
   - Alport
   - Pendred
   - Jervell and Lange-Nielsen

8. Neurodegenerative disorders, such as Hunter syndrome, or sensory motor neuropathies, such as Friedreich ataxia and Charcot-Marie-Tooth syndrome

9. Culture-positive postnatal infections associated with sensory-neural hearing loss, including confirmed bacterial and viral (especially herpes viruses and varicella) meningitis

10. Head trauma, especially basal skull/temporal bone fractures that requires hospitalization

11. Chemotherapy

frequency region important for speech recognition (approximately 500 through 4000 Hz). As would be expected, the greater the degree of hearing loss and the older the age of the child, the more parents notice that their children do not exhibit developmentally appropriate language and auditory-related behaviors. In short, all professionals should heed parent's intuition that something is wrong, and they should refer to a center specializing in the evaluation of pediatric communicative disorders whenever parent/caregiver concerns are raised.

SUMMARY

In value-added practice, we will no longer be afforded the luxury of having a child return for annual audiological testing without reason or data to support such follow-up. Permanent hearing loss is a "chronic" health condition and needs to be addressed as such. Even with appropriate intervention (e.g., hearing aids, cochlear implant, and communication therapy), the child will always have listening challenges in diverse listening environments. However, in the healthcare system of the past (fee for service), hearing loss has not received the same attention as other chronic healthcare issues in children such as asthma or juvenile diabetes. In the healthcare system of the future (health promotion through prevention of chronic health issues), it is incumbent on the profession of audiology to collect and disseminate data that supports EHDI as a preventative and cost effective public policy as well as the need for ongoing audiological care and effective surveillance in children. For example, strong evidence has been collected and published that documents the progressive nature of hearing loss in children who have congenital cytomegalovirus and the need for ongoing, frequent audiological follow-up (Fowler, 2013; Fowler et al., 1997). However, this same level of evidence does not exist for other causes of hearing loss and in turn, reimbursement for justifiable and necessary audiological care may not be supported in the future. Audiologists and hearing scientists need to take the lead on collecting and publishing data on the outcomes of *any* etiology of hearing loss that could place a child at risk for even slight educational performance deficits.

While the audiologist may know what caused the hearing loss in about 60% of the pediatric patients served, he or she may not know the cause for the remaining 40%. Once thresholds have been obtained and are stable, a child should only have his or her pure tone thresholds obtained when there is an observed concern by relevant care givers (e.g., pediatrician, parent, therapists, and/or child) or, to determine eligibility for appropriate support services in the school. If the hearing loss is progressive, thresholds should be checked at least once a year.

Parents and physicians should look for signs/symptoms of changes in hearing status and must be advocates for referrals to audiologists. One of these signs/symptoms could be the child complaining that he can't hear as well as he has in the past. This could be due to changes in hearing status or changes in the functioning of his amplification. In either case, the child would need to be seen by an audiologist for determination of the cause of the complaint. Any time a child reports a difference in the way he or she hears, or the parent notices a change in how a child reacts to sound or speech, it would be prudent to seek consultation and testing by the managing audiologist.

REFERENCES

Allen, S. (2008). *Auditory Perception Test for the Hearing Impaired*. San Diego, CA: Plural.

Allum, J., Greisinger, R., Staubhaar, S., & Carpenter, M. (2000). Auditory perception and speech identification in children with cochlear implants tested with the EARS protocol. *British Journal of Audiology, 34*(5), 393–303.

American Academy of Family Physicians, American Academy of Otolaryngology–Head & Neck Surgery, & American Academy of Pediatrics Subcommittee on Otitis Media with Effusion. (2004). Otitis media with effusion. *Pediatrics, 113*(5), 1412–1429.

American Academy of Pediatrics Task Force on Newborn and Infant Hearing. (1999). Newborn and infant hearing loss: Detection and intervention. *Pediatrics, 103*(2), 527–530.

American Speech-Language-Hearing Association (ASHA). (2006). *Roles, knowledge, and skills: Audiologists providing clinical services to infants and young children birth to five years of age [Knowledge and skills]*. Retrieved from http://www.asha.org/policy

American Speech-Language-Hearing Association (ASHA). (2011). *National outcomes measurement system*. Retrieved from http://www.asha.org/NOMS/

Anderson, I., Philips, L., Robert, L., Jamieson, L., Costa, A., & Cross, S. (2004, May). *TeenEARS: Development of a test battery for teenagers.* Presented at ESPCI 2004, Geneva, Switzerland.

Anderson, K. (1989). *Screening Instrument for Targeting Educational Risk (SIFTER).* Retrieved from http://successforkidswithhearingloss.com/tests

Anderson, K. (2002). *Early Listening Function (ELF).* Retrieved from http://successforkidswithhearingloss.com/tests

Anderson, K. (2004). *Secondary Screening Instrument for Targeting Educational Risk (Secondary SIFTER).* Retrieved from http://successforkidswithhearingloss.com/tests

Anderson, K., & Matkin, N. (1996). *Preschool Screening Instrument for Targeting Educational Risk (Preschool SIFTER).* Retrieved from http://successforkidswithhearingloss.com/tests

Anderson, K. L., & Smaldino, J. J. (1996). *Listening Inventory for Education; An efficacy tool (LIFE).* Retrieved from http://successforkidswithhearingloss.com/tests

Anderson, K. L., & Smaldino, J. J. (2000). *Children's Home Inventory for Listening Difficulties (CHILD).* Retrieved from https://successforkidswithhearingloss.com/uploads/child_questionnaire.pdf

Anderson, K. L., Smaldino, J. J., & Spangler, C. (2011). *Student Listening Inventory for Education–Revised (LIFE-R).* Retrieved from http://successforkidswithhearingloss.com/tests

Bamford, J., Fortnum, H., Bristow, K., Smith, J., Vamvakas, G., Davies, L, . . . Hind, S. (2007). Current practice, accuracy, effectiveness and cost-effectiveness of the school entry hearing screen. *Health Technology Assessment, 11*(32), 1–168.

Centers for Disease Control and Prevention (CDC). (2013). *Summary of 2011 national CDC EHDI Data.* Retrieved from http://www.cdc.gov/ncbddd/hearingloss/2011-data/2011_ehdi_hsfs_summary_a.pdf

Centers for Medicare & Medicaid Services (CMS). (2013). *Bundled payments for care improvement (BPCI) initiative: General information.* Retrieved from http://innovation.cms.gov/initiatives/bundled-payments/

Centers for Medicare & Medicaid Services (CMS). (2014). *Quality initiatives—general information.* Retrieved from http://www.cms.gov/Medicare/Quality-Initiatives-Patient-Assessment-Instruments/QualityInitiativesGenInfo/index.html

Ching, T., & Hill, M. (2005). The parents' evaluation of aural/oral performance of children (PEACH) scale: Normative data. *Journal of the American Academy of Audiology, 18*, 220–235.

Ching, T. C., Hill, M., & Psarros, C. (2000, August). *Strategies for evaluation of hearing-aid fitting for children.* Paper presented at the International Hearing Aid Research Conference, Lake Tahoe, CA.

Coninx, F., Weichbold, V., Tsiakpini, L., Autrique, E., Bescond, G., & Tamas, L. (2009). Validation of the LittlEARS® Auditory Questionnaire in children with normal hearing, *International Journal of Pediatric Otorhinolaryngology, 73*, 1761–1768.

Curry, A., & Gaffney, M. (2010). *MPH Directors of Speech and Hearing Programs in State Health and Welfare Agencies (DSHPSHWA): Overview and summary of 1999–2004 DSHPSHWA data.* Retrieved from http://www.cdc.gov/ncbddd/hearingloss/documents/1999-2004_dshpshwa-summary.pdf

Elliott, L. L., & Katz, D. (1980). *Development of a new children's test of speech descrimination* [Technical manual]. St. Louis, MO: Auditec.

Estrabrooks, W. (1994). *Auditory-verbal therapy for parents and professionals.* Washington, DC: Alexander Graham Bell Association for the Deaf and Hard of Hearing.

Etymotic Research. (2005). *BKB-SIN Speech-in-Noise Test.* Retrieved from http://www.etymotic.com/pro/bkbsin.aspx

Finitzo, T., Albright, K., & O'Neal, J. (1998). The newborn with hearing loss: Detection in the nursery. *Pediatrics, 102*, 1452–1460.

Fowler, K. B. (2013). Congenital cytomegalovirus infection: Audiologic outcome. *Clinical Infectious Disease, 57*(S4), S182–184.

Fowler, K. B., McCollister, F. P., Dahle, A. J., Boppana, S., Britt, W. J., & Pass, R. F. (1997). Progressive and fluctuating sensorineural hearing loss in children with asymptomatic congenital cytomegalovirus infection. *The Journal of Pediatrics, 130*(4), 624–630.

Gravel, J. S. (2002). Potential pitfalls in the audiological assessment of infants and young children. In R. C. Seewald & J. S. Gravel (Eds.), *A sound foundation through early amplification 2001. Proceedings of the second international conference* (pp. 85–101). Stafa, Switzerland: Phonak AG.

Hagan, J. F., Shaw, J. S., & Duncan, P. M. (2008). *Bright futures: Guidelines for health supervision of infants, children and adolescents* (3rd ed.). Elk Grove Village, IL: American Academy of Pediatrics.

Harrison, M., Roush, J., & Wallace, J. (2003). Trends in age of identification and intervention in infants with hearing loss. *Ear and Hearing, 24*(1), 89–95.

Haskins, H. (1949). *A phonetically balanced test of speech discrimination for children* (Unpublished Master's thesis). Northwestern University, Evanston, IL.

Institute of Medicine (IOM). (2001). *Executive summary. Crossing the quality chasm: A new health system for the 21st century.* Washington, DC: National Academies Press.

Joint Committee on Infant Hearing (JCIH). (2007). Year 2007 position statement: Principles and guidelines for early hearing detection and intervention. *Pediatrics, 120*(4), 898–921. doi:10.1542/peds.2007-2333

Joint Committee on Infant Hearing (JCIH). (2013). Supplement to the JCIH 2007 position statement: Principles and guidelines for early intervention after confirmation that a child is deaf or hard of hearing. *Pediatrics, 131*(4), e1324–e1349. doi:10.1542/peds.2013-0008

Kemp, D. T. (1978). Stimulated acoustic emissions from the human auditory system. *Journal of the Acoustical Society of America, 64*, 3566–3576.

Kirk, K. I., Pisoni, D. B., & Osberger, M. J. (1995). Lexical effects of spoken word recognition by pediatric cochlear implant users. *Ear and Hearing, 15*(5), 470–481.

Klein, J. O. (1989). Epidemiology of otitis media. *Pediatric Infectious Diseases Journal, 8*(Suppl. 1), S9.

Lin, F. R., Ceh, K., Bervinchak, D., Riley, A., Miech, R., & Niparko, J. (2007). Development of a communicative performance scale for pediatric cochlear implantation. *Ear and Hearing, 28*(5), 703–713. Retrieved from http://www.hopkinsmedicine.org/otolaryngology/specialty_areas/listencenter/pediatric_cochlear_implants/download_fapci.html

Ling, D., & Ling, A. H. (1978). *Aural habilitation: The foundation of verbal learning.* Washington, DC: Alexander Graham Bell Association for the Deaf and Hard of Hearing.

Lins, O. G., & Picton, T. W. (1995). Auditory steady-state responses to multiple simultaneous stimuli. *Electroencephalography and Clinical Neurophysiology, 96*, 420–432.

Matkin, N. (1977). Assessment of hearing sensitivity during the preschool years. In F. Bess (Ed.), *Childhood deafness* (pp. 127–134). New York, NY: Grune and Stratton.

Mendel, L. L. (2009). Subjective and objective measures of hearing aid outcome. *Audiology Online.* Retrieved from http://www.audiologyonline.com/articles/subjective-and-objective-measures-hearing-891

Meinzen-Derr, J., Wiley, S., Creighton, J., & Choo, D. (2007). Auditory skills checklist: Clinical tool for monitoring functional auditory skill development in young children with cochlear implants. *Annals of Otology, Rhinology, & Laryngology, 116*(11), 812–818.

Moog, J., & Biedenstein, J. (1998). *Teacher assessment of spoken language.* Retrieved from http://www.moogcenter.org/Bookstore.aspx

Moog, J., & Geers, A. (1990). *Early Speech Perception (ESP) Test.* St. Louis, MO: Central Institute for the Deaf.

Newcomer, P. L., & Hammill, D. D. (2009). *Pragmatic Language Observation Scale (PLOS).* Austin, TX: Hammill Institute on Disabilities.

Nilsson, M. J., Soli, S. D., & Gelnett, D. J. (1996). *Development and norming of a hearing in noise test for children.* Los Angeles, CA: House Ear Institute Internal Report.

Oates, P., & Stapells, D. R. (1997). Frequency specificity of the human auditory brainstem and middle latency response to brief tones. I. High-pass noise masking. *Journal of the Acoustical Society of America, 102*(6), 3597–3608.

Olsho, L. W., Koch, E. G., Carter, E. A., Halpin, C. F., & Spetner, N. B. (1988). Pure-tone sensitivity of human infants. *Journal of the Acoustical Society of America, 84*, 1316–1324.

Perigoe, C. B., & Paterson, M. M. (2015). Understanding auditory development and the child with hearing loss. In D. R. Welling & C. A. Ukstins, (Eds.), *Fundamentals of audiology for the speech-language pathologist* (pp. 173–193). Burlington, MA: Jones & Bartlett Learning.

Purdy, S. C., & Abbas, P. J. (2002). ABR thresholds to tone bursts gated with Blackman and linear windows in adults with high frequency sensorineural hearing loss. *Ear and Hearing, 23*(4), 358–368.

Robbins, A. M. (1993). *Mr. Potato Head Test.* Indianapolis, IN: Indiana University School of Medicine.

Robbins, A. M., Renshaw, J. J., & Berry, S. W. (1991). Evaluating meaningful auditory integration in profoundly hearing-impaired children. *American Journal of Otology, 2*(Suppl.), 144–150.

Ross, M., & Lerman, J. W. (1971). *Word Intelligibility by Picture Identification (WIPI)*. Pittsburgh, PA: Stanwix House.

Roth, D. A., Hildesheimer, M., Bardenstein, S., Goidel, D., Reichman, B., Maayan-Metzger, A., & Kuint, J. (2008). Preauricular skin tags and ear pits are associated with permanent hearing impairment in newborns. *Pediatrics, 122*(4), 884–890. doi:10.1542/peds.2008-0606

Sininger, Y. S., Grimes, A., & Christensen, E. (2010). Auditory development in early-amplified children: Factors influencing auditory-based communication outcomes in children with hearing loss. *Ear and Hearing, 31*(2), 166–185.

Smoski, W. J., Brunt, M. A., & Tannahill, J. C. (1992). Listening characteristics of children with central auditory processing disorders. *Language, Speech, and Hearing Services in Schools, 23*, 145–152. doi:10.1044/0161-1461.2302.145

Stapells, D. R. (2011). Frequency-specific threshold assessment in young infants using the transient ABR and the brainstem ASSR. In R. Seewald & A. M. Tharpe (Eds.), *Comprehensive handbook of pediatric audiology* (pp. 409–448). San Diego, CA: Plural.

Stredler-Brown, A., & Johnson, C. D. (2001). *Functional auditory performance indicators: An integrated approach to auditory skill development.* Retrieved from https://www.mariondowns.com/assessment-tools

Tsiakpini, L., Weichbold, V., Kuehn-Inacker, H., Coninx, F., D'Haese, P., & Almadin, S. (2004). *LittlEARS. Auditory Questionnaire.* MED-EL, Innsbruck, Austria.

van Zon, A., van der Heijden, G. J., van Dongen, T. M., Burton, M. J., & Schilder, A. G. (2012). Antibiotics for otitis media with effusion in children [Review]. *Cochrane Database System Review, 9*, CD009163.

Wilkes, E. (2001). *Cottage Acquisition Scales for Listening, Language, & Speech (CASLLS).* Retrieved from http://sunshineorders.org/index.php/educational_products/our_products/caslls/

Williams, C. (2003). The Children's Outcome Worksheet (COW)—an outcome measure focusing on children's needs (Ages 4–12). *News from Oticon.* Retrieved from http://www.oticonusa.com/~asset/cache.ashx?id=10833&type=14&format=web

Yoshinaga-Itano, C., Baca, R. L, & Sedey, A. L. (2010). Describing the trajectory of language development in the presence of severe-to-profound hearing loss: A closer look at children with cochlear implants versus hearing aids. *Otology & Neurotology, 31*(8), 1268–1274.

Zimmerman-Phillips, S., Robbins, A. M., & Osberger, M. J. (2000). Assessing cochlear implant benefit in very young children. *Annals of Otology, Rhinology, & Laryngology, 109*(Suppl. 12), 42–43.

CHAPTER 5

Speech Production Assessment

Marietta M. Paterson and Christina Barris Perigoe

KEY POINTS

- A clear relationship exists between speech perception and speech production in all children, especially those with hearing loss who are acquiring spoken language.
- For a child with hearing loss who is learning to speak, various aspects of speech production must be appropriately assessed to capture the child's capabilities.
- The speech characteristics of children with hearing loss are specific and can be assessed with a comprehensive approach and with specific instruments.
- Assessments of speech production in children with hearing loss should include both the phonetic and phonologic levels, and clinicians and teachers must understand how to integrate the assessment data to select speech targets for teaching and remediation.
- An informal unpublished instrument with an emphasis on the evaluation of suprasegmentals and prosody developed in 1992 by Paterson and Cole is presented.

INTRODUCTION

This is an exciting period of change and new trends in the early childhood learning and education of children with hearing loss. How do these trends and current view of the field inform our approach to speech production assessment? Early detection and subsequent diagnosis of hearing loss of all degrees and types is now common. Almost monthly advances in assistive hearing technology have increased the availability of powerful hearing aids, cochlear implants, bone conduction hearing aids, and FM systems (Cole & Flexer, 2011; Flexer, 2013). Fitting of hearing aids on infants in the first weeks of life is happening as a matter of course in many programs, and early cochlear implantation by the end of the first year of life is increasingly common. Also, the Joint Commission on Infant Hearing (JCIH) has recognized that early auditory-based intervention provided by professionals with specialized knowledge to develop listening and spoken language is desirable and urgently needed (JCIH, 2007, 2013).

Earlier and emerging research indicates that, as anticipated, the earlier children with hearing loss receive appropriate amplification and intervention, the more likely they will mirror typical speech sound development and possibly sequences (Eriks-Brophy, Gibson, & Tucker, 2013; Ertmer, 2011; Ertmer & Inniger, 2009; Paterson, 1992, 1997; Warner-Czyz, Davis & Morrison, 2005; Wiggins, Sedey, Awad, Bogle, & Yoshinaga-Itano, 2013). It is important for early intervention providers to encourage and monitor speech sound acquisition and to expect more typical speech production and vocal quality.

At the same time, up to 40% of infants with hearing loss are lost to follow-up in the early hearing detection and intervention (EHDI) process (JCIH 2007, 2013; NCHAM & AG Bell Association, 2012). This means some children with hearing loss are late to listening and late to speech acquisition. These children will be as diverse as in the past and may have learning trajectories more similar to the patterns of the past. In addition, it is estimated that there are approximately 40% of young children with hearing loss who are considered multihandicapped with respect to their learning (Gallaudet Research Institute, 2008; Perigoe & Perigoe, 2004). The challenge for the **early interventionist** is to be able to discern what speech production issues are related to the hearing loss and what may be individual to the child or the child's environment. It may or may not be evident that an infant will be a learner with additional needs, but as intervention progresses, these children may demonstrate difficulty in auditory processing, speech sound production, integrative learning, or have a spoken language disability that is not accounted for by deafness/degree of hearing loss.

Therefore, in developing a speech assessment protocol, the teacher or clinician needs to include informal and formal assessments appropriate for each child's age and relative stage of development and consider concomitant issues that may impact auditory spoken language and speech development.

FACTORS THAT IMPACT SPEECH PRODUCTION IN CHILDREN WITH HEARING LOSS

Impact of Hearing Loss: The Relationship Between Speech Perception and Speech Production

Children with hearing loss speak the way they hear. While this may sound simple, the direct link between **speech perception** and **speech production** has been clearly demonstrated (Boothroyd, 1982, 1986; Ling, 1989). If an infant hears normally, the auditory signal received by the brain initiates the neuronal development that permits increasingly greater capacity to use the innate speech perception ability that humans are born with (Cole & Flexer, 2011; Dornan, 2012; Owens, 2012; Perigoe & Paterson, 2013; Robertson, 2013). Daniel Ling, a noted professor, teacher, and researcher, wrote and spoke eloquently about the potential for even a child with a profound loss to be able to acquire intelligible speech (Ling, 1989, 2002). He stressed that the older the child and the less well the child uses hearing, the more formal our assessment and teaching need to be. Conversely, the earlier the child is aided and the better the child uses listening, the more informal our assessment and teaching can be.

Thus, the first step in assessment of speech production development in a child with hearing loss begins with a consideration of the speech perception potential of the individual child; it is essential to determine exactly what a child with hearing loss *can* and *cannot* hear (Cole & Flexer, 2011; Cole & Paterson, 1984; Flexer, 2013; Ling, 2002). This includes ongoing, appropriate audiologic assessment and an informed interpretation of the child's listening potential and limits, based on hearing aid targets and real ear measures or an aided audiogram and cochlear implant map. This should include not only what the child can detect but what he or she can discriminate, identify, and comprehend (Cole & Flexer, 2011; Erber, 1982; Flexer, 2013; Hirsch, 1970). Speech assessment is not useful if the professional is not informed about the listening status of the child, including auditory access and the child's auditory learning environment (Cole & Flexer, 2011; Perigoe & Paterson, 2013).

Speech Acoustics and the Ling Six–Sound Test

Perhaps the most useful and enduring contribution by Daniel Ling was the development of *The Six-Sound Test* (Ling, 2006). These six sounds, /u/, /m /, /a/, /i/, "sh" and /s/, cover the range of speech from the lowest to the highest in frequency. Some professionals also include a period of "silence" (Cole & Flexer, 2011). *The Six-Sound Test* is used to determine whether the child's hearing technology is functioning and whether the child can hear across the entire frequency range of speech. Parents and professionals working with children with hearing loss should perform this as a daily listening check. In addition, this is a necessary check of listening that should be done prior to any and all speech or language testing and intervention.

The skilled teacher or clinician is not only able to interpret audiometric results for the family and explain aided and unaided hearing levels, but is able to use knowledge of speech acoustics to determine whether the child's hearing technology is providing optimal access to the speech signal. Given the range of available hearing technologies currently available, most children with hearing loss should be able to hear across the entire range of speech. In addition, the professional needs to be able to supplement traditional audiological measures with a functional assessment of the child's listening abilities (Flexer, 2013; Perigoe & Paterson, 2013). This will give a more complete picture of what the child can discriminate and understand via audition alone. For example, if a child cannot discriminate two speech sounds, it is unlikely that he or she will be able to produce them adequately without intervention. By the same token, by maximizing hearing, the teacher or clinician is able to have the child use hearing to develop speech, rather than visual or tactile methods. Hearing is powerful; it is the most suitable modality for the acquisition speech.

Ling was expert at demystifying speech acoustics. In Figure 5–1, Ling and Ling (1978, p. 69) produced a visual representation of first (F1) and second (F2) formant frequencies for vowels, with a simple sentence to remember the progression from back to front vowels. Unstressed vowels are in parentheses.

"Who would know more of art must (**a**gain) learn (moth**er**) and then take his ease."

By examining the trajectory of F2, one can easily see that a child with limited access to frequencies above 1000 Hz will

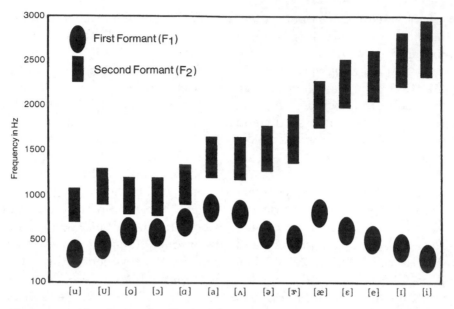

Figure 5–1. Vowel acoustics. Used with permission by AG Bell Association for the Deaf and Hard of Hearing.

likely confuse vowels with similar first formants (F1), such as /u/ and /i/. This child would also have poor responses to "sh" and /s/ on the Ling Six-Sound Test, indicating that he or she will have difficulty detecting, discriminating, and perhaps producing high-frequency speech sounds.

Here are some examples of how we might apply information of speech acoustics from the Ling Six-Sound Test to our understanding of what the child can perceive, and possibly produce.

Child A has a severe hearing loss, sloping to profound in the high frequencies. With her bilateral hearing aids, she detects /u/, /m/, /a/, and /i/, and discriminates /u/, /m/, and /a/ from each other. She cannot discriminate /u/ from /i/. She can only hear "sh" when using her FM system. She does detect /s/, even with the FM. She responds well to her mother's voice (because she hears the

low frequencies). It is not surprising that this child has difficulty producing /s/ and most other high frequency sounds, because she does not hear them. At 6 years of age, this child is already working on some phonemes using a remedial model. Although aided early, her hearing technology has not provided her with the input necessary to acquire speech along a typical developmental pathway. Despite the fact that we have better audiology and better hearing technology than we did 20 years ago, children like this, with inadequate access to speech and spoken language, are still seen in our schools today.

Child B has a profound hearing loss and has been wearing bilateral cochlear implants since 12 months of age. This child's cochlear implant is well-programmed, enabling her to detect and discriminate all the Ling sounds in quiet and at a distance of 20 feet. The teacher or clinician can feel confident that this child will be able to hear the full range of speech in a quiet room during speech training (but will still need an FM in a classroom situation). This child, at 6 years of age, has a natural sounding voice, good vowel system, most consonants (including high frequency sounds, such as /s/ and /f/) and is making appropriate progress developmentally.

This demonstrates how speech perception—what the child can detect, discriminate (and process)—influences speech production. For additional information on speech components relative to the speech frequencies between 125 and 8000 Hz, see Table 5–1 (Ling, 1989, p. 69).

In addition to the issue of what the child can perceive is the notion of a critical

Table 5–1. Speech Acoustics

125 Hz	250 Hz	500 Hz	1000 Hz	2000 Hz	4000 Hz	8000 Hz
F_0 of most adult male voices	Voicing cues	Primary cues on manner of production, most consonants	Additional cues on manner of consonant production	Primary cues on place of consonant production	Secondary cues on place of consonant production	Turbulent noise of all fricatives and affricates
	F_0 of most female and child voices	Harmonics of most voices	The harmonics of most voices	Additional cues on manner of consonant production	The upper range of harmonics, most voices	
	The low harmonics of adult male voices	F_1 and T_1 of most vowels	T_1 of the laterals /l/ and /r/	The harmonics of most voices	The noise bursts of plosives and affricates	
	The nasal murmur (F_1 of /m/, /n/, and ng)	Noise bursts of plosives in back vowel contexts	F_2 of nasal consonants	F_2 and T_2 of front vowels	Turbulent noise of voiced and unvoiced fricatives	
	F_1 of high back and high front vowels	T_1 of the semivowels	F_2 and T_2 of back and central vowels	The noise bursts of most plosives and affricates		
		F_1 of the laterals /l/ and /t/	The noise bursts of most plosives	Turbulent noise of fricatives sh, /f/, and th		
			T_2 of the semivowels	T_2 and T_3 of /l/ and /r/		

Source: Courtesy of Alexander Graham Bell Association for the Deaf and Hard of Hearing.

period for speech development. The typically developing child has acquired foundational spoken language skills and most speech sounds by the age of six years. Different tables of consonant acquisition by hearing children show similar ranges in ages for phoneme mastery (Owens, 2012; Sander, 1972; Shipley & McAfee, 2008, pp. 208–209). For example, some children may start to produce /s/ around 3 years of age with the range extending to 7.6/8 years of age. Some people think of /s/ as a later preschool to school aged production problem (Bleile, 2006). For a child with hearing loss and appropriate prerequisite speech skills, early acquisition of /s/ is important, as this phoneme is so crucial to early morphological marking and meaning in spoken language. Hence, demographic timetables of typical development should be applied with caution to children with hearing loss. Although we are expecting children who start early to be developing typically, professionals should not be targeting speech based solely on demographic tables, but on individualized assessment. Those children with hearing loss who have not mastered **suprasegmental patterns**, vowels, **diphthongs** and the majority of consonant **phonemes** by school age will require systematic and intensive speech intervention (Cole & Paterson, 1984; Paterson, 1994).

> ## DIFFERENTIATING ARTICULATION AND PHONOLOGICAL PROCESSES AND POTENTIAL ERRORS

Historically, due to poor access to the auditory signal, individuals with hearing loss have manifested speech characterized

as "deaf speech" (Ling, 2002). This section provides an overview of the characteristics and potential errors of speakers with hearing loss across the production of the following: voice, vowels and diphthongs, consonants, consonant clusters, phonological processes, and connected speech. This information highlights why assessing and targeting speech production with this population goes far beyond just articulation errors.

Differentiating Voice Production Characteristics

The seminal, landmark study of adult deaf speakers by Hudgins and Numbers (1942), defined the characteristics of "deaf speech" that we still use as a reference today (Table 5–2). Note, that all but one of the characteristics below (omission and misarticulation of some phonemes) is

Table 5–2. Voice Production Characteristics of Deaf Speakers (Adapted From Hudgins and Numbers, 1942)

Inadequate breath control
Excessive and inappropriate pausing
Inappropriate pitch register
Hypernasality
Excessive tenseness or harshness
Inappropriate duration of syllable articulation
Inappropriate duration of vowels
Inappropriate duration of both stressed and unstressed syllables

Note. Omission and misarticulation of some phonemes is not related to the control, coordination, and timing of the respiratory, laryngeal, and articulatory systems to support the creation of speech.

related to the control, coordination, and timing of the respiratory, laryngeal, and articulatory systems to support the creation of speech (Cole & Paterson, 1984; Ling, 2002).

Of specific note is that production of any or all of these characteristics is evidence of some degree of poor timing and control of breath flow and air pressure, control of onset and offset of phonation to support the articulators in the rapid production of manner, place, and voicing contrasts. These vocal production features are produced as suprasegmentals or aspects of **prosody** (Cole & Paterson, 1984; Paterson, 1986). Prosody is an enormous component of speech perception and speech production and spoken language. Assessment, targeting, and intervention with children or students with hearing loss who evidence combinations of these voice characteristics must take this into account so that speech session plans include listening practice; phonetic level practice; and phonologic level practice, including conversation, where aspects of prosody occur naturally.

The child with hearing loss is born with normal physiological potential for speech production (except for some children with additional disabilities). Today, the majority of children with hearing loss are not expected to manifest these voice production characteristics. It is quite common to encounter very young children with advanced hearing aids or cochlear implants who are developing intelligible speech with natural voice patterns (Cole & Flexer, 2011; Flexer, 2013). Children who have not had consistent auditory access or whose training may have focused solely on visual systems, however, continue to present with characteristics of "deaf speech."

Preventing Deaf Speech Characteristics

A number of researchers have been interested in the early vocalization to verbal development of infants and toddlers with hearing aids (Oller, 1986; Paterson, 1990, 1992; Stoel-Gammon & Kehoe, 1994) and those with early cochlear implants (Paterson, 1997). In the past 15 years and currently, as a result of very early cochlear implantation and technological advances, more comparative information on early vocalization quality and vocal to verbal production is emerging (Bass-Ringdahl, 2010; Ertmer & Goffman, 2011; Ertmer, Young, & Nathani, 2007; Saffran, Werker, & Werner, 2006). There are several systems for assessing speech perception and tracking early vocal production (Ertmer, 2001; Kishon-Rabin, Taitelbaum-Swead, & Segal, 2009; Nathani, Ertmer, & Stark, 2006; Uhler, Yoshinaga-Itano, Gabbard, Rothpletz, & Jenkins, 2011). The **LENA** (Language **EN**vironment **A**nalysis) **system** is based on the Oller acoustic model of vocalization development in the first of year of life of hearing children (Oller, 1986; Oller et al., 2010). The LENA recording and software analysis system shows great promise for data collection and longitudinal tracking of vocal to verbal development in the home environment (Morrison & Lew, 2012). To date, results suggest that early access to audition allows the child to develop typical voice features.

Pathophysiology in Past Studies

Physiological changes in the speech production system can develop with years of improper vocal production related to auditory sensory pathology, late access to sound, late vocalization development, or poor teaching of speech (Paterson, 1994; Table 5–3).

These physiological changes continue to be studied in older speakers with hearing loss, but our goal is to prevent this from happening. Early encouragement of speech production to automaticity should prevent actual physiologic changes; however, the authors still encounter school-aged students with habituated speech output patterns clearly influenced by some of the above (usually nasality, poor

tongue control, and poor control of breath flow).

Differentiating Characteristics of Vowels, Diphthongs, and Errors

Vowels are so easily acquired by hearing children that few standardized tests evaluate them adequately for those with hearing loss. For children with hearing loss, ensuring good vowel perception and production is crucial to the develop-

Table 5–3. Pathophysiology in Speakers With Hearing Loss, Historically

Velopharyngeal insuffiency	Velum (soft palate) does not function normally to close and open the velopharyngeal port efficiently. Results in nasal overtone to vocal/oral quality and production confusions between oral and nasal phonemes—/ba/ from /ma/.
Poor control of breath stream	Poor "breath control or breath support" is identified as one of the major voice problems of HI speakers. Caused by poor use of flow of the breath stream to support speech. Important to be careful, is this really physical abnormality or just poor coordination of the use of airflow typical in some deaf/hard of hearing speakers?
Partial vocal fold atrophy	Inability to change or make pitch changes at will.
	Inability to maintain appropriate vocal pitch register. Major cause: poor control of changes in vocal fold tension and air pressure.
Inappropriate high voice pitch or loud voice	Production of high voice instead of loud voice.
	Production of loud voice instead of high voice. Major cause: inability to produce appropriate adjustments of subglottal pressure and vocal fold tightening.
Voice loudness	Inability to maintain or to adjust voice loudness.
	Inability to make appropriate stress patterns in syllables, multisyllabic words and phrases. Major cause: poor control of subglottal pressure and interaction with vocal fold tension.
Poor tongue control	Inability to automatically locate tongue targets.
	Poor tongue control and movement in phoneme production has been one of the commonest problems for many speakers with hearing loss. Tongue held or moved in abnormal ways. What are some clues that the speaker is not achieving appropriate tongue targets? If assessment indicates: poor diphthongization, poor alveolar plosives, poor fricatives, poor retro-flexion.

ment of speech. Table 5–4 summarizes the historical findings of studies on vowel production errors of individuals with hearing loss.

Why Are Vowels and Diphthongs Crucial to Speech Production?

The characteristics of vocal production in speakers with hearing loss and pathophysiology noted above are preventable and remediable (Cole & Paterson, 1984; Ling, 1976, 1989, 2002). Vowels and diphthongs are the essence of vocalization. Vowel production must be assessed up the speech chain for the speaker's ability to coordinate: breath flow from the lungs; initiation and maintenance of phonation; resonance (nasal–oral contrasts); and articulation through changing the shape and position of articulators in the vocal tract. There are 15 vowels and 4 diphthongs in standard American English. Diphthongs are combinations of two vowels and require tongue movement from one vowel position to the next, for example /a/ + /u/ = /aʊ/ (e.g., /aʊ/). Ling classified /w/ and /j/ as "semivowels" because they can be conceptualized (and developed) similarly, for example, /u/ + /a/ = /wa/; /i/+/u/ = /ju/. In diphthongs, the emphasis is on the first vowel or element and in semivowels it is on the second element.

What Is the Role of the Vowel in Connected Speech?

The vowel is the nucleus of the syllable; without a vowel-like sound, there is no syllable. Good vowel articulation contributes greatly to speech intelligibility. The principal articulators for vowels are the tongue, the jaw, and the lips. The tongue plays the most important role in vowel formation and poor tongue movement to vowel targets is the most common cause of poor vowel articulation (Ling, 2002; Paterson, 1994). As stated earlier, the impact of hearing loss is that the formants needed for vowel identification may not both be audible and usable for the child. Today, we can differentiate vowel perception expected across those children or students wearing hearing aids and those with cochlear implants. While vowel perception and production may continue to be problematic for students who wear hearing aids, we expect students who use cochlear implants and who have a good perceptual result to have very good vowel and diphthong production (Paterson, 1997; Werner-Czyz, Davis, & Morrison, 2005).

Table 5–4. Vowel Production Characteristics of Speakers With Hearing Loss

1. Neutralization to a schwa-like vowel	6. Nasalization
2. Substitutions of vowels close together on the vowel quadrilateral	7. Excessive diphthongization
	8. Prolongations
3. Tense–lax errors	9. Exaggeration
4. Unidentifiable distortion	10. Multiple faults
5. Context-dependent pitch	11. Omissions

Consonants:
Differentiating Characteristics

Historically, consonant studies of school-aged children with hearing loss found similar patterns of error in consonant production (Monson, 1983). There is general agreement that typical consonant errors may reflect the following kinds of problems (Table 5–5).

These consonant errors can still occur and a deep phonetic level evaluation and a phonologic evaluation would identify the contexts of the errors. It is not sufficient to identify the error and count occurrences. To be useful to the student with hearing loss, the practitioner needs to understand why the error is occurring and what the commonalities are across the errors. When these errors are present in consonant production, there is usually a concomitant problem with vowel and diphthong production in coarticulation and speech intelligibility issues. By school age, these are either learned or acquired error patterns that are now habitual and more difficult to change.

Consonants are sounds made with complete or partial constriction of the vocal tract and defined by the type and the place of constriction. They can occur in English syllables relative to the vowels and diphthongs in three positions: prevocalic, postvocalic, and intervocalic (Small, 2008). Consonants may be categorized by manner of production, place of production, and voicing (Table 5–6).

The role of consonants is to release, arrest, or interrupt vowels. There is a useful consonant–vowel coding system that can be used to analyze speech productions at word and interword level (Table 5–7). Using this notation system, teachers and clinicians can track the accuracy of production of the phoneme or syllabic elements of speech. Teacher-made assessments of this type could be developed and used with a student to record and analyze

Table 5–5. Consonant Errors in School-Age Speakers With Hearing Loss

Problem		Cause
Voiced–voiceless distinctions Cannot maintain /b/ versus /p/ differences	→	Cause: poor earlier patterns; and inadequate timing and control or phonation and creation of intraoral pressure for plosive
Substitutions of one consonant for another; voiced for voiceless; nasal instead of oral; fricative instead of stop	→	Cause: poor control and coordination of the air flow, air pressure, phonation and constrictions in the vocal tract; poor automaticity
Omission of initial and final consonants	→	Cause: poor automaticity in consonant production coupled with audibility issues; linguistic knowledge
Distortions (nasal emission; too great or too little plosive effort)	→	Poor coordination of speech mechanisms
Inappropriate nasalization of consonants	→	Velopharyngeal insufficience; habitual production
Final consonant deletions (e.g., /s/ deletions)	→	Cause: /s/ in final position is very soft to hear and is often not perceptible in connected speech even though child or student may produce well

Table 5–6. Consonant Classification

Manner of production	How consonant is made	Plosive, stop, fricative, affricate, nasal glide, liquid
Place of production	Where consonant is made	Bilabial, labiodental, linguadental, alveolar, palatal, velar, glottal
Voiced/voiceless production	Made with/without vocal fold vibration	Voiced consonants Voiceless consonants

Table 5–7. CV Coding System

VC	= at	/aet/	CCVC	= sleep	/slip/
CV	= to	/tu/	CCVCC	= squeak	/skwik/
CVC	= cat	/kaet/	VCCVC	= I'm sad	/aɪmsaed/

a particular pattern or error or production or omission and then to analyze.

Today it is possible for young children with hearing loss to develop consonant and cluster production following the same sequences of consonant development that have been suggested for children with normal hearing. Recent longitudinal studies, case studies, and consonant inventories of children with cochlear implants and hearing aids are providing evidence of more similarities to typical children, although more studies are needed (Eriks-Brophy, Gibson, & Tucker, 2013; Nicholas & Geers, 2006; Spencer & Guo, 2013; Warner-Czyz, Davis, & Morrison, 2005; Wiggins, Sedy, Awad, Bogle, & Yoshinaga-Itano, 2013).

Phonological Processes and Children With Hearing Loss

In the 1980s to the 1990s, research revealed that typical hearing children advance their speech production in early childhood through a system of "practice makes perfect." Children demonstrate systematic and logical speech errors as they work through the establishment of their phonological system. A recent study compared the Khan-Lewis Phonological Procedure with hearing children and children with hearing loss (Eriks-Brophy, Gibson, & Tucker, 2013; Khan-Lewis, 2002) and found some similarities and differences to typical children.

Older and newer tools exist for assessing phonological processes for children with hearing (Khan-Lewis, 2002; Levitt, Youdelman, & Head, 1990) and for children with hearing loss (Grunwell, 1985; Paden & Brown, 1992; Vardi, 1991). However, using a **phonological process** approach for speech assessment and teaching of children with hearing loss needs further understanding. With these children, the "error" may more likely be due to, or at the very least entangled with, speech perception (Ling, 2002). For example, if a child with amplification is not able to perceive sound above 4000 Hz, that child will not hear /s/. Thus, reporting an /s/ deletion as a phonological process problem or final consonant deletion does not adequately explain the cause for the error. That is why knowledge of the acoustics of speech is fundamental.

Speech assessment and teaching purely through a phonological process approach may not be a sufficient treatment approach to ensure that the child with hearing loss develops a complete phonetic and phonologic repertoire by entry to school (Cole & Paterson, 1984; Ling, 2002; Paterson, 1994).

Coarticulation is the phenomenon of combining the segmentals and suprasegmental in connected spoken discourse. Coarticulation skill is a challenge for children with hearing loss if the foundational systems are poorly developed and coordinated. Yet, coarticulatory skill is the requirement to achieve intelligible speech with the goal of expressing meaning in spoken language.

The differentiating characteristics of "deaf speech" and challenges discussed above, while appearing overwhelmingly complex, are preventable and/or remediable. This complexity is the reason why a thorough in-depth assessment protocol is needed in working with children with hearing loss.

OVERVIEW OF ASSESSMENT PROCESS: ARTICULATION AND PHONOLOGICAL ASSESSMENT

What does the professional need to know, understand, and monitor in order to select an appropriate set of tools to determine speech production performance and make sense of the individual child's capacity and speech performance in connected discourse?

Who are we assessing? The first consideration is to determine what factors may be influencing the child's speech production abilities. These interrelated factors

may be intrinsic or extrinsic to the child (Ling, 1989; Paterson, 1994). Table 5–8 is by no means a complete list, but gives the reader some insight into the complexity of assessing the speech production of a child with hearing loss.

How these various factors combine will produce circumstances for speech assessment unique to each child with hearing loss. Four types of situations may lead to different choices in informal and formal speech assessments:

1. The early-starting child with hearing loss (otherwise typically developing);
2. The late-starting child with hearing loss (with no other special needs);
3. The early-starting child with hearing loss and additional special needs; and
4. The late-starting child with hearing loss and additional special needs. For children with additional speech needs, these needs may be obvious quite early on, or may become evident during the observation and assessment process, and will influence treatment options. (Perigoe, 2013)

However, regardless of individual learner characteristics, a thorough assessment of speech perception and production is needed, using a variety of assessments. These should include: assessments of auditory function; oral-peripheral sufficiency; speech production across suprasegmentals/prosodic and voice features; phonetic (syllable) level production of vowels, consonants and blends; phonologic level speech production in words and spontaneous speech; and an estimate of intelligibility. No single assessment tool can provide the teacher or clinician with all of this information; thus, a battery of assessments is necessary (Shipley & McAfee, 2008).

Table 5–8. Intrinsic and Extrinsic Factors to Consider in Assessment

Intrinsic (Child) Factors	Extrinsic (Environmental) Factors
1. Age of onset of hearing loss (congenital/acquired; prelingual/postlingual).	1. Age at fitting of hearing technology (hearing aids, cochlear implant(s), bone anchored hearing aids, FM systems).
2. Age at detection of hearing loss.	2. Appropriateness of hearing technology for full access to the range of speech.
3. Degree of hearing loss/level of hearing sensitivity (mild, moderate, severe, profound, total).	3. Amount of consistent hearing technology use; (e.g., full-time wearing of hearing technology).
4. Type of hearing loss (intermittent conductive loss, permanent conductive, permanent sensorineural, progressive, central, etc.).	4. Age at initiation of intervention.
5. Etiology of hearing loss (environmental; disease-related; genetic, syndromic/nonsyndromic; some causes may be associated with additional handicapping conditions).	5. Method/type and quality of early intervention program.
6. Individual response to the use of assisted hearing through hearing technology.	6. Parental ability to cope with diagnosis, participate productively in early education, styles of interaction, talk and communication skills.
7. Cognitive, psychosocial abilities, learning style.	7. Consistency and appropriateness of individual educational planning and treatment.
8. Other special needs or concomitant organic factors (visual impairment; autism; dyspraxia; motor disorders, such as cerebral palsy; syndromes, such as Waardenburg syndrome; etc.).	8. Knowledge and skill of the professionals in the integration of knowledge of audition, amplification, communication, speech and language development and assessment.
9. Individual ability to exploit sensory input: use of residual hearing (where available), vision, and touch.	9. Degree of coordination between all professionals and parents or caregivers.

Types of Tests

Tests of speech and speech production may be classified in a number of ways. They may be formal or informal; observational or task-oriented; norm-referenced or criterion-referenced; commercial or teacher-made. Most require a subjective assessment of how close the speech produced by the child is to the desired target sound (or adult model).

Norm-referenced tests are standardized, formal tests in which the child is compared to a larger group. These are commercially available tests. Norm-referenced test results usually provide a standard score, percentile rank, stanine and age-equivalency score. Standardized tests, such as the Goldman-Fristoe Test of Articulation-2 (2005), can be used to determine age-equivalency scores and sometimes help the child meet eligibility requirements for services. For children with hearing loss who are following a developmental trajectory of speech skill acquisition, it is useful to compare their speech results to those of their hearing peers. However, word tests should be used with caution and never on their own with children with hearing loss. Attention to phoneme production in words (especially the emphasis on consonants and /s/ blends in some tests) can put undue importance on that level of production and ignore bigger-picture issues, such as voice and prosody. Word-level tests also do not give the tester information about whether the child can produce the phoneme in nonmeaningful syllables (e.g., at the phonetic level). An argument for the use of standardized speech assessment tools on hearing children is that they can supply an age-equivalency measure, which may be necessary in order to establish a rationale for intervention services for the child.

Criterion-referenced tests allow the teacher or clinician to monitor the child's performance over time by comparing the child's speech production to his or her own previous performance. The child is not compared to other children. The majority of speech assessments developed for children with hearing loss are criterion-referenced tests and many can be administered formally or adapted to be administered informally. For example, information about the child's phonetic level repertoire can be gathered through the use of vocal play, speech babble, or imitation of sound-object associations (such as "moo" for the cow) when informally assessing younger children or children with additional disabilities. Criterion-referenced assessments, such as the Ling Phonetic Level Evaluation (Ling, 1976), do not require the teacher or clinician to start at the beginning of the test each time. The teacher or clinician can start at the point at which the child had inconsistent or incorrect responses. Informal and formal speech assessments that are criterion-based can be used to chart progress and monitor acquisition of phonemes and phonology.

While speech of children with hearing loss can be observed, subjective reports are less reliable than assessing what the child can do on a speech task where speech performance is specifically assessed. In some cases, teacher-made tests, which target specific skills of an individual child, can be quite useful, especially for very young children or children with multiple disabilities. At any age or stage, a video or digital recording of spoken language is recommended. The sound quality of video or digital recordings can be quite good at capturing speech in spoken language in real-life conversational exchanges, allowing the evaluator to assess speech skills (and spoken language) in authentic social situations. A combination of assessments is necessary for establishing targets for Individual Family Service Plans (IFSPs) and Individualized Education Plans (IEPs).

What are we assessing and why? Table 5–9 presents a rationale for what areas should be assessed and why test results might be used to develop a learner profile and to set appropriate targets for speech development and/or remediation. The next section highlights tools the authors have found useful in assessing the speech production abilities of children with hearing loss.

TRADITIONAL ASSESSMENT PROCEDURES

Traditionally, teachers and clinicians trained to work with children with hearing loss use a combination of phonetic and phonologic assessment procedures. This section will present details about the use of an oral-peripheral evaluation, the Ling Phonetic Level Evaluation (PLE), some selected word tests, the Ling Phonologic Evaluation (Ling, 1976) and a procedure being published for the first time, the Paterson-Cole Phonologic Evaluation Procedure (PC-PEP; Appendix 5–A).

Table 5–9. What to Consider in a Comprehensive Assessment Protocol

Aspects	Speech Perception and Speech Production
Information on audition Child's ability to hear and listen	• Determine auditory access through: hearing aids, cochlear implants, bone conduction aids and FM systems (Cole & Flexer, 2011; Perigoe & Paterson, 2013). • Interpret the aided audiogram and understand speech perception results. • Understand cochlear implant map and need for adjustments in the case of noticeable changes in quality of voice and speech production. • Perform the Ling Six-Sounds Test routinely. • Relate results of the Six-Sounds Test to the "speech banana" aided hearing. • Based on acoustic phonetics knowledge, predict the expected ease and difficulty of phoneme and phonologic perception.
Auditory/speech perception	• Assess detection and discrimination of phonemes across the distinctive features of manner, place, and voicing. • Assess ability to identify and comprehend words auditorily. • Assess discrimination of suprasegmental information: voice/voiceless, intensity, duration, and pitch differences. • Assess ability to discriminate and use linguistic aspects of prosody for language comprehension (Paterson, 1986; Perigoe & Paterson, 2013). • Assess the ability to predict sentence meanings in connected speech, using semantic and syntactic knowledge "to fill in the gaps." • Assess ability to follow conversational turns.
Integration of all sense modalities	• Understand the child's or student's use of each sense modality: audition; visual awareness and speech-reading ability; understanding and use of tactile and orosensory cues.
Oral-peripheral exam	Observe and note: • Integrity of oral speech production mechanisms. • Extraneous and interfering facial movements. • Excess effort such as jaw dropping, tongue contortions, overexaggerated lip-rounding.
Oro-motor assessment	For those children with hearing loss who may have concomitant cranio-facial anomalies or other reason to suspect an oral-motor problem in addition to hearing loss. *Note: Children with hearing loss do not all have oro-motor problems. Tongue practice external to the oral cavity does not improve proprioception.
Phonetic repertoire evaluation (syllables)	• Motor speech evaluation of the phonetic repertoire. • Vowels and diphthongs (tongue flexibility & tongue targeting). • Consonants by manner, place and voice/voiceless features. • Consonant clusters/blends. • Noting of distinctive feature errors, substitutions, and distortions.
Aspects of prosody	• Assess voice and suprasegmental features and voice in linguistic context: • Ability to sustain phonation and vocal quality. • Ability to initiate, control, and release the breath stream for control of phrase duration. • Ability to make intensity changes in overall voice production and the ability to make stress differentiation within words and phrases. • Ability to maintain an age- and sex-appropriate pitch register and the ability to vary intonation contour to mark discourse functions and to indicate affect. • The linguistic aspects of prosody should be assessed in at least sentence length context.

continues

Table 5–9. *continued*

Aspects	Speech Perception and Speech Production
Word tests	• Assess articulation of phonemes in a word test to supplement Phonetic & Phonologic Evaluation: • Standardized, formal test: will assess selected words and phonemes. • Teacher-made test; will assess speech production in any context deemed appropriate to show changes, growth, and to track development.
Sentence tests	• Assess articulation and coarticulation of phonemes in sentence context: • Standardized, formal test: will assess phonemes in standard sentence context; not able to evaluate all possible coarticulatory contexts. • Teacher-made sentence test: will assess speech production in any context deemed appropriate to show changes, growth, and to track development.
Phonological processes	For those children for whom it is appropriate: • Assess phonologic processes from conversational sample or test.
Phonologic level evaluation (from spoken language sample)	From connected discourse: • Assess ability to speak across sentences with appropriate juncture, rhythm, intonation, and stress patterns. • Note examples of coarticulation break-down. • Assess ability to self-repair.
Intelligibility rating	• Rate conversational intelligibility with observational tool. • Note features impacting listener comprehension of the spoken message.
Conversational skills	• Assess child's or student's conversational competency: • Assess auditory turn-taking and taking a conversational turn. • Assess ability to use speech to backchannel. • Assess ability to ask clarification questions. • Assess ability to repair communication breakdown. • Assess knowledge of speaker role and listener role in communication.
Student self-evaluation and participation in assessment	• Assess the motivation of child or student and awareness of own speech production issues: (inventory, questionnaire) • Student confidence level, self-esteem. • Child's awareness of own problem areas in speech and spoken language production. • Self-analysis of comfortable and uncomfortable conversational situations. • Knowledge of conversational frame, conversational mechanisms, and paralinguistic features. • Extended script knowledge. • Use of different sense modalities to monitor the speaker partner. • Elements of speech that the student would like to work on. • Knowledge and skill with self-repair/correction strategies.
Spoken language sampling	• Analysis of pragmatics/discourse, semantics, and syntax will highlight areas where articulation and/or prosodic problems are affecting the child's or student's ability to orally communicate.

Oral–Peripheral Evaluation

Most texts in speech pathology describe administration of a basic oral-peripheral examination. Ling includes a brief evaluation, adequate for most children, in his text (2002). A more extensive evaluation can be found in Shipley and McAfee (2008), and can be used with any child about whom there is a concern. Key areas to be assessed with respect to symmetry, range of motion, strength, any abnormal movements, or unusual color are the face, jaw, lips, frenulum, teeth/dentition, tongue, hard palate, soft palate, pharynx, and tonsils. Some also include information on posture at rest, breathing (e.g., mouth), and diadochokinetic rate (/p^t^k^/).

Phonetic Inventory Assessment: "Phonetic Level Evaluation"

A number of test instruments have been developed specifically for use with students with hearing loss, some as in-house research tools and others tools that are more widely used. Ling's Phonetic Level Evaluation (PLE) has been possibly the most widely used articulation test created for use with students with hearing loss. The PLE components have been adapted by other programs serving children and students with hearing loss (Central Institute for the Deaf, Sunshine Cottage School for the Deaf, CREC-Soundbridge) and are seen in many versions, often in a reduced format, so that evaluation time to establish speech targets is reduced. Ling himself revised his original PLE in the second edition of his text, *Speech and the Hearing-Impaired Child: Theory and Practice* (2002), to include a Phonologic Level Evaluation and a rating scale, thus eliminating some

elements. It is the authors' view that in attempting to provide a rating, the power of obtaining a more complete picture of a child's phonetic repertoire was lost. The authors prefer the original (Ling, 1976) version of the PLE for speech assessment to be done along with the Ling Phonologic Evaluation. The new Paterson-Cole Phonologic Level Evaluation, PC-PEP (Appendix 5–A), can be done in lieu of the Ling Phonologic Level Evaluation or used to replace the nonsegmental section of the PLE.

Before discussing the components of the PLE and how it is administered, it is necessary to understand the concept of automaticity and its importance in speech development and, therefore, speech assessment. Automaticity in speech production is a key concept in Ling's (2002) model of speech assessment and teaching. The four components of automaticity are: accuracy; speed; economy of effort; and flexibility. Thus, automaticity is a set of interactive skills, which are necessary for the speaker to produce fluent, coarticulated speech. Automaticity allows the speaker to focus on the message without thinking about how to make each individual phoneme. These are extremely useful constructs when determining how to avoid the characteristics of "deaf speech." Table 5–10 presents the four parameters of automaticity and explanatory notes.

Typically developing children develop automaticity in speech production over time. In the early stages of speech development, the neural and mechanical response times are longer as the child is still developing control. As normal children develop and as they become more sophisticated in using feedback and feedforward mechanisms, they also acquire the ability to produce fast and

Table 5–10. Automaticity Parameters in Speech Production

Accuracy	• Precision in producing the target: accurate in place, manner, and voiced/voiceless features.
	• Precision in moving from the target to other sounds, as in tongue transitions in diphthongs.
	• Precision in anticipatory and perseveratory coarticulation.
	• Precision in control of onset and offset of phonation.
	• Good use of feedback and feedforward.
Speed	• Rate of phoneme production = at least 3 syllables per second.
	• Speed requires control and accuracy of **anticipatory coarticulation**.
	• Speedy vowel transitions are required for diphthongization and CV formations.
	• Requires feedforward skills.
Economy of Effort	• Accurate and speedy production of syllables requires economy in motor activity.
	• There should be no evident "struggle" behaviors: excessive jaw dropping or movement, excessive lip rounding, nasality, or tongue contortions.
	• Ability to sustain at least 12 syllables on one breath.
Flexibility	• Ability to alternate the target syllable with other syllables with accuracy, speed, and economy of effort.
	• Good anticipatory and perseveratory coarticulation.
	• Good overall coarticulation abilities with variations in intensity, duration, and pitch (prosody).

clear speech. That is, they have mastered phoneme coarticulation to the point that they can plan what to say and express the utterance without having to think about how to say the next sounds. The motor speech center is on "automatic"—like a car—and the child's brain does not have to painstakingly shift gears to produce phonemes, words, or phrases. The children also have learned to think ahead; the brain anticipates what is coming and they develop **metaphonologic** ability to laugh at, recognize, and repair their speech production errors. This is *automaticity* in speech production. Clinicians and teachers want these abilities for the child or student with hearing loss.

The auditory–vocal loop: Children with hearing loss must establish the auditory–vocal loop. By working on speech through audition, children with hearing loss can learn that "what comes out of my mouth has something to do with

what I am hearing." Children with hearing loss who are late to talking may have slower response times that affect both feedback and feedforward skills. These longer response times will introduce distortions of timing in running speech, which will affect fluency and coarticulation (Ling, 2002). External feedback systems, visual (such as mirrors or computer systems), tactile or written aids, may act as crutches and prevent automaticity from developing (Cole & Paterson, 1984; Ling, 2002; Paterson, 1994). Any such crutches should be used only briefly to help attain a goal, then removed to ensure that the student is developing internal feedback and feedforward mechanisms and proprioception.

The Phonetic Level Evaluation (PLE) is an evaluation of motor speech ability and neuro-motor coordination (Ling, 2002). This tool allows the professional to make a perceptual, subjective judgment of the child or student's skill at producing consonant-vowel syllables with automaticity (Table 5–11). It is a more flexible and authentic tool to use to evaluate articulation than a standardized test and unlike a standardized test can be administered in sections and at intervals. The PLE is a criterion-referenced test intended to be used systematically over time as the child or student progresses through acquiring speech targets in a diagnostic teaching approach. The PLE is *NOT* a test of speech production in words and if it is used with word prompts, this negates the value of the test as a test of motor speech ability.

This test is meant to be a living tool and not to be used once a year for IEPs.

Test administration and sense modalities: The PLE is not a test of speech perception. It is a test of feedforward skill and automaticity of speech production. The evaluator should give the student with hearing loss access to maximum auditory and visual (e.g., speechreading) information during the test. It is meant to be a measure of an individual's best effort in production of speech syllables on the day of the evaluation.

The PLE is arranged to follow Ling's sequential interpolated model although the sections are separate (Table 5–12). The test begins with attention to assessing nonsegmental aspects of speech, and follows with a detailed vowel and diphthong section. The consonants are organized in a relatively developmental order and include the distinctive features of manner, place, and voicing.

The PLE scoring system has three levels that include: (1) a check mark [✓] for well produced, meaning that the phoneme in syllables is produced with automaticity; (2) a plus sign [+] for present

Table 5–11. What Questions Does the PLE Answer?

1. Is the child capable of differentiated speech sound production to the extent required? (Automaticity)

2. Can speech patterns be reliably repeated?

3. Can patterns be alternated with other patterns at an acceptable rate? (rate of production of 3 syllables per second)

4. Can segments be varied in duration, intensity, and pitch?

Table 5–12. Components of the Ling (1976) PLE

Nonsegmentals	Vocalization, duration, intensity, pitch
Vowels and Diphthongs	a, i, u, aʊ, aɪ ɔ, ɔɪ, ɛ, u, ɪ æ, ʌ, a, o, oʊ, e, eɪ ɝ, ə, ɚ
Step One Consonants	b, p, m, f, v, θ, ð, h, w, stop b, stop p
Step Two Consonants	d, t, n, ʃ, ʒ , s, z, j, l, stop d, stop t
Step Three Consonants	g, k, ŋ, tʃ, dʒ, r, stop g, stop k
Step Four Consonants	voiced–voiceless and diadokinetic rate
Word–Initial Blends	
Word–Final Blends	

but not quite right [could be slow rate of production, substitution, or slight distortion]; and (3) a minus sign [–] to indicate that the target is missing or not able to be produced at all. Substitutions are noted and targets for instruction listed to the right.

A degree of ear training on the part of the evaluator is required. Some teachers and clinicians find that they can tune their ears more easily than others, so most evaluators need practice in scoring a variety of children at various levels of speech performance

Rate of syllable production is an element of the PLE that the rater needs to monitor. The goal is for the child or student to be able to automatically repeat syllables at the rate of 3 syllables per second. This approximates the rate of typical speech production (Ling, 2002). Therefore, if the child or student cannot produce some consonant-vowel combinations at that rate, he or she would receive a [+] for that sound and rate of production would be a target. There is a misunderstanding that 3 per second means that, when selected as a target, speech is practiced only in 3-syllable sets. In fact, rehearsing productions of multiple syllables in strings of varying length is the goal.

Parent and student participation in the PLE is helpful. Parents can and should be present at the evaluation of young children, so that they can participate and become effective promoters of their child's speech improvement. School-aged students who have done the PLE before will notice you scoring and may become concerned. It is recommended that school-aged students be included in the process by having the evaluator do a student inventory with them.

Order of evaluation issues: Ling recommended a relatively strict order of evaluation, starting with nonsegmentals and continuing with vowels, diphthongs, and consonants until the child has made about six or seven errors, which become the six to seven teaching targets. There are some misunderstandings about what to include in targeting that are discussed in the next section of the chapter. The authors agree on some variations of the original evaluation approach and those are summarized in Table 5–13.

Does the order of evaluation of sections imply a strict teaching order? No, in fact, the order of the PLE for assessment purposes absolutely does not infer a teaching order. The PLE is not a lesson plan and is not meant to be used as such. The teacher or clinician must prioritize a logical set of targets that must include vowels and/or diphthongs and consonants that will be practiced with suprasegmental variation (prosody). There has long been some misunderstanding that the Ling model suggests that you start with (and only) practice the nonsegmentals first until the student can do them. Yet, how can that be logical? Suprasegmentals must be practiced within the context of vowels. It is also useful to release vowels with a consonant that the child can produce easily. When assessing short vowels, such as /ɪ/ or repeated vowels, whether short (e.g., /bɪbɪbɪ/) or long (e.g., /bababa/), releasing with a consonant helps avoid tension, glottalization or other poor speech productions. Table 5–13 asks and answers some common questions about the PLE. A summary of relevant speech acoustics is provided in Figure 5–1 (Ling, 1989, p. 69).

Suggested variations on PLE administration: When Ling recommended assessing /b/ or /p/ (for example), it was before the current era of advanced hearing technologies and early detection for most children.

Table 5–13. Questions About Administration of the PLE

Is it necessary to complete the entire evaluation?	NO. Stop when the child has about 6–7 targets. However, make sure that suprasegmentals, some vowels and diphthongs, and some early consonants are assessed. You should not have only suprasegmentals and vowels selected as targets. Exception: child with almost complete repertoire where blends are focus (do all).
How quickly should you go through the PLE?	Administering the PLE is not a speed trial. Take your time to really listen and watch the child's production.
How long should the PLE take?	For most children, 15 or 20 minutes is sufficient. For the student with more speech ability (who will get further in the test) it will take longer for the first administration, but be brief on reassessment (since you need not reassess well-developed skills). Also, the PLE can be done in sections over more than one session.
How often should I give the PLE?	As a criterion-referenced test, the PLE can be used as frequently as it makes sense to do so.
Is the suprasegmental section a complete enough assessment?	The PLE suprasegmental section gives a gross measure and is insufficient for analysis if child has suprasegmental problems. Analysis of what the child does in connected speech is needed. The PC-PEP was developed to address this area.
Why should I use a consonant to release the vowels and diphthongs?	Ling (1976) recommends that vowels should be evaluated by being released from the plosive /b/ instead of in isolation. Releasing vowels with a consonant helps avoid poor speech productions.
Do I need to assess vowels in four contexts? S — single production R — repeated syllables A — alternated syllables P — with pitch variation	Start with *repeated* syllables. Only go back to single syllables if the child cannot do well in repeated syllables. Variation: do not assess all of the SRAP conditions while doing the vowel system. If in your chat with the child, prosody is of concern, it is not useful to spent time assessing all vowels in the alternated and pitch condition. It is adequate to assess in the S & R condition only, as you will test alternations with the consonants and pitch through the suprasegmentals.
Why am I asking the child to imitate production at the *rate* of three syllables per second?	The rate of three syllables per second represents typical syllable speed production. This rate allows us to assess speed and accuracy of production.
Why am I evaluating the consonants in three different vowel contexts /a/, /u/, and /i/?	These are the three "cornerstone" vowels (as you can also see from Ling's vowel sentence presented earlier). They represent the vowel with the highest constriction at the front of the mouth /i/, the loudest mid vowel /a/, and the vowel made with highest constriction at the back of the mouth /u/. Deaf/HH children may be able to produce consonants with some vowels, but not others. For example, a child may be able to produce /gagagagaga/, but not be able to produce the /g/ at all when asked to imitate /gigigigi/. In addition, it helps to identify other related errors, such as "context dependent pitch" or "nasalization." For example, some children may have a normal sounding voice for /dadada/, but their pitch may go up for /dididi/ or /dududu/ because of inappropriate vocal fold tension. A child may produce /mamama/ well, but have a very nasalized vowel when attempting /mimimi/. If consonants are only assessed with one vowel, these important productions can be missed.

continues

Table 5–13. *continued*

Why did Ling pick those particular Step One Consonants?	Step One Consonants: Most of the <u>manner of production</u> distinctions are established as well as *voiced and voiceless differences.* Manner of consonant production is carried by low and mid-frequency acoustic information (see Ling table [Table 5–1]) and accessible to most. Also, most Step One consonants are produced at the front of the mouth, so they provide more visual cues (speechreading). Most (not all) are early developing and more easily produced. These consonants lay the foundation for later developing phonemes.
Variation for all Steps	Notice on the Ling (1976) form that he originally recommended assessing /b/or /p/ etc. We now assess /b/ and /p/ as voiced-voiceless distinction can be achieved early for most d/hh speakers.
Why did Ling pick those particular Step Two Consonants?	Step Two Consonants: *Place of consonant production is key* as well as manner and voiced and voiceless differences. Place of consonant production is carried by high frequency and transitional acoustic cues (see Ling table [Table 5–1]). Most of these consonants are made on or around the alveolar ridge, and palate. These are the middle of the mouth consonants and less visible than Step One Consonants.
Why did Ling pick those particular Step Three Consonants?	Step Three Consonants: Place of consonant production is key as well and manner and voiced and voiceless differences. Place of consonant production is carried by mid and high frequency acoustic cues (see Ling table [Table 5–1]). Most of these consonant phonemes are made centrally or at the back of the mouth and the least visible through speechreading.
What is the purpose of assessment at the level of Step Four Consonants?	The main feature of Step Four is voiced–voiceless distinctions. Diadochokinetic rate is also recorded. Ling felt that these distinctions could wait until the basic manners and places were mastered. Variation: With today's hearing technology, most children master voiced–voiceless distinctions (cognate pairs) as they acquire the consonants in the Steps.
When do I assess Word Initial Consonant Blends (clusters)? Ling (1976) called these "blends." Today they are referred to more commonly as consonant clusters	There is a misconception that you wait to assess consonant blends until you reach this page of the PLE. In fact, consonant cluster production begins developmentally in early speech and several phonological processes are related to cluster production. In fact (Ling, 2002) includes /s/ production in blends as a strategy for teaching the /s/. Recommendation: Once the child or student is producing *any* of the blending consonants (e.g., s, l, r, w), it is fine to assess and work on the related blends.
When do I assess word-final blends?	They are on the last page, but are they really last? No. They should be assessed (and taught) concurrently with word-initial blends and should be assessed when a child is producing any of the blend components. Again, some word final blends occur in early phonology, depending upon linguistic context. Recommendation: Assess final blends in word contexts for children who are struggling.

Source: Created by Perigoe and Paterson, 2014 (adapted from Ling,1976, and Perigoe, 1981, 1995, 2001, 2007).

The authors recommend assessing the voiced and voiceless plosives with the simple consonants at each stage as the ability to produce one voiced–voiceless contrast facilitates development of the other. The authors still recommend assessing only the voiceless fricatives in Step One Consonants if the child cannot easily produce /f/ and /v/. In phonology, when we are producing connected speech, the voiced fricatives sometimes reduce to voiceless, in order for us to keep speaking quickly. So, the authors would assess only the voiceless fricatives, which are also easier to teach (Cole & Paterson, 1984; Paterson, 1994), if fricative production is problematic.

Phonologic Level: Word Tests

Articulation is arguably one of the easiest aspects of speech to describe (Paterson, 1994) and there are a variety of tools standardized on hearing children that are used to assess articulation of school-aged deaf and hard of hearing children. Standardized tests, such as the Goldman-Fristoe Test of Articulation-2 (2005), are commonly used by speech pathologists when it is necessary to obtain a rating that compares the child with hearing loss to typically developing hearing children and to establish eligibility for speech services. This instrument and others, however, only provide a limited description of the articulation capacity. Such tests typically do not include all vowel and diphthong productions, do not assess the suprasegmentals of speech, or co-articulated speech in running conversation. Target phonemes are evaluated in a limited representative set of words and sentences and may only be evaluated in initial, medial, or final positions. A child

with hearing loss may be able to produce a speech sound in some words but not others, and be unable to consistently produce the target phoneme in all the varying contexts in conversational speech. Word tests are, therefore, only one small part of the complete picture of what the child can and cannot do.

In addition to tests for typically developing hearing children, there are some word tests for children with hearing loss worth discussing. *Identifying Early Phonological Needs* in *Children with Hearing Loss* (Paden & Brown, 1992) is a useful test for children with limited vocabularies as it uses only 25 words. This makes it suitable for young children or children with additional special needs. It is relatively easy to give, but scoring takes some practice. That said, it gives excellent data for emerging speech at the word level for word patterns, vowels, and consonants by manner, place, and voicing. The authors recommend that scores for individual categories (e.g., fricatives) be kept separate, rather than using the summary scores, as the summary scores obscure the rich data collected in the analysis.

The *CID Picture Spine* (Central Institute for the Deaf, 1988) has the advantage of giving a sense of control to the students; they feel like they are the teacher. The student looks at the cards (without letting the evaluator see them), says the name of the picture aloud, and the teacher or clinician listens and takes the test. It looks like a spelling test for the teacher, but it is really a test of speech intelligibility of the student. There are four decks of 50 cards (25 pictures, each appearing twice), which get progressively more difficult. One disadvantage is that the cards have words printed on them, so it is important that the child does not perceive this as a test of reading. The assessment can be done in different sessions to maintain interest. The authors also have found that the test is more authentic if the listener is not provided with a word bank for each section. In addition, we have found it helpful to compare scores from listeners familiar with the child (e.g., a parent) with scores from an unfamiliar listener.

The value of word tests is to help bridge the gap between phonetic level assessment and spontaneous speech. They should not be used, however, to the exclusion of phonetic level testing and a spontaneous speech sample.

Phonologic Level: Speech In Connected Language

In order to assess speech production in connected spoken language, it is necessary to obtain a spoken language sample. In some cases, this can be video or digitally recorded in play or conversational situations that are authentic representations of the child's spoken language. In other instances, spoken language may be elicited to obtain a representative sample. Perigoe and Ling (1986) recommend eliciting a language sample in five areas of discourse, with the objective of obtaining a wider variety of language constructions and speech usage than conversation alone can provide. The teacher or clinician can also "load the deck" by asking the child to retell a story with potential speech targets. For example, if the teacher suspects that /s/ and /s/ blends are problematic, the child might be asked to retell the story of "Cinderella." For /dg/ and /r/, "The Gingerbread Man" is a good choice. The tasks selected must be suited to the age and language level of the child. Table 5–14 provides only a small sample of the differences in language and speech elements that might be evidenced through such elicited language sampling.

Once the language sample is collected, it needs to be transcribed orthographically (in English). Then the teacher or clinician listens to the recording (perhaps several times) and makes note of any problems the child may have with prosodic elements, as well as with segmental patterns (vowels, diphthongs, consonants and consonant blends). The child's speech production is transcribed phonetically above the orthographic transcription. A variation which the authors have found works extremely well for students with hearing loss who have good vocal quality and prosodic patterns, good vowel production and only consonant errors, is to transcribe ONLY the errors above the phonemes in question. This takes less time than a full phonetic transcription and has the advantage of making the error analysis much easier.

The Ling Phonologic Level Evaluation (1976) was originally used for analyzing the spoken language sample. Later, Ling incorporated it into a combined version, the Phonetic-Phonologic Level Evaluation (2002). The authors prefer the first version and also the initial scoring system, which mirrors Ling's PLE of correct (✓), inconsistent (+) and incorrect/missing (−) with space at the right to record errors and speech targets. The authors have used this successfully with students who have satisfactory suprasegmentals and vowels and who are primarily working on consonants and consonant blends/clusters. For students who have challenges in prosodic features, the authors prefer *The Paterson-Cole Phonologic Evaluation Procedure, (PC-PEP)*, which is now presented and discussed in detail.

Table 5–14. Discourse Types With Potential Linguistic and Speech Elements

Discourse Type	Potential Linguistic Elements	Potential Speech Elements
Conversation	Topic initiation/closure, e.g., Hi, bye	h, b
	Topic maintenance	
	Use of names, places, pronouns, me, you, etc.	m, /j/, w
Narration	Use of sequences, e.g., first, then, before, after	f, "th," b
	Use of character names and places	(various)
Explanation	Command language and verbs, e.g., push, pull, open, cut, spread, etc.	p, k
	Sequences, e.g., first, second, etc.	
Description	Prepositions, e.g., in, on, under, beside, behind, next to, over	n, b, s, v
	Modifiers, colors, numbers	
Question Formation	Question forms e.g., "wh" questions	w, h, d
	"Does it, did it, has it, is it," etc.	final z, t

The Paterson-Cole Phonologic Evaluation Procedure (PC-PEP) was first developed in 1992, as a procedure to analyze suprasegmental production and to assess how the child uses prosodic components in spoken language and as a quick phonetic evaluation. Dr. Elizabeth Cole is a former professor and the current director of the CREC Soundbridge program serving children with hearing loss, birth through high school, in Connecticut. In past writings and presentations on assessing and teaching speech, the authors (Paterson & Cole) discussed the overattention to articulation assessment and syllable level practice, and the unfortunate neglect of the crucial area of prosody in spoken language (Cole & Flexer; 2011; Cole & Paterson, 1984; Paterson, 1986 , 1992, 1994). The prosodic components of speech that Ling included in his PLE are noted as vocalization, duration, intensity, and pitch. However, evaluation of these suprasegmentals

(nonsegmentals) of speech from the PLE exclusively does not guide the professionals sufficiently to target improvement of those aspects in spoken language or phonologic level practice (Cole & Paterson, 1984; Paterson, 1982, 1986; Table 5–15). In addition, the nonsegmentals of speech are very difficult if not impossible to work on in isolation. They are best assessed and worked on in connected spoken language or discourse. Paterson (1986) presented a table that connected the suprasegmentals with their corresponding elements of prosody in spoken language that is the basis of the PC-PEP. (See Appendix 5–A.)

As noted above, hearing loss can impact the development of clear, melodic sounding speech. These prosodic acoustic cues are what the infant listens to (**motherese**) and they provide information for discrimination of male versus female voice, tone of voice (angry, happy, sad, etc.) and early cues for conversa-

Table 5–15. Basic Relationship of Prosodic Features in Language to Suprasegmentals

Suprasegmental Aspects of Speech	Linguistic Occurrence of Prosody
Vocalization: Ability to produce voicing	Oral sounding vocal quality
Duration: Ability to control length of voicing; onset and offset	Timing, rhythm, pausing, marking juncture
Intensity: Ability to vary subglottal pressure	Stress patterns in words (meaning differences: con'duct vs. 'conduct), phrases, and across sentences and overall voice loudness variation
Pitch: Ability to vary vocal fold tension and subglottal pressure	Overall voice pitch and the intonation patterns in English that differentiate: statements, commands, negative, question types; affect and tone of voice

Source: Adapted from Cole and Paterson, 1984; Paterson 1986.

tional turn-taking. Prosodic components of spoken language are an acoustic phenomenon and not discernable through the visual sense (Paterson, 1986, 1994).

The PC-PEP can be used to evaluate conversational speech or a spoken language sample, either live or from a recorded sample. The overall goal is to be a specific as possible about the elements of prosody that assist or detract from intelligibility. There are two columns. In column one, the assessor is directed to listen for how well the speaker produces prosodic features in connected discourse and intelligibility of the message. For example: Does the speaker mark normal sentence boundaries (control of duration)? Does the speaker produce the appropriate stress marking in multisyllabic words (intensity change)? Does the speaker produce the intonational contour appropriate for the meaning and syntax of the utterance (pitch contour)? Then, in column two the assessor makes a perceptual judgment of the speaker's quality of phonation and ability to produce duration, intensity and pitch changes at the physiologic level.

For example, if the child or student has demonstrated poor ability to mark

appropriate word and sentence stress patterns, the underlying cause is likely to be physiological. This could be an interaction of a poor ability to sustain phonation over a breath phrase coupled with a poor ability to coordinate a change in subglottal pressure. A rapid increase in subglottal pressure results in an intensity change, which the listener hears as a stress pattern. English is a stress-timed language (Ling, 2002; Small, 2008) and the ability to mark stress patterns appropriately contributes enormously to the listener's rating of a deaf or hard of hearing speaker's intelligibility. Column two is more difficult for most assessors while column one, with a focus on key components of prosody in spoken language, is easier.

The PC-PEP allows a tester to identify areas that impact conversational intelligibility. Useful phonologic targeting can be achieved through this process. Then, through listening practice and the use of spoken language, a professional can more safely have a student practice appropriate prosodic patterns such as word or sentence stress in planned conversational contexts. Not only is this is useful for diagnostic purposes, it leads to more appropriate developmental or remedial strategies that are conversationally based.

The PC-PEP has been presented in numerous workshops, is used as an assessment procedure in graduate training courses and used clinically by both authors, although it has never been published until now. A table aligning the PC-PEP elements with their relevant speech acoustics is found in Perigoe and Paterson (2013). Since the emphasis of the PC-PEP is on prosodic elements, rather than on articulation of specific phonemes in connected speech (which was addressed by Ling, 1976, in the Phonologic Level Evaluation), the PC-PEP is ideal for analyzing the speech of children or students with hearing loss who clearly do not have typical vocal quality or use of prosodic patterns. In addition, the authors have found it extremely useful for young children with hearing loss who are late starters and for students who have additional special needs. It has also been used successfully with adults who have had long-term poor auditory access, especially those receiving cochlear implants later in life.

INTEGRATING ASSESSMENT DATA

Speech is a complex event. As stated earlier, whatever the particular characteristics of the learner, a thorough and complete assessment of the child's speech perception and speech production abilities is required in order to select targets for teaching and monitor the child's progress. The authors have discussed the importance of assessing the child's oral mechanism, his or her suprasegmental production or control over prosodic features, his or her production of phonemes in syllables, words, and connected discourse, as well as the child's overall speech intelligibility.

It is essential for the teacher or clinician to compare results across assessments to get a better picture of whether the child is developing along a typical speech acquisition trajectory or whether the child needs remedial help. By comparing phonetic and phonologic level performance, the professional can see whether the child generalizes phonetic (syllable) level skills to words and to spontaneous speech. Then targets for training can be selected at both the phonetic and phonologic levels to move the child forward on his or her developmental or remedial pathway.

Target Setting From the Phonetic Level Evaluation

The purpose of a phonetic level evaluation is to identify speech production errors at phonetic level, to understand the nature of those speech production errors and then to select appropriate targets for development or remediation. To achieve this Ling recommended that the teacher or clinician establish or exploit precursory skill. For example, if the student produces any voiced plosive, this ability to produce plosion is precursory to learning other voiced plosives. An example of more complicated targeting would be the teacher or clinician's knowledge that targeting the "ch" phoneme is pointless until the student has near automaticity in the production of the two elements of "ch"— that is the stop /t/ and the "sh." This is an also an example of another Ling principle that holds true: "work from the simple to the difficult and work from the known to the unknown" (Ling, 2002).

How many targets should be set at any one time? Ling recommended selecting approximately six or seven targets to be worked on concurrent currently. Speech is a dynamic, inter-related process. An analogy might be that it is easier to weave a quilt if there are more threads on the loom. Working on multiple targets helps the child learn to contrast manner of articulation (e.g., /m/ versus /b/), place of articulation (e.g., /p/ versus /t/), and voicing (e.g., /p/ versus /b/). In addition, it can assist when developing sounds that are similar in any of these parameters (e.g., such as working on several fricatives in Step One consonants to develop a sense of breath flow). This use of multiple targets also helps both the child and teacher maintain motivation and increases the potential for success.

Mastery of phonetic production is a complicated concept and there are some misconceptions. A student does not need 100% mastery at the phonetic level to work on carryover to words and phrases at the phonologic level. Phonetic and phonologic practice go hand in hand both for assessment and then in teaching (Ling, 2002; Perigoe, 1992). Typically developing children use approximations in their pathway towards mastery of spoken language. The goal of the teacher or clinician is to improve the student's ability to self-monitor and self-correct their speech productions. The student's goal is to achieve automaticity in coarticulated connected speech with appropriate prosodic features.

Comparing Results From Phonetic and Phonologic Level Evaluation

The blank form of the *Speech Target Summary* (Appendix 5–B) is useful to record your judgments from the PLE, any word

tests, and your phonologic evaluation (Ling or PC-PEP). It is ideal to put your speech targets from each assessment onto the summary, use it to prioritize teaching targets, and then add and progress to additional targets as the child achieves mastery. The child's errors should be recorded in the same relative order that they appear on the evaluation forms in order to line them up. Next, analyze the data to understand patterns and relationships. You are seeking to understand more about why a phoneme is produced correctly, incorrectly, or is missing. Briefly, describe or characterize the speech problem. Here are some guiding questions:

- How does this phoneme relate to other sounds? For example, are they all fricative sounds? Are the errors all tongue-tip or alveolar sounds?
- Does the child have adequate auditory access to hear the sound? For example, are the sounds all high-frequency and does the child then require better or different amplification or a new cochlear implant map?
- What is the fundamental physiologic problem?

Analyzing the errors in this way helps the teacher or clinician to develop a treatment plan and monitor progress. Appendix 5–C is a sample of the *Speech Target Summary* for a school-aged student with hearing loss, with a rationale about *why* particular targets were chosen for remediation.

By determining whether the child is following a developmental trajectory or requires a more remedial approach, the teacher or clinician will prioritize the speech targets at both phonetic and phonologic levels. Speech targets that are inconsistently produced will be more amenable to acquisition than those that have not yet started to be acquired.

Student Motivation: A student might be asking themselves, "Why should I make the effort to practice all of this speech when I can communicate just the way I am?" Motivation to do "speech practice" can be a big issue for school-aged students. Children or students sometimes change speech production despite speech teaching, as they are able to do incidental learning from the environment. Some school-age children continue with impoverished speech production systems despite regular speech sessions or classroom correction. Time is spent in speech "work" with less change than desired (Paterson, 1994). In early childhood, children are more willing to engage in speech practice and their vocal production systems are more flexible. For all ages, keep the speech sessions fun, start with something the child can do well, embed the hard part in the middle, and end with success. Engage the child or student and keep practice meaningful. Sessions should combine phonetic and phonologic level practice so that target(s) can be practiced in language that is meaningful to the child. Have the student help in setting goals and charting progress.

Timetable for improvement: It is important to consider how long it should or could take to achieve the targets in speech practice. You are selecting a first set of six or seven targets to give you an entry point into the speech remediation system of the student. In what period of time will you evaluate the progress of the student towards mastery? The authors suggest that this should be thought of in terms of weeks, not months, and months, not a year. The expectation is to notice the

child or student using speech in language and transfer to phonology. Some challenges in targeting and prognosis may be related to the IEP process where too few targets are selected, targeting is too nonspecific, the time frame for change is too long, and there may be too little ongoing evaluation and resetting of targets. Paterson (1994) cited a number of specialists who were concerned that speech improvement for the school-aged student seemed to be considered a lifelong, extended school goal. When we recall that a child with normal hearing has mastered phonology by around 7 to 8 years of age, why is speech an IEP goal into the middle and high school years?

Today time is precious and professionals want "quick and easy" ways to assess. It is possible to learn to administer the PLE relatively quickly but it is not easy to make sense of the findings, prioritize a sequence of targets, and predict the next targets. One caution relates to establishing speech goals for a student's IEP. The essence of the Ling approach is excellent evaluation, targeting, flexible and informed speech teaching, and then moving on. As stated previously, the goal is to have students enter school with a complete phonetic repertoire. A student must have more than one set of targets in a school year or something is missing in the speech support.

In addition to selecting speech targets for long and short-term goals, continued ongoing assessment allows the teacher or clinician to determine whether the child meets speech goals and makes adequate progress. For children following a developmental path, we are expecting that they make one year of growth in one year. For those starting late, we need to work at closing the gap between their hearing age and chronological age. To do that, they need to make more than one year of speech progress in a year. More important than a gauge of age-equivalency, however, is the importance of the child becoming a confident spoken language communicator.

SUMMARY

Ling's model, guiding principles, and writings (Ling, 1976, 1989, 2002), as well as writings and presentations of those influenced by his work (some represented in this chapter), continue to offer guidelines for the most comprehensive and useful approach to the assessment and teaching of speech to children with hearing loss. In this chapter, the model has been expanded to include explanations, variations, consideration of word tests, and phonologic processes. The authors have also added a new assessment tool called the PC-PEP. Information has been presented on

- the impact of speech perception on speech production,
- the need for a comprehensive assessment battery, and
- the integration of speech perception and speech assessment data to create individualized speech teaching plans.

The task of the professional is not only to accurately assess the child's speech production, but to set appropriate speech targets and implement an intervention program designed to prevent, reduce, and remediate the impact of the hearing loss on the child's speech and spoken language development to the greatest

degree possible. In order to do that, the next step is to become a flexible, knowledgeable teacher or clinician with a deep understanding of how to develop speech in children with hearing loss.

REFERENCES

Bass-Ringdahl, S. M. (2010). The relationship of audibility and the development of canonical babbling in young children with hearing impairment. *Journal of Deaf Studies and Deaf Education, 15*(3), 287–311. doi:10.1093/deafed/enq013

Bleile, K. (2006). *The late eight.* San Diego, CA: Plural.

Boothroyd, A. (1982). *Hearing impairments in young children.* Englewood Cliffs, NJ: Prentice Hall.

Boothroyd, A. (1986). *Speech acoustics and perception.* Austin, TX: Pro-Ed.

Cole, E., & Flexer, C. (2011). *Children with hearing loss: Developing listening and talking, birth to six* (2nd ed.). San Diego, CA: Plural.

Cole, E., & Paterson, M. M. (1984). Assessment and treatment of phonologic disorders in the hearing-impaired. In J. Costello (Ed.), *Speech disorders in children: Recent advances* (pp. 93–127). San Diego, CA: College Hill Press.

Dornan, D. (2009). *Hearing loss in babies is a neurological emergency.* Washington, DC: Alexander Graham Bell Association for the Deaf and Hard of Hearing.

Erber, N. (1982). *Auditory training.* Washington, DC: Alexander Graham Bell Association for the Deaf and Hard of Hearing.

Eriks-Brophy, A., Gibson, S., & Tucker, S. (2013). Articulatory error patterns and phonological use of preschool children with and without hearing loss. *The Volta Review, 113*(2), 87–125.

Ertmer, D. J. (2001). Interactive website for instruction in prelinguistic vocal development of young cochlear implant recipients. Retrieved from http://www.vocaldevelopment.com

Ertmer, D. J. (2011). Assessing speech intelligibility in children with hearing loss: Toward revitalizing a valuable clinical tool. *Journal of Speech, Language, and Hearing Research, 42*(1), 52–58.

Ertmer, D. J., & Goffman, L. (2011). Speech production accuracy and variability in young cochlear implant recipients: Comparison with typically developing age-peers. *Journal of Speech, Language, and Hearing Research, 54,* 177–189. doi:10.1044/1092-4388

Ertmer, D. J. & Inniger, K. I. (2009). Characteristics of the transition to spoken word in two young cochlear implant recipients. *Journal of Speech, Language, and Hearing Research, 52,* 1579–1594. doi:10.1044/1092-4388

Ertmer, D. J., Young, N. M., & Nathani, S. (2007). Profiles in vocal development in young cochlear implant recipients. *Journal of Speech, Language, and Hearing Research, 50,* 393–407.

Flexer, C. (2013). Technology and listening. In L. Robinson (Ed.), *Literacy and deafness: Listening and spoken language* (2nd ed., pp. 43–65). San Diego, CA: Plural.

Gallaudet Research Institute. (2008, November). *Regional and national summary report of data from the 2007–08 Annual Survey of Deaf and Hard of Hearing Children and Youth.* Washington, DC: GRI, Gallaudet University.

Goldman, R., & Fristoe, M. (2000). *Goldman-Fristoe 2 Test of Articulation manual.* Minneapolis, MN: NCS Pearson.

Grunwell, P. (1985). *PACS: The Phonological Assessment of Child Speech.* Windsor, UK: NFER-Nelson.

Hirsh, I. J. (1970). Auditory training. In H. Davis & S. Silverman, (Eds.), *Hearing and Deafness.* (pp. 346–359). New York, NY: Holt, Rinehart & Winston.

Hudgins, C. V., & Numbers, F. C. (1942). An investigation of the intelligibility of the speech of the deaf. *Genetic Psychology Monographs, 25,* 289–392.

Joint Committee on Infant Hearing (JCIH). (2007). Year 2007 position statement: Principles and guidelines for early hearing detection and intervention programs. *Pediatrics, 120,* 899–921.

Joint Committee on Infant Hearing (JCIH). (2013). Supplement to the JCIH 2007 position statement: Principles and guidelines for early intervention after confirmation that a child is deaf or hard of hearing. *Pediatrics, 131*(4), 1324–1349. doi:10.1542/peds.2013-0008

Khan, L. M., & Lewis, N. P. (2002). *KLPA-2: Khan-Lewis phonological analysis* (2nd ed.). Circle Pines, MN: American Guidance Service.

Kishon-Rabin, L., Taitelbaum-Swead, R., & Segal, O. (2009). Prelexical infant scale evaluation: from vocalization to audition in hearing and hearing-impaired infants. In L. Eisenberg (Ed.), *Clinical management of children with cochlear implants.* San Diego, CA: Plural.

Levitt, H., Youdelman, K., & Head, J. (1990). *Fundamental speech skills test.* Englewood, CO: Research Point, a division of Cochlear Corporation.

Ling, D. (1976). *Speech and the hearing-impaired child: Theory and practice.* Washington, DC: Alexander Graham Bell Association for the Deaf and Hard of Hearing.

Ling, D. (1989). *Foundations of spoken language for hearing impaired children.* Washington, DC: Alexander Graham Bell Association for the Deaf and Hard of Hearing.

Ling, D. (2002). *Speech and the hearing-impaired child: Theory and practice* (2nd ed.). Washington, DC: Alexander Graham Bell Association for the Deaf and Hard of Hearing.

Ling, D. (2006). The six-sound test. In W. Estabrooks (Ed.), *Auditory-verbal therapy and practice.* Washington, DC: Alexander Graham Bell Association for the Deaf and Hard of Hearing.

Ling, D., & Ling, A. (1978). *Aural habilitation.* Washington, DC: Alexander Graham Bell Association for the Deaf and Hard of Hearing.

Monsen, R., Moog, J. S., & Geers, A. E. (1988). *CID Picture SPINE: Speech intelligibility evaluation.* St. Louis, MO: Central Institute for the Deaf (CID).

Monson, R. B. (1983). General effects of deafness on phonation and articulation. In J. Hochberg, H. Leavitt, & M. J. Osberger, *Speech of the hearing-impaired.* Baltimore, MD: University Park Press.

Morrison, H., & Lew, V. (2012). *An analysis of the natural language environment of children with hearing loss: The impact of home language and maternal education level.* Poster session at the Alexander Graham Bell Association for the Deaf and Hard of Hearing Convention, Orlando, FL.

Nathani, S., Ertmer, D. J., & Stark, R. E. (2006). Assessing vocal development in infants and toddlers. *Clinical Linguistics and Phonetics, 20,* 351–369.

National Center for Hearing Assessment and Management (NCHAM), & The Alexander Graham Bell Association for the Deaf and Hard of Hearing. (2012). *Early hearing detection and intervention programs: A blueprint for success.* Retrieved from http://www.agbell .org

Nicholas, J. G., & Geers, A. E. (2006). Effects of early auditory experience on the spoken language of deaf children at 3 years of age. *Ear and Hearing, 27*(3), 286–298.

Oller, D. K., Nigogi S., Gray, S., Richards, J. A., Gilkerson, D., Xu, D., . . . Warren, S. F. (2010). Automated vocal analysis of naturalistic recordings from children with autism, language delay, and typical development. *Proceedings from the National Academy of Natural Sciences of the United States of America, 107*(30).

Oller, K. (1986). Metaphonology and infant vocalizations. In B. Lindblom & R. Zetterstrom (Eds.), *Precursors of early speech.* New York, NY: Stockton Press.

Owens, R. E. (2012). *Language development: An introduction* (8th ed.). Needham Heights, MA: Allyn & Bacon.

Paden, E., & Brown, C. (1992). *Identifying early phonological needs in children with hearing loss.* Durham, NC: MED-EL Group.

Paterson, M. M. (1986). Maximizing the use of residual hearing with school-aged hearing-impaired students: A perspective. *Volta Review, 88*(5), 93–106.

Paterson, M. M. (1992). *Teaching speech to the deaf: MORE than an articulation problem.* Invited short course at the Alexander Graham Bell Association for the Deaf and Hard of Hearing Convention, San Diego, CA.

Paterson, M. M. (1994). Articulation and phonological disorders in hearing-impaired school-aged children with severe and profound sensorineural losses. In J. E. Bernthal & N. W. Bankson (Eds.), *Assessment and intervention with special populations.* New York, NY: Thieme.

Paterson, M. M. (1997). *Analysis of vocalisation development in hearing-impaired children between 18 months and 30 months of age, pre-and post-cochlear implantation.* Invited paper of research in progress at International Symposium on Cochlear Implants, Melbourne, Australia.

Perigoe, C. (1992). Strategies for the remediation of speech of hearing-impaired children. *Volta Review, 88*(7), 351–366.

Perigoe, C. (2013). Developing speech skills: Part of the Ling legacy. *Volta Voices, 20*(6), 24–27.

Perigoe, C., & Ling, D. (1986). Generalization of speech skills in hearing-impaired children. *The Volta Review, 88,* 351–365.

Perigoe, C., & Perigoe, R. (2004). Multiple challenges—multiple solutions: Children with hearing loss and special needs. *The Volta Review Monograph, 104*(4).

Perigoe, C. B., & Paterson, M. (2013). Understanding auditory development and the child with hearing loss. In C. A. Ukstins & D. R. Welling (Eds.), *Fundamentals of audiology for the speech-language pathologist* (pp. 173–204). Burlington, MA: Jones and Bartlett Learning.

Robertson, L. (2013). *Literacy and deafness: Listening and spoken language* (2nd ed.). San Diego, CA: Plural.

Saffran, J. R., Werker, J. F., & Werner, L. A. (2006). The infant's auditory world: Hearing, speech, and the beginnings of language. In D. Kuhn, R. S. Siegler, D. William, & R. M. Lerner (Eds.), *Handbook of child psychology: Vol 2. Cognition, perception, and language* (6th ed., pp. 58–108). Hoboken, NJ: John Wiley and Sons.

Sander, E. (1972). When are speech sounds learned? *Journal of Speech and Hearing Disorders, 37,* 55–63.

Shipley, K. G., & McAfee, J. G. (2008). *Assessment in speech-language pathology: A resource manual* (4th ed.). Independence, KY: Cengage Learning.

Small, L. H. (2005). *Fundamentals of phonetics: A practical guide for students* (2nd ed.). Boston, MA: Pearson Education.

Spencer, L. J. & Guo, L. (2013). Consonant developments in pediatric cochlear implant users who were implanted before 30 months of age. *Journal of Deaf Studies and Deaf Education, 18*(1), 93–109.

Stoel-Gammon, C., & Kehoe, M. M. (1994). Hearing impairment in infants and toddlers: Identification, vocal development and intervention. In J. E. Bernthal & N. W. Bankson (Eds), *Assessment and intervention with special populations.* New York, NY: Thieme.

Uhler, K., Yoshinaga-Itano, C., Gabbard, S. A., Rothpletz, A. M., & Jenkins, H. (2011). Longitudinal infant speech perception in young children. *Journal of the American Academy of Audiology, 22*(3), 129–142.

Vardi, I. (1991). *Phonological profile for the hearing impaired: Manual.* Australia: Edith Cowan University.

Warner-Czyz, A. D., Davis, B. L., & Morrison, H. M. (2005). Production accuracy in a young cochlear implant recipient. *Volta Review, 113*(2), 151–173.

Wiggin, M, Sedey, A., Awad, R., Bogle, J. M., & Yoshinaga-Itano, C. (2013). Emergence of consonants in young children with hearing loss. *Volta Review, 113*(2), 127–148.

PC–PEP, Paterson–Cole Phonologic Evaluation Procedure

A. Instructions: Record spoken language sample or listen to live connected speech. Listen for and make perceptual judgments about the quality of utterances as "thought groups" or "breath phrases." As you listen, check off the subelements for each category. Then, rate your overall impression of each major category: Scale 1–5 (1 = least appropriate or clear to 5 = most appropriate and clear).

1. Evaluate Prosodic Features in Spoken Language Through Listening	Rating	2. Analyze Suprasegmental Production: Analyze Underlying Physiological and Biomechanical Correlates of Speech	Rating
Intelligibility: Overall Impression of Conversational Intelligibility			
Vocal Quality		**Vocalization**	
___ Pleasant and unremarkable ___ Some features noteworthy ___ Overall nasal tone ___ Monotone		___ Able to phonate ___ Appropriate use of breath to support speech ___ Speech sounds oral [control of oral-nasal contrast] ___ Able to produce relaxed voice, not tense ___ Able to produce smooth voice, not harsh ___ Tense vocal production ___ Harsh vocal production	
Rhythm, Pause, Timing		**Duration**	
___ "Thought groups" [utterances] marked with appropriate pausing ___ Rate of conversational speech typical ___ Able to pause appropriately to mark word boundaries ___ Able to pause appropriately at sentence boundaries		___ Able to control length of phonation ___ Able to control onset/offset of phonation ___ Vowel duration at ends of words or sentences is appropriate ___ Produces run-on vowels ___ Appropriate rate of utterance ___ Inappropriate rate of utterance ___ Stops and starts at awkward phonation junctures	
Stress Marking		**Intensity**	
___ Stress marking produced on correct syllable in words ___ Stress produced on correct word in phrase ___ Conversational voice loudness appropriate		___ Able to vary subglottal pressure to create loudness contrasts ___ Able to flexibly make changes in voice loudness ___ Able to whisper ___ Able to produce loud voice ___ Able to produce soft voice	

Intonational Contour		Pitch	
___ Able to produce correct SS pattern for Statements		___ Able to vary degree of vocal fold tension	
___ Able to produce correct SS pattern for Questions		___ Pitch register appropriate for age	
___ Able to produce correct SS pattern for Imperatives		___ Able to modulate pitch over a range of tones	
___ Able to produce correct SS pattern for Negatives		___ Monotone vocal production	
___ Able to produce SS pattern to express tone of voice and mood differences			

Paterson-Cole Phonologic Evaluation Procedure (PC-PEP), 2014; From Paterson-Cole (1992); Adapted by Paterson (1995, 2005, 2007).

B. While listening to the prosodic elements above, note main features of phoneme production in connected speech.

Articulation / Coarticulation of Phonemes   **Examples**

Vowels

_____ able to mark extremes of the range of vowels [a,u,i]

Diphthongs

_____ vowel transitions audible to listener

Consonants

Manner contrasts marked:

_____ oral/nasal contrast e.g., ba–ma

_____ fricative

_____ plosive

_____ stop

_____ affricate

Voiced/voiceless distinction: e.g.,

_____ ba–pa _____

_____ fa–va _____

_____ "tha"–"tha" _____

_____ da–ta _____

_____ sa–za _____

Place differentiation:

_____ ba ___ da ___ ga ___

_____ pa ___ ta ___ ka ___

_____ fa ___ "tha"___ "sha"___

_____ ma ___ na ___ "ng"___

NOTES:

Paterson-Cole Phonologic Evaluation Procedure (PC-PEP), 2014; From Paterson-Cole (1992); Adapted by Paterson (1995, 2005, 2007)

127

Speech Target Summary

Name: _____ Date: _____ Teacher/Therapist: _____

	Phonetic Level	Phonologic Level		Target
	Syllables (Ling PLE)	Words (Word Level Test)	Phrases/ Sentences (Spontaneous Speech Sample)	Teaching Order
Suprasegmentals				
Vowels & Diphthongs				
Step 1 Consonants (Manner of artic.)				
Step 2 Consonants (Place of artic.)				
Step 3 Consonants (Place of artic.)				
Step 4 Consonants (Voicing, occurs earlier for most)				
Initial Blends				
Final Blends (Concurrent with initial blends)				

Estimated % Intelligibility: familiar listener: _____ naïve listener: _____

Source: Created by Perigoe and Paterson, 2014 (adapted from Ling, 1976, and Perigoe, 1981, 1995, 2001, 2007).

Speech Target Summary Example

Name: _____ Date: _____ Teacher/Therapist: _____

	Phonetic Level	Phonologic Level		Target
	Syllables (Ling PLE)	Words (Word Level Test)	Phrases/ Sentences (Spontaneous Speech Sample)	Teaching Order
Suprasegmentals				
Vowels & Diphthongs	short /I/ "schwar" (+) Stressed "er" (+)	short "u" as in book (+) /e/ (+) "schwar" (+) "e" as in bed	/e/ (+) "schwar" (+) Stressed "er" as in bird (+)	#1 #2 #3
Step 1 Consonants (Manner of artic.)	no targets	no targets	final /s/	
Step 2 Consonants (Place of artic.)	/di/ and /du/ (+) "shi" and "shu" (+) /si/ and /su/ (+) /j/ no gliding (+) /l/ all vowels (−) stop /d/ (−)	/di/ and /du/ (+) "shi" and "shu" (+) /si/ and /su/ (+) /j/ no gliding (+) /l/ all vowels (−) stop /d/ zh" as in beige "z"	/di/ and /du/ (+) "shi" and "shu" (+) /si/ and /su/ (+) /j/ no gliding (+) /l/ all vowels (−) stop /d/	#4 #5 #6 #7

continues

	Phonetic Level	Phonologic Level		Target
	Syllables (Ling PLE)	Words (Word Level Test)	Phrases/ Sentences (Spontaneous Speech Sample)	Teaching Order
Step 3 Consonants (Place of artic.)	/g/ (+) all vowels "ch" all vowels "ng" all vowels /r/ Stop /k/			
Step 4 Consonants (Voicing, occurs earlier for most)				
Initial Blends				
Final Blends (Concurrent with initial blends)				

Estimated % Intelligibility: familiar listener: _____ naïve listener: _____

Source: Created by Perigoe and Paterson, 2014 (adapted from Ling, 1976, and Perigoe, 1981, 1995, 2001, 2007).

Initial Targets and Rationale

#1	short "oo" PH	Mastered at Phonetic Level. Nearly mastered in phonologic use in words and sentences. Check for how close to automaticity at phonetic level in varied alternations, check auditory discrimination and then practice in words.
#2	/e/ PH	Important cardinal vowel; check how close to automaticity, check auditory discrimination, practice in words.
#3	Short /I / P, PH	Short /I/ able to produce but not consistent in phonology. Revisit phonetic level repetitions in reduplicated syllable context before moving on to alternations to stabilize place of production.
#4	/d/ P	Errors at both phonetic and phonologic level. Not consistent with [u,a,i] vowels but is present in repertoire. Child has /b/ at mastery, therefore voiced plosive manner established; is this a place or production problem? Work at phonetic level, stabilize single production across three vowels then repetitions, continue with stages of practice. It is important to analyze why voiced plosive manner is a problem for this student.
#5	/s/ P	Step one fricatives (unvoiced) are mastered. Therefore, fricative manner well established. Present at phonetic level but not with /a,i,u/ vowels. Stabilize in single production with the three vowels and stabilize at repeated syllable practice. Strategies would included comparison and contrast of place of production with /f/ and "sh." /s/ crucial for grammar.
#6	"sh" P	Phonetic level as for /s/.
#7	/j/ P, PH	Diphthongization not happening. Treat /j/ as a semivowel and stabilize manner of production in single syllables with three vowels, then repetitions. Important phoneme in daily school language contexts asap, e.g., you, yes, yellow, yesterday. Strategies for evoking would include comparison and contrast with known, well-produced diphthongs.

Note. P= Phonetic target; *PH*= Phonological target.

continues

Probable next targets:

As some of our first set of targets move from evoking and early stabilization, more targets can be added:

1. "e" as in bed

2. /l/ once /j/ is stable

3. Step three consonants:
   a. /g/ phonetic level by analogy from /b/ and /d/
   b. /r/ by contrast acoustically to /l/ and /j/
   c. ch
   d. Stop /k/ in contrast to unvoiced stops p and t

Wait on stressed "ir" and unstressed "er" until /r/ is appropriately developed.

CHAPTER 6

Language Assessment of Children With Hearing Loss

Hannah Eskridge and Kathryn Wilson

KEY POINTS

- The types of formal and informal measures used will vary depending on a child's age, stage of development, purpose of assessment, and presence or absence of additional learning challenges.
- Detailed working knowledge of typical language development, components of language assessment, and a variety of approaches are necessary to effectively assess children with hearing loss, interpret results, and develop intervention plans.
- Selection and utilization of appropriate strategies and techniques for children with hearing loss is an important factor in conducting effective language assessment.

INTRODUCTION

Assessment of language and vocabulary is one of the most basic and essential services provided to children with hearing loss and their families. The impact of hearing loss on language development and acquisition among children with hearing loss is well documented (ASHA, 2014a; Nott et al., 2009; Prezbindowski & Lederberg, 2003; Tur-Kaspa & Dromi, 1999). Because it is the child's level of oral language and vocabulary that serves to determine early literacy and later success in school (Beck, McKeown, & Kucan, 2002; Robertson, 2009; Sarant et al., 2009; Trelease, 2006; Waterman, 1994), it is vital that professionals understand and implement preferred practices for assessment of all facets of language and vocabulary.

What, then, are the various purposes of language and vocabulary assessment? Why is assessment essential? What are the reasons practitioners must conduct language and vocabulary assessment? There are at least four primary purposes:

1. Eligibility Determination

In order to receive early intervention or public school services, a child must meet eligibility criteria. In accordance with the Individuals with Disabilities Act (IDEA,

2004), following a referral, an initial evaluation takes place. The evaluation includes individual assessments and observations. IDEA defines evaluation and assessment differently. Evaluation is the process of determining eligibility while assessment refers to the specific tools practitioners use to gather relevant information about a child (IDEA, 2004).

2. Identification of Strengths And Weaknesses

Appropriate selection, administration, and interpretation of language assessments allows practitioners to determine a child's present level of performance in receptive and expressive language and vocabulary. This process serves to inform the practitioner about a given child's areas of strength and weakness, and forms the foundation for the development of appropriate intervention and educational plans and programs.

3. Develop Long- and Short-Term Plans

Practitioners rely on assessment results to construct plans such as the Individual Family Service Plan (IFSP) or Individual Education Program (IEP). These plans incorporate specific goals and objectives focused on a child's needs in language and vocabulary development. A typical long-term plan includes annual goals and objectives; while a short-term plan usually includes targets to be addressed in a 3 to 6 month timeframe. An IEP (long-term) must be reviewed periodically—at least annually—and be revised as appropriate (IDEA, 2004). An IFSP (short-term) must also be formally reviewed on an annual

basis with the family at least every six months (IDEA, 2004).

In addition to an IEP, there is another type of long-term plan that relies on comprehensive assessment. For children who are delayed more than a year in language and vocabulary acquisition, a multiyear plan is needed to guide parents and professionals in closing the gap between a child's language/vocabulary age and chronological age (Walker & Wilson, 2011). This type of plan, like others described in this section, is based on appropriate and thorough assessment of language and vocabulary.

4. Monitor Progress

Monitoring language and vocabulary growth on a regular and frequent basis is necessary to determine if a child with hearing loss is making adequate progress. Progress monitoring is accomplished through the use of both standardized tests and various tracking tools and informal measures.

This chapter provides a brief overview of normal language development, followed by a discussion related to assessment approaches and the components of appropriate language assessment for children with hearing loss. Strategies specific for assessing children with hearing loss are examined. A case study approach is used to analyze assessment practices and protocols for the young child, the school-age child, and children with hearing loss who have additional challenges. Finally, existing resources to assist practitioners in the planning, execution, and interpretation of language and vocabulary assessment measures are provided.

NORMAL DEVELOPMENT

If children with hearing loss are expected to develop in close parallel to their hearing peers, it is critical to use information from typical development to guide our assessment and intervention practices. Without knowledge of typical language development, professionals cannot determine if the child with hearing loss is making adequate progress or if he or she is closing the gap between his or her language and the language of their typically hearing peers. This information allows us to determine the need for services, to ascertain when changes to those services are needed, as well as to provide the information parents need to best advocate for their child.

While formal study of normal language development began in the 19th century (Brisbane, 2005), theories regarding the acquisition of language have continued to evolve among linguists, speech-language scientists, and practitioners. Currently, several theories exist for the purpose of explaining and understanding how typically developing children acquire spoken language. These theories include the behaviorist, psycholinguistic, and the interactionist theories (Bui, 2003). The seemingly effortless language-learning process develops as a result of frequent, meaningful interactions among children, their caregivers, and others in the home and community. Regardless of the theory or combination of theories that best fits one's beliefs about how young children acquire language and vocabulary, there is consensus regarding several key factors (Brisbane, 2005):

- Children grow and develop at different rates. What is "normal" for one child looks different from that of another child.
- Children pass through the same developmental milestones, acquiring skills that build on each other, during predictable time periods (Eliot, 1999). For example, a child must babble single syllables at about 4 to 6 months before babbling multiple syllables at 7 to 9 months, before speaking 2-word sentences at 18 to 24 months of age.
- Developmental domains are interrelated. For example, as a child becomes more mobile, he or she will begin to learn more about the world which will in turn impact language development.
- Development is influenced by family, socioeconomic status, ethnicity, culture and history.
- While significant developmental changes take place in childhood, we continue to expand our language and vocabulary throughout our lifespan.

PRECURSORY SKILLS

Before children start talking, they demonstrate many ways to communicate their wants and needs with their caregivers through a variety of precursory language and communication skills. Precursory skills develop in infants between the chronological ages of birth to 18 months (Heerboth, 2014). During this time, infants acquire cognitive and play skills, gestures, social interaction abilities, and speech sounds for the purpose of communication. "Infants develop the capacities for learning language as they learn to see, hear, and do" (Bloom & Lahey, 1978, p. 73).

Cognition and Play Development

Even the very young infant likes to play. Prior to 3 months of age, children can anticipate during an activity such as nursing and can communicate excitement to their caregivers. They begin to explore the use of objects and enjoy play through tickling, bouncing, and interaction with caregivers prior to 6 months of age. Feeding and early play also constitute the beginning of turn-taking. Turn-taking is a skill essential for the later development of conversational skills. During this time, infants also experiment with cause and effect through activities like shaking a rattle. The 6- to 9-month-old baby shows emerging object permanence by searching for a partially hidden object. Object permanence is generally mastered by 12 months of age.

Gestures

Gestures begin as early as 3 to 6 months when infants start to reach for objects. From 6 to 9 months they give, point and show objects of interest, imitate arm movements, reach to request, and respond with appropriate arm gestures to familiar phrases like "bye bye." Before their first birthday, children can shake their head "no" and push away undesired objects. Gestural communication develops to represent functional words such as "bye-bye," "no," "up," "hi," "so big," "more," and "all gone" in the second 6 months of life (Pollack, Goldberg, & Caleffe-Schenck, 1997).

Social Interaction

Children are naturally social beings and begin to interact with those in their environment from birth. During the first 3 months of life, infants begin to develop a social smile and attend to a speaker's mouth and eyes. By 6 months of age, they can maintain appropriate eye contact and share in joint attention. Between 6 to 9 months of age, children call to gain attention.

Speech and Vocal Expression

Children begin cooing as early as 3 months, and by 3 to 6 months, they are vocalizing to express a variety of feelings. By the time they are a year old, typically developing toddlers are babbling with intonation to scold, state, exclaim, and greet. Through the use of gestures and vocalizations, the infant learns to engage in joint attention and reference. This is critical for the ability to establish a topic and provides the infant with the ability to engage in communication to share information (Owens, 1996, 2005, 2012).

The development of the skills previously described is important because they enable a child to learn language. In early development, the parents' response to these infant behaviors is more important than the behaviors themselves. Social communication through the use of precursory skills in an infant's first 24 months of life provides the semantic structure and pragmatic function needed for language development (Owens, 1996, 2005, 2012).

Regardless of when a child with hearing loss first has access to sound, it is critical that he or she develop these precursory skills. Without the ability to demonstrate skills such as turn-taking, vocal play, and joint attention, children are missing the key first steps to understand and produce meaningful spoken language.

VOCABULARY

Vocabulary is the knowledge and use of words and their meanings (Pikulski & Templeton, 2004). Development begins very early and is significantly impacted by a child's environment. Hart and Risley (1999) studied how many words children hear from birth to 3 years of age. The number of words heard per hour was vastly different depending on the education level and socioeconomic status of the parents. Children of parents who were professionals heard on average 2,100 words per hour. Children in working-class families heard 1,200 words per hour, and those in a welfare family heard on average 600 words hourly. Outcomes indicated "the first 3 years of experience put in place a trajectory of vocabulary growth and the foundations of analytic and symbolic competencies that will make a lasting difference to how children perform in later years" (Hart & Risley, 1999, p. 193).

Children typically acquire between 30 to 60 expressive vocabulary words before forming two-word combinations. They use approximately 900 words by the age of three and will need to acquire a minimum of 2,500 words expressively before formal reading instruction is initiated. The exact number of words a child uses at a given age varies due to the fact that children grow and develop at different rates. What is *"normal"* for one child looks different from another child. In Table 6–1, a general guide for *expressive* vocabulary use is depicted.

LANGUAGE

Language is composed of both receptive and expressive components. Receptive language refers to one's understanding and develops prior to expressive use of language. Children around the world, speaking different languages, follow the same general pattern of development. Children progress from early prelinguistic communication skills to the use of complex sentences by their fifth birthday (Brisbane, 2005; Eliot, 1999; Owens, 1996, 2005, 2012).

Specifically, following acquisition of precursory language skills, expressive use of single words, and comprehension of longer utterances, children begin to combine words. For most children, this occurs around 18 months of age. Eliot's (1999)

Table 6–1. General Guide for Expressive Vocabulary

Age	Vocabulary	Syntax
12 months	1st word emerges	One word
18 months	20–50 words	Maybe 2-word combinations
2 years	200–300 words	Average 2-word phrases
3 years	900–1000 words	Average 3–4 word sentences
4 years	1500–1600 words	Average 4–5 word grammatically correct sentences

Source: Owens, 1996, 2005, 2012.

description of the transition from growth in infancy to the onset of expressive language is beautifully stated:

> [Expressive] language lies quietly in wait during the first twelve to eighteen months of a child's life. Though you can see only the merest hints of it in infancy, it grows like an air bubble submerged deep in the sea, rising and expanding until finally, somewhere in the middle of the second year, it explodes for all to hear. (p. 368)

Early two-word combinations appear to follow predictable patterns and generally follow correct word order. The examples in Table 6–2 represent how young children combine words to express a variety of thoughts and ideas in different semantic categories (Bloom & Lahey, 1978; Pollack, Goldberg, & Caleffe-Schenck, 1997).

Following the two-word phase, preschoolers between the ages of 3 and 5 enter the syntactic stage of language acquisition. This stage is often referred to as the telegraphic stage, because many function words (or, to, the, am, do,) are omitted in short sentences that convey meaning. Children begin to sort out the rules of language and often over generalize. They begin to use plurals, verb tenses, prepositions, and conjunctions (Pollack, Goldberg, & Caleffe-Schenck, 1997). They are able to follow two- and three-step commands, use sentences with increasing complexity, and ask questions to learn more about their environment. By age five, 90% of the grammar used to produce language has been acquired (Owens, 1996, 2005, 2012).

The school-aged child continues to acquire language through vocabulary, refined conversational skills, and figurative language. During the elementary school period, children further expand their language in the following ways (ASHA, 2014c):

- Answer more complex yes/no questions.
- Demonstrate narrative mastery including telling stories with increased detail in a logical order.

Table 6–2. Semantic Categories

Existence:	A ball.
Nonexistence/Denial (negation):	No ball. Not tired.
Questions:	What's that?
Attribution (noun plus modifier):	Big ball.
Recurrence:	More ball. Another car.
Action (verbing):	Throw ball.
Possession:	Mommy ball. My car.
Quantity:	Two ball.
Locative/Locative Action:	Up ball. Sit down. Right there!
Adverbs:	Too late! All wet.
Commands:	Help me. Open door.
Demands:	Want more. Come here.

- Use most grammatical structures correctly by the end of first grade.
- Stay on topic, take turns, and initiate conversations.
- Give directions that increase in the number of steps and accuracy.
- Ask and answer all "wh" questions.
- Use language for a variety of purposes such as to persuade, entertain, clarify, and inform.

By age 12 years, children have mastered many of the language skills of an adult (Owens, 1996, 2005, 2012).

APPROACHES TO LANGUAGE ASSESSMENT

For both initial evaluations and ongoing progress monitoring, clinicians create a plan to identify the measures they will use to obtain information about the child's present level of performance, strengths, and needs. IDEA (2004) requires that multiple types of tools, tests, and procedures are used to determine eligibility for services, rather than reliance on a single test or procedure. The latter is not acceptable under the law. Professionals responsible for language and vocabulary assessment of children with hearing loss will want to be familiar with a variety of assessment approaches and the advantages and limitations of various approaches.

Formal

Formal assessment is comprised of standardized tests, norm-referenced tests, and criterion-referenced measures. Standardized tests rely on specific administration, scoring, and interpretation meth-

ods. Norm-referenced instruments allow for comparison of a child's performance to others in a normative sample. Criterion-referenced assessments are those designed to determine if an individual has mastered specific skills or content. With a criterion-referenced assessment, there is no comparison of performance to other individuals or groups.

Some formal assessments address multiple aspects of language and vocabulary. The *Clinical Evaluation of Language Fundamentals, 5th Edition* (Semel, Wiig, & Secord, 2013) is an example of a standardized test designed to assess several different aspects of receptive and expressive language and vocabulary. Other measures —such as the *Expressive Vocabulary Test, 3rd Edition* (Williams, 2007)—only evaluate a particular language feature. The *Rossetti Infant-Toddler Language Scale* (Rossetti, 2006) is a criterion-referenced instrument appropriate for assessing language and other communication skills in children birth to 3 years of age. It is important to note that the majority of measures used with children with hearing loss are not designed specifically for children with hearing loss. Furthermore, it is vital that clinicians consider the potential impact of cultural bias in the selection, administration, and interpretation of assessment instruments since many measures are not normed on racially and linguistically diverse populations (ASHA, 2014b).

Informal

Informal measures are content rather than data-driven (Weaver, n.d.) and allow practitioners to obtain valuable information about a child's language and vocabulary using instruments other than standardized, formal measures. In order to obtain a complete representation of a child's language and vocabulary functioning, clinicians can opt to use informal assessments such as checklists, parent interviews, observations, and diagnostic teaching. The latter type of assessment—diagnostic teaching—is especially useful in working with children with hearing loss. Caleffe-Schenck (2012) describes diagnostic teaching as a process of individualized interactions. When listening and spoken language specialists employ diagnostic teaching, they engage in functional, authentic assessment. Based on the child's performance, the professional can adjust session targets in real time, as well as use the assessment information to make adjustments in long- and short-term plans.

Structured Language Analysis

Perhaps one of the most valuable approaches is that of language sampling accompanied by a structured analysis. This approach requires a practitioner to engage a child in activities such as conversation, description, narration, explanation, and questioning (Ling, 1989) for the purpose of collecting spontaneous utterances. Once the child's utterances are recorded and transcribed, an analysis is conducted to determine the length and complexity of the child's utterances (**syntax**/grammar), the number of different words and word types (**semantics**), and social (**pragmatic**) aspects. Although the approach is regarded as valuable and informative, it is not frequently used by many clinicians (Heilman, 2010). Reasons cited for infrequent or nonuse include the length of time required to analyze the data and difficulties in learning how to conduct proper language sampling and analysis. Presently, the *Systematic Analysis*

of Language Transcripts or SALT (Miller & Iglesias, 2008) is available—as a software program—to streamline the process of data collection, transcription, analysis, and interpretation.

COMPONENTS OF LANGUAGE ASSESSMENT

Language can be assessed according to three primary components: form, content, and use (Bloom & Lahey, 1978). Language form includes syntax, **morphology** and **phonology**; while language content refers to semantics (the meaning underlying what we say). Language use or pragmatics is another component of language. These components are separate and distinct; practitioners must understand the contribution of each dimension individually, while recognizing that these components are overlapping and interrelated. This understanding of the singular and collective contributions of form, content, and use sets the stage for proper and appropriate holistic language assessment.

Morphological

Morphology is the study of the internal structure of words (Owens, 1996, 2005, 2012). Words consist of smaller units called morphemes. A morpheme is the smallest unit of a word that contains meaning (Payne, 1997). A morpheme that can stand alone is referred to as a *free* morpheme while those that cannot stand alone are referred to as *bound* morphemes (Gleason, 2001). For example, the word "horses" has two morphemes; *"horse"*—which refers to a large animal that you can ride, and often lives on a farm—is a free morpheme and "*s*"—to indicate there is more than one—is a bound morpheme. The potential influence of hearing loss on morphological development is worth noting here. Historically, some children with hearing loss have experienced difficulty with auditory access of certain morphological features including plurals, possessive -*s*, and regular past tense -*ed*. Limited auditory access has, in turn, resulted in incomplete morphological development for some children. Additionally, it is important to note that given today's technology, even children with profound hearing loss have the auditory potential to access and develop difficult-to-hear morphological features.

One method to assess a child's level of morphological development is a calculation of the mean length of utterance (MLU). The MLU is calculated by obtaining a language sample of 100 utterances and dividing the total number of words and morphemes by 100 (the number of utterances). The work of Brown (1973), summarized in Table 6–3, can function as a tool to analyze a child's morphological development according to MLU and Brown's 14 Grammatical Morphemes.

Semantic

Semantics refers to the underlying meaning of language including complex use of vocabulary and figurative language. Children can demonstrate semantic difficulties when they display limited vocab-

Table 6–3. Morphological Development According to Brown (1973)

Stage	MLU	Approximate Age (Months)	Grammatical Morphemes
I	1.0–2.0	12–26	Pronouns (I, you, me), familiar names, nouns (food, toys), verbs (eat, wash), and adjectives (hot, big, dirty) produced as single words and in combination to utterances such as: daddy eat, doggie bed, mommy throw ball
II	2.0–2.5	27–30	Present progressive (ing), regular Plurals, prepositions (in, on), and possessive pronoun (my)
III	2.5–3.0	31–34	Irregular past tense, uncontractible copula, possessives, prepositions (under, with, of, for, to), and pronouns (he, she, him, her, your)
IV	3.0–3.75	35–40	Regular past tense, modal verbs (can, will), prepositions (around, behind), prepositional phrases, pronouns (they, we, them, us, hers, his)
V	3.75–4.5	41–46	Uncontractible and contractible auxiliary, contractible copula, third person singular (He walks and He does), modals (could, would), prepositions (beside, between), wh questions + inverted auxiliary/copula, possessive pronouns (its, our, ours, their, theirs), and reflexive pronouns (myself, herself, himself, yourself, ourselves, themselves)
V+	4.5+	47+	Morphological development is complete at the end of Stage V or V+

ulary, longer response time in selecting vocabulary, and figurative language problems. Informal assessment of semantics can include (Shipley & McAfee, 2009):

- defining words;
- giving synonyms and antonyms for words;
- determining common theme/ category in a group of words (i.e., water, milk, orange juice);
- listing words in a given category (i.e., vegetables);
- explaining the meaning of phrases and figurative language; and
- making comparisons between two words.

Syntactic

Syntax is the study of the rules that govern how words are organized into phrases and sentences. It differs from morphology in that it deals with rules related to putting words together versus the rules

of formulating those words. Like morphology, syntax follows a clear pattern of development based on age, as indicated in Table 6–4.

There are many standardized language assessments that look specifically at the development of syntax and that can be used when assessing a child with hearing loss. Comprehensive language assessment measures that examine syntax include the *Oral and Written Language Scales*, 2nd Edition (Carrow-Woolfolk, 2011); *Clinical Evaluation of Language Fundamentals*, 5th Edition (Semel, Wiig & Secord, 2013) and the *Comprehensive Assessment of Spoken Language* (Carrow-Woolfolk, 1999).

Pragmatic

The knowledge of appropriate use of language is known as pragmatics. Hymes (1972) introduced the term "communicative competence" or the concept that we have to not only know what to say (vocabulary) and how to say it (syntax,

Table 6–4. Syntactic Development

Stage	Approximate Age (Months)	Stage Characteristics
One-word/holophrastic stage	12–18	Children use one word to convey a sentence; they often overgeneralize words (doggie is any four-legged animal).
Two-word stage	18–24	Two word phrases to impart various semantic meanings from categories such as recurrence (more water) and action (throw ball).
Telegraphic stage	24–30	Children use just enough to get their meaning across. May include 3 to 4 word utterances and begin to overgeneralize their language use ("mouses" instead of "mice"), utterances contain mostly nouns, verbs and adjectives.
Later multiword stage	30+	Function words begin to appear and clauses are linked ("When will Mommy cook dinner?").

morphology) but also when, where, and why to say it.

After the early childhood years and children learn the "rules" of the what and how of language, their language continues to develop through the learning of pragmatic rules. Children demonstrate increased use of conversation, narratives, idioms, figurative language, and jokes. Many aspects of pragmatic development require "overhearing" others in our environment as well as things such as tone to detect sarcasm. Children with hearing loss are at a disadvantage for these things and sometimes may need to be taught certain pragmatic elements that other children pick up on their own. Therefore, it is important to assess them so they can be incorporated into regular therapy and carry over at home.

CONSIDERATIONS AND STRATEGIES

Listening and spoken language specialists must demonstrate knowledge and application of many different strategies. In intervention, strategies are used to promote the auditory learning of targets in speech, language, audition, and cognition. Selection and use of strategies is equally important in the assessment process. The following considerations and strategies will be described within the context of language assessment: technology check, positioning, attention, environment, wait time, visual processing time, and **acoustic highlighting**:

- Technology check: Before any assessment of a child with hearing loss, a technology check must be performed to ensure that the equipment (hearing aids, cochlear implants, FM system) is functioning properly. This should include both checking the device(s) and the child's responses to the Ling Six-Sound Test. (See Chapters 9, 10, and 11 for more discussion.)

- Positioning: A preferred practice in intervention sessions calls for adults to sit *beside* the child to minimize visual clues. During assessment, sitting *across* from the child is beneficial. This approach allows the administrator to more easily manipulate test materials, read test instructions, and record responses on test protocols outside of the child's visual range. Sitting across from the child also provides the added benefit of speechreading, if necessary. When we conduct standardized language and vocabulary testing, our goal is to obtain the most reliable and valid information possible; therefore, we ensure that the child has access to both speechreading and auditory cues.

- Attention: Prior to the presentation of stimuli, the clinician should obtain the child's auditory attention. Many formal measures do not allow the test administrator to repeat items; therefore, it is vital that the child is attending before questions are asked or directions are given. A few ways to obtain auditory attention include saying: "here we go," "ready," or "next one." Waiting for the child to look at the examiner and providing frequent breaks are other ways to gain and maintain optimal attention.

- Environment: Children with hearing loss require a favorable listening environment (Cole & Flexer, 2011).

This means that care needs to be taken to minimize background noise, speak close to the microphone of the child's hearing technology, and use a regular speaking voice (Estabrooks, 2012). If the child has personal FM technology, it should be used during assessment. Using a small, portable table-top sound field system can enhance the listening environment as well (Flexer, 2012).

■ Wait time: Tobin (1987) defines wait time as a silent-pause between adult initiation and learner response. To optimize language assessment outcomes, sufficient wait time is necessary for the child to process the meaning of the stimulus and formulate a response. Age, cognition, language level, and task complexity are all variables that influence wait-time (Rhoades, 2013). Carey-Sargeant and Brown (2003) propose that children with hearing loss need longer pause lengths for sufficient processing. Although, it is not possible to state precisely how long one should wait for a response, anecdotal information obtained from listening and spoken language specialists suggest that practitioners employ wait times ranging from 10 to 45 seconds (Rhoades, 2011).

■ Visual processing time: It is helpful to provide a brief period of time for children to visually inspect test items before questions or instructions are stated, especially if the child has a tendency to respond impulsively. The examiner can encourage the child to first look at all the pictures or graphics. This can be done by simply stating, "Let's look at all the pictures first" and subsequently touching each item for the child to examine.

■ Acoustic Highlighting: Acoustic Highlighting refers to techniques employed to enhance audibility in speech, language, and auditory learning (Daniel, 2012; Simser & Estabrooks, 2001). Examples include repetition, increased rhythm and pitch variation, emphasis on key words (Simser & Estabrooks, 2001), and prolongation of phonemes (Daniel, 2012). In assessment, examiners may find it helpful to use acoustic highlighting to ensure optimal audibility of stimuli. For example, in asking a child to identify an item for plural /s/, the examiner might emphasize plurality in the following way: "Show me cats*sssss* vs cats." Using a slightly slower rate and/or a sing-song voice can facilitate attention in children with hearing loss. Placing emphasis on a keyword, for example, "The dog is *in* the box," serves to ensure that a child has appropriate access to the target test item.

ASSESSING THE YOUNG CHILD

Name: Nick

Age: 20 months

CI Age: 11 months

History:

Nick is a 20-month-old male with a bilateral profound hearing loss. His hearing loss was identified at three months of age and he was subsequently fitted with Phonak Naida VSP bilateral hearing aids. Early intervention services began when

Nick was four months of age. He received a right N5 cochlear implant at 9 months of age. Nick's parents chose the auditory-verbal approach. He lives at home with both parents and is seen in his home three to four times monthly for parent participation sessions. Nick's parents are very involved in his care and his development of listening and spoken language.

A comprehensive evaluation was conducted when Nick was initially referred for early intervention services. In keeping with recommendations specified by the Joint Commission on Infant Hearing (2013), Nick was assessed every six months following his initial evaluation. The purpose of the current assessment was to obtain present level of performance in language and vocabulary in order to monitor progress, and revise Nick's treatment plan for the next six months. Nick's mother was present during the assessment sessions which occurred over the course of two home visits.

Assessment Instruments

- The Rossetti Infant-Toddler Language Scale (Rossetti, 2006)
- Preschool Language Scale, 5th Edition (PLS-5; Zimmerman, Steiner, & Pond, 2011)
- The MacArthur-Bates Communicative Development Inventories: Words and Sentences (Fenson et al., 2007)

Findings

The Rossetti Infant-Toddler Language Scale

The Rossetti Infant-Toddler Language Scale (Rossetti, 2006) is an instrument designed to assess both preverbal and verbal areas of communication in children from birth to 36 months of age. The Rossetti (Rossetti, 2006) is composed of six areas. A definition of each area and results are described below:

Interaction–Attachment. This section assesses the relationship and patterns of interaction between the child and caregiver. Nick passed all items through the 15 to 18 months level. There are no test items beyond 15 to 18 months.

Pragmatics: Skills in this area reflect the way a child uses language to communicate with others. Nick demonstrated mastery of skills through 15 to 18 months and all but one skill through the 18 to 21 months level. There are no items beyond 18 to 21 months. Nick received credit for the following:

- Engages in adult-like dialogue.
- Uses vocalizations and words during pretend play.
- Uses words to interact with others.

Nick is not yet taking turns talking during conversation.

Gestures. Children use gestures to express their thoughts and intentions prior to their use of spoken language. This section evaluates the child's use of gestures. Nick passed items through 12 to 15 months. There are no items at 18 to 21 months. He also passed 4/5 items at 21 to 24 months and 3/4 items at 24 to 27 months. The following behaviors were either observed or reported by the parents:

- Gestures to request action (to get others to sit).
- Pretends to pour from a container.
- Flies a toy airplane.

- Pretends to write or type.
- Wipes hands and face.
- Slaps a palm in response to "give me five."

Nick is not yet gesturing to indicate toileting needs (21–24 months) or pretending to talk on the telephone (24–27 months).

Play. As a child grows, many changes in play skills take place. This section evaluates a child's individual play skills as well as play with others. Nick demonstrated mastery of all skills through 27 to 30 months, with the exception of two items (see below*). Nick received credit for the following;

- Puts away toys on request.
- Stacks and assembles toys and objects.
- Shares toys with other children.
- Demonstrates parallel play with other children.
- Performs many related activities during play.

*Nick does not yet demonstrate the following skills:

- Groups objects in play (18–21 months).
- Talks and verbalizes more in play around other children.

Language Comprehension. The language comprehension component assesses a child's understanding of verbal language. Nick passed all items through 21 to 24 months with the exception of "identifies objects by category." He was credited with two items at 24 to 27 months, that is, "recognizes family member names and points to four action words in pictures." He demonstrated the following skills:

- Identifies four body parts and clothing items on self.
- Identifies pictures when named.
- Chooses one object from a group of five upon verbal request.
- Points to four action words in pictures.
- Recognizes family members names (Mama, Daddy, Max).
- Understands new words rapidly.

Skills that have not yet been demonstrated include:

- Identifies objects by category.
- Understands the concept of one.
- Understands size concepts.

Language Expression. This section examines a child's use of both preverbal and verbal skills. Nick passed all items at 12 to 15 months and demonstrated scattered skills through 24 to 27 months. He is able to do the following:

- Uses single words frequently.
- Uses sentence-like intonational patterns.
- Uses two-word phrases occasionally.
- Uses new words regularly.
- Imitates two numbers or unrelated words upon request.
- Uses action words.

Skills that have not yet been demonstrated include:

- Asks, "What's that?"
- Imitates words overheard in conversation.
- Imitates environmental noises.
- Refers to self by name.
- Uses early pronouns occasionally.
- Uses two-word phrases frequently.

Preschool Language Scale, 5th Edition (PLS-5)

The PLS-5 (Zimmerman, Steiner, & Pond, 2011) is a standardized test that provides information about a child's understanding and use of language. There are two subtests, that is, Auditory Comprehension and Expressive Communication. For each subtest, a standard score, percentile rank, and age equivalent are obtained. A Total Language Score is also obtained reflecting combined performance of the two subtests. Standard scores between 85 to 115 are in the average range for a child of Nick's age. Results are as follows:

Auditory Comprehension:

Standard Score: 120

Percentile Rank: 91

Age Equivalent: 2 years, 3 months

Expressive Communication

Standard Score: 116

Percentile Rank: 86

Age Equivalent: 2 years, 3 months

Total Language

Standard Score: 120

Percentile Rank: 91

Age Equivalent: 2 years, 3 months

The MacArthur-Bates Communicative Development Inventories: Words and Sentences (Fenson et al., 2007)

The first portion of this tool, Part A— Vocabulary Checklist, is used to gain an inventory of words children use, regardless of pronunciation. Based on the parents' responses, Nick uses a total of 95 different words. Most of Nick's vocabulary clusters around the following categories (including 9 or more words): sound

effects and animal sounds, animals, food and drink, action words, (e.g., hug, help, blow), games and routines (e.g., bath, night night), and descriptive words (e.g., all-gone, high, stuck). Word use was scattered among the other categories (including 1–5 words): vehicles, toys, clothing, body parts, small household items, furniture/rooms, outside things, places, people, time, pronouns, question words, prepositions/locations, and quantifiers/articles. No helping verbs (e.g., am, be) or connecting words (and, but) were noted. Nick's word use falls within the 38th percentile for boys his age, and the 30th percentile for 20-month-old boys and girls combined.

Summary of Nick's Assessment

Both informal and formal measures were used to obtain information regarding Nick's present level of performance. Results of the Rossetti (Rossetti, 2006) indicate that Nick has made significant gains in all areas since previous testing. Skills in the Play domain are a relative strength for him. Since activation of his cochlear implant about one year ago, Nick has not only made a year's progress in a year's time but has demonstrated accelerated (catch-up) growth.

The PLS-5 (Zimmerman, Steiner, & Pond, 2011) was used to obtain information regarding receptive and expressive language. Nick scored in the above average range for the Auditory Comprehension area and slightly above average in the Expressive Communication component for a child his age. Nick was credited with use of 95 different words on the MacArthur-Bates Communicative Development Inventories: Words and Sentences (Fenson et al., 2007). Nick's parents maintain a vocabulary list of words he is heard to say that are not listed on the MacArthur-Bates (Fenson et al., 2007). Nick has made excellent progress in his understanding and use of new words since receiving his cochlear implant. His present level of vocabulary acquisition is more advanced than his cochlear implant age but not yet at the level of the typical 20-month-old.

Recommendations

- Continue regular audiological management.
- Continue regular sessions of auditory-verbal therapy.
- Provide a favorable listening environment.
- Provide a minimum of 1 hour daily to carry-over goals established in therapy during a structured play session, and a minimum of 4 to 5 hours daily to embellish goals during the course of daily routines.
- Continue reading several books each day to develop language, vocabulary, attention span, and interest in books.
- Continue ongoing monitoring of progress in all areas of development.

ASSESSING THE SCHOOL–AGE CHILD

Name: Sarah

Age: 6 years, 6 months

CI Age: 3 years. 8 months

History:

Sarah is a six-year, six-month-old girl with a bilateral sensorineural hearing loss of unknown etiology, identified through newborn hearing screen. She received hearing aids at 3 months of age and began receiving early intervention services at that time. At 3 years of age, she received a cochlear implant in her right ear. She continues to wear a hearing aid in her left ear. She began auditory-verbal therapy at the time of her implant. She currently attends a mainstream first grade classroom with a language facilitator. She also receives services with a teacher of the deaf for 1 hour each day. She was discharged from speech-language therapy at the end of her kindergarten year. She continues to attend private auditory-verbal parent participation sessions bimonthly.

This evaluation was conducted to evaluate current speech, language, and audition skills and to follow-up on the recommendation to remove the language facilitator from her mainstream classroom.

Assessment Instruments

- The Oral and Written Language Scales, 2nd Edition (OWLS-II; Carrow-Woolfolk, 2011)
- Expressive Vocabulary Test, 2nd Edition (EVT 2; Williams, 2007)
- Peabody Picture Vocabulary Test, 4th Edition (PPVT 4; Dunn & Dunn, 2007)

Findings

Oral and Written Language Scales

Oral and Written Language Scales, Second Edition (OWLS-II; Carrow-Woolfolk, 2011) is a norm-referenced assessment to measure receptive and expressive language communication skills in children ages 3 to 21. Standard scores are based on a mean of 100 and a standard deviation of 15. Therefore, standard scores between 85 and 115 are considered within normal limits. Results are as follows.

Areas of strength:

- Understands complex sentences (i.e., The boy she waved to was sitting).
- Understands prepositions.
- Understands irregular present perfect tense (i.e., Show me the girl who has eaten her apple.).

Areas of need:

- Understands inferences related to world knowledge (i.e., Show me the picture in which Dad is thinking, "Too bad she can't be in the race.").
- Understands adverbs (i.e., hurriedly).
- Understands present progressive in a negative sentence (e.g., Which girls have not been raking?).

Oral Expression

Standard score: 101

Percentile rank: 53

Areas of strength:

- Understands complex sentences (i.e., The boy she waved to was sitting).
- Understands prepositions.
- Understands irregular present perfect tense (i.e., Show me the girl who has eaten her apple.).

Areas of need:

- Use of 3rd person plural personal pronoun (theirs).

- Use of passive voice.
- Use of irregular past tense.

Oral Composite

Standard score: 96

Percentile rank: 39

Expressive Vocabulary Test

The Expressive Vocabulary Test, 2nd Edition (EVT-2; Williams, 2007) is a norm-referenced assessment to measure expressive vocabulary and word retrieval for individuals from ages 2.6 to 90+. Standard scores are based on a mean of 100 and a standard deviation of 15. Therefore, standard scores between 85 and 115 are considered within normal limits. Results are as follows:

Standard score: 101

Percentile rank: 53

Peabody Picture Vocabulary Test

Peabody Picture Vocabulary Test, 4th Edition (PPVT-4; Dunn & Dunn, 2007) is a norm-referenced assessment to measure receptive vocabulary comprehension for individuals from ages 2.6 to 90+. Standard scores are based on a mean of 100 and a standard deviation of 15. Therefore, standard scores between 85 and 115 are considered within normal limits. Results are as follows:

Standard score: 94

Percentile rank: 34

Summary of Language Assessment

Sarah is a 6-year-old girl with a bilateral sensorineural hearing loss. The results of these language assessments indicate that she has continued to demonstrate language progress with her cochlear implant. Her current receptive and expressive language and vocabulary skills are within normal limits for her age when compared to her typically hearing peers. However, her scores do not equal those of her cognitive abilities and therefore do not meet her potential language abilities. She has continued needs within the areas of vocabulary, and receptive and expressive language use to match the language of her typical hearing such as the skills listed in this evaluation.

Recommendations

Based on these needs, Sarah needs to continue receiving the following services:

- Bimonthly auditory-verbal therapy parent sessions with daily carryover at home.
- Individual sessions with the teacher of the deaf to preteach vocabulary and language that will be used in the mainstream classroom as well as age-appropriate language targets she is not comprehending or using.
- It is appropriate at this time to begin to transition her away from the use of a language facilitator in the classroom.
- Parents should continue to read aloud at home for 30 minutes per day.
- Sarah should continue to wear the cochlear implant device all waking hours and pursue aggressive audiological management.
- Parents, therapists, teachers, and other caregivers should continue to provide extensive language stimulation in all settings.

ASSESSING CHILDREN WITH HEARING LOSS AND ADDITIONAL CHALLENGES

Name: Miguel

Age: 4 years, 1 month

History:

Miguel is a 4-year, 1-month-old Hispanic male. He was born prematurely at 28 weeks, weighed 4 pounds and required two weeks in an incubator. His early history is significant for breathing problems, jaundice, excessive crying, feeding difficulties, hearing problems, ear infections, eye/visual problems, colic, and allergies. Miguel was diagnosed with auditory neuropathy in his left ear at 13 months of age.

Miguel currently lives at home with his parents and younger brother. He attends a special needs preschool classroom. Miguel has a current Individualized Education Program (IEP) under developmental delay. Miguel's preschool teacher reports concerns with doing what is asked, responding to simple commands, social skills with peers and adults, lack of interest in toileting, drawing/handwriting, understanding language, social use of language, problem solving, and early literacy skills.

Miguel was referred to a university specialty clinic to gain a better understanding of his language delays and to determine if he meets criteria for an autism spectrum disorder.

Assessment Instruments

- Test of Auditory Comprehension of Language, 3rd Edition (TACL-3; Carrow-Woolfolk, 1998)

- Aided Language Stimulation Activities (Drager, 2009)
- Autism Diagnostic Observation Schedule, Module 1 (ADOS; Lord et al., 2000)
- Parent Interview

Findings

Test of Auditory Comprehension of Language

Administration of the Test of Auditory Comprehension of Language (TACL-3; Carrow-Woolfolk, 1998) was attempted to assess Miguel's understanding of language. Miguel was asked to identify common words by pointing to pictures, which did not require him to use spoken language; however, the TACL-3 (Carrow-Woolfolk, 1998) was discontinued due to difficulty engaging Miguel in the task.

In an effort to gain an estimate of receptive vocabulary, the clinicians tried using tangible objects, such as a book, spoon, cup, duck, and a frog. Objects were presented two at a time, and Miguel was asked "Show me ___?" The clinicians modeled how to reach for the corresponding item. This informal assessment was also discontinued because Miguel appeared to reach indiscriminately or toward a preferred object.

Aided Language Activities

Miguel was further assessed for stimulability using aided language boards with a bubble activity and a balloon activity. This strategy involved using a communication board that contained related vocabulary and picture symbols (or pictures) to communicate during an activity. For example, during the bubble activity, a communication board with symbols for actions (e.g.,

open, blow, pop) and a symbol for *bubbles* was used. Although Miguel attended to the symbols on the board as the examiners modeled its use during the bubble activity (i.e., pointing to pictured vocabulary as they spoke), he only once spontaneously pointed to the board to communicate a request.

During a requesting and choice-making activity, the clinicians took turns modeling holding out their hands to request a cookie. Miguel appeared to observe these interactions and began to request another cookie the same way, and on one occasion used the sign for "more." Miguel's request time decreased as the interaction progressed, which is important because it demonstrates that with a highly motivating item (such as a cookie), modeling and direction, along with wait time, Miguel will initiate expressive communication in an appropriate and meaningful way.

Communication

Autism Diagnostic Observation Schedule, Module 1 (ADOS; Lord et al., 2000). Miguel's communication attempts were limited throughout the assessment. He produced minimal verbalizations, which were rarely directed toward others. Miguel used few gestures during the ADOS (Lord et al., 2000), although he demonstrated an open-handed reach to request and to push undesired items away. These gestures were rarely coordinated with eye gaze. Miguel used his mother's hand as a tool and pulled her hand to other desired objects; for example, he placed her hand on the bubble gun to activate it.

Social Interaction

Miguel's social interaction skills were limited compared to other children his age.

Although he used eye contact to check in with others on his own terms, he did not use it in combination with other behaviors, such as vocalizations or gestures within social interactions. Although he showed shared enjoyment by occasionally smiling toward the examiner and his mother during peek-a-boo and tickling games, it was difficult for both the examiner and his mother to get him to produce a purely reciprocal social smile just by smiling at him. Other than an occasional smile, Miguel demonstrated rather flat affect and did not direct facial expressions toward others. He did not look toward the examiner after his name was called several times, but he did respond to his name being called by his mother on her second attempt. The best examples of requests during the ADOS (Lord et al., 2000) generally included reaching without eye contact or verbalization or pulling an adult's hand to a desired item. Overall, Miguel demonstrated a slightly unusual quality of social interaction because his interactions are mainly limited to his interests or personal demands; however, he did initiate a peek-a-boo game with a clinician.

Summary of Language Assessment

Although the examiners were unable to use formal testing to assess language skills, based on previous evaluation reports and informal observation, it was evident that Miguel presented with delayed receptive and expressive language skills. Based upon the ADOS (Lord et al., 2000) and the parental report, the assessment team concluded that Miguel demonstrates communication, social interaction, and behaviors consistent with the criteria for a diagnosis of autistic disorder. Miguel was stimulable for aided

language communication strategies, which provide him visual support for receptive input of language, while providing him with a model of alternative means to communicate with available vocabulary.

Recommendations

- Continue current speech and language services to address overall delays in communication development. The following communicative functions that emerge before words should be targeted: behavior regulation (requesting/protesting objects and actions), social interaction (requesting routines, calling, showing off), and joint attention. The following communicative means are also important for Miguel to develop: contact gestures, distal gestures, and vocalizations.
- Implement an aided language communication approach.
- Sing songs and read books with repetitive lines to encourage Miguel to initiate communication. After singing or reading the same song or book several times, begin to pause at the repeated line and wait expectantly for him to fill in the line by vocalizing or by activating a speech-generating switch on which the repeated line is recorded.
- Encourage engagement with others or joint attention by pointing out objects and events that interest him.
- Due to communication, social, and behavioral challenges, Miguel is likely to benefit from a classroom setting that includes a structured and organized environment, a

predictable schedule of activities, visual supports, and a low teacher–student ratio.

- An *Object Exchange Communication System* might also be beneficial for Miguel in teaching him to communicate. Use objects for communication in order to help Miguel understand that the objects are symbolic of a request for another object, for an action, or for an event to take place.

THE ROLE OF PARENTS IN LANGUAGE ASSESSMENT

Parents play a crucial role in the assessment process. They act as historians and informants. Parents must provide an accurate history of their child's hearing, medical, and educational history. They must act as informants regarding the child's current language use, educational, and therapeutic services, and voice any concerns they have regarding their child's progress. Parents must also provide the clinician with information regarding their child's performance (i.e., Is this typical behavior?), the need for breaks, and potentially regulate the child's behavior during testing. They provide any relevant information needed to support the comprehensive assessment of language for the child with hearing loss.

CONCLUSION

Assessing the language and vocabulary of infants, toddlers, and children with hearing loss is necessary to fulfill both legal directives and to provide essential information to determine eligibility, facilitate intervention planning, and monitor progress. Effective and comprehensive assessment requires practitioners to demonstrate knowledge and application of normal language development, as well as a variety of formal and informal approaches designed to measure all facets of language form, content, and use. Selection and use of specific strategies and techniques serves to optimize the assessment process and results. Parents play an important role in planning and conducting language assessment for children with hearing loss.

REFERENCES

American Speech-Language-Hearing Association (ASHA). (2014a). *Effects of hearing loss on development.* Retrieved from http://www.asha.org/public/hearing/Effects-of-Hearing-Loss-on-Development

American Speech-Language-Hearing Association (ASHA). (2014b). *IDEA part B issue brief: Culturally and linguistically diverse students.* Retrieved from http://www.asha.org/Advocacy/federal/idea/IDEA-Part-B-Issue-Brief-Culturally-and-Linguistically-Diverse-Students

American Speech-Language-Hearing Association (ASHA). (2014c). *Your child's communication development: Kindergarten through fifth grade.* Retrieved from http://www.asha.org/public/speech/development/communicationdevelopment.htm

Beck, I. L., McKeown, M. G., & Kucan, L. (2002). *Bringing words to life: Robust vocabulary instruction.* New York, NY: Guilford Press.

Bloom, L., & Lahey, M. (1978). *Language development and language disorders.* New York, NY: MacMillan.

Brisbane, H. (2005). *The developing child.* Peoria, IL: McGraw-Hill. Retrieved from http://highered.mcgraw-hill.com/sites/dl/free/007231639x/45070/papch01.pdf

Brown, R. (1973). *A first language: The early stages.* London, UK: George Allen & Unwin.

Bui, Y. (2003). *Language and communicative development. Theories and patterns of language development.* Retrieved from http://elearndesign.org/teachspecialed/modules/ocada7081_norm2/23/24_2/35.html

Caleffe-Schenck, N. (2012). How do parents and practitioners use children's literature for auditory development? In W. Estabrooks (Ed.), *101 Frequently asked questions about auditory-verbal practice: Promoting listening and spoken language for children who are deaf and hard of hearing and their families* (pp. 325–329). Washington, DC: Alexander Graham Bell Association for the Deaf and Hard of Hearing.

Carey-Sargeant, C. L., & Brown, P. M. (2003). Pausing during interactions between deaf toddlers and their hearing mothers. *Deafness and Education International, 5,* 39–58.

Carrow-Woolfolk, E. (1998). *Test of Auditory Comprehension of Language* (3rd ed.). Austin, TX: Pro-Ed.

Carrow-Woolfolk, E. (1999). *Comprehensive Assessment of Spoken Language.* Austin, TX: Pro-Ed.

Carrow-Woolfolk, E. (2011). *Oral and Written Language Scales* (2nd ed.). Torrance, CA: Western Psychological Services.

Cole, E. B., & Flexer, C. (2011). *Children with hearing loss: Developing listening and talking—Birth to six* (2nd ed.). San Diego, CA: Plural.

Daniel, L. (2012). What is acoustic highlighting? In W. Estabrooks (Ed.), *101 Frequently asked questions about auditory-verbal practice: Promoting listening and spoken language for children who are deaf and hard of hearing and their families* (pp. 108–112). Washington, DC: Alexander Graham Bell Association for the Deaf and Hard of Hearing.

Drager, K. D. R. (2009). Aided modeling intervention for children with autism spectrum disorders who require AAC. *SIG 12 Perspectives on Augmentative and Alternative Communication, 18,* 114–120. doi:10.1044/aac18.4.114. Retrieved from http://sig12perspectives.pubs.asha.org/article.aspx?articleid=1765977

Dunn, L. M., & Dunn, D. M. (2007). *Peabody Picture Vocabulary Test* (4th ed.). San Antonio, TX: Pearson.

Eliot, L. (1999). *What's going on in there? How the brain and mind develop in the first five years of life.* New York, NY; Bantam Books.

Estabrooks, W. (Ed.) (2012). What is auditory-verbal practice? In W. Estabrooks (Ed.), *101 Frequently asked questions about auditory-verbal practice: Promoting listening and spoken language for children who are deaf and hard of hearing and their families* (pp. 31–34). Washington, DC: Alexander Graham Bell Association for the Deaf and Hard of Hearing.

Fenson, L., Marchman, V., Thal, D., Reznick, J., & Bates, E. (2007). *MacArthur-Bates Communicative Development Inventories* (2nd ed.). Baltimore, MD: Paul H Brookes.

Flexer, C. (2012). How does a child with hearing loss benefit from an FM system and/or a sound field system in the classroom? In W. Estabrooks (Ed.), *Frequently asked questions about auditory-verbal practice: Promoting listening and spoken language for children who are deaf and hard of hearing and their families* (pp. 93–97). Washington, DC: Alexander Graham Bell Association for the Deaf and Hard of Hearing.

Gleason, J. B. (2001). *The development of language* (5th ed.). Needham Heights, MA: Allyn & Bacon.

Hart, B., & Risley, T. (1999). *The social world of children learning to talk.* Baltimore, MD; Brookes.

Heerbooth, J. (2014). *Normal development of language precursors.* Retrieved from http://www.robinbest.com/normal_dev_language.html

Heilmann, J. (2010). Myths and realities of language sample analysis. *SIG 1 Perspectives on Language Learning and Education, 17,* 4–8. doi:10.1044/lle17.1.4. Retrieved from http://sig1perspectives.pubs.asha.org/article.aspx?articleid=1767671&resultClick=1

Hymes, D. (1972). On communicative competence. In J. B. Pride & J. Holmes (Eds.), *Socialinguistics* (pp. 269–293). New York, NY: Penguin Books.

Joint Committee on Infant Hearing (JCIH). (2013). Supplement to the JCIH 2007 position statement: Principles and guidelines for early intervention after confirmation that a child is deaf or hard of hearing. *Pediatrics, 131*(4), e1324–e1349. Retrieved from http://www.audiology.org/resources/documentlibrary/Documents/JCIH_PositionStatement_2013.pdf

Ling, D. (1989). *Foundations of spoken language for hearing-impaired children.* Washington, DC: Alexander Graham Bell Association for the Deaf and Hard of Hearing.

Lord, C., Rutter, M., Dilavore, P., & Risi, J. (2000). *Autism Diagnostic Observation Schedule.* Torrance, CA: Western Psychological Services.

Miller, J. F., & Iglesias, A. (2008). Systematic analysis of language transcripts (SALT). [Computer software]. Madison, WI: SALT Software.

Nott, P., Cowan, R., Brown, P. M. & Wigglesworth, G. (2009). Early language development in children with profound hearing loss fitted with a device at a young age: Part I, The time period taken to acquire first words and first word combinations. *Ear and Hearing, 30*(5), 526–540.

Owens, R. E. (1996). *Language development: An introduction* (4th ed.). Needham Heights, MA: Allyn & Bacon.

Owens, R. E. (2005). *Language development: An introduction* (6th ed.). Boston, MA: Pearson/ Allyn & Bacon.

Owens, R. E. (2012). *Language development: An introduction* (8th ed.). Boston, MA: Allyn & Bacon.

Payne, T. E. (1997). *Describing morphosyntax: A guide for field linguists.* New York, NY: Cambridge University Press.

Pikulski, J. J., & Templeton, S. (2004). *Teaching and developing vocabulary: Key to long-term reading success.* Retrieved from http://www.eduplace .com/marketing/nc/pdf/author_pages.pdf

Pollack, D., Goldberg, D., & Caleffe-Schenck, N. (1997). *Educational audiology for the limited-hearing infant and preschooler: An auditory-verbal program* (3rd ed.). Springfield, IL: Charles C. Thomas.

Prezbindowski, A. K., & Lederberg, A. R. (2003). Vocabulary assessment of deaf and hard-of-hearing children from infancy through the preschool years. *Journal of Deaf Studies and Deaf Education, 8*(4), 383–400.

Rhoades, E. A. (2011). Listening strategies to facilitate spoken language learning among signing children with cochlear implants. In R. Paludneviciene & I. W. Leigh (Eds.), *Cochlear implants: Evolving perspectives* (pp. 142–171). Washington, DC: Gallaudet University.

Rhoades, E. A. (2013). Interactive silences: Evidence for strategies to facilitate spoken language in children with hearing loss. *The Volta Review, 113*(1), 57–73.

Robertson, L. (2009). *Literacy and deafness: Listening and spoken language.* San Diego, CA: Plural.

Rossetti, L. (2006). *The Rossetti Infant Toddler Scale.* Moline, IL; LinguiSystems.

Sarant, J. Z., Holt, C. M., Dowell, R. C., Rickards, F. W., & Blamey, P. J. (2009). Spoken language development in oral preschool children with permanent childhood deafness. *Journal of Deaf Studies and Deaf Education 14*(2), 205–217.

Semel, E., Wiig, E. A., & Secord, W. (2013). *Clinical Evaluation of Language Fundamentals* (5th ed.). Toronto, CA: Pearson.

Shipley, K. & McAfee, J. (2009). *Assessment in speech-language pathology: A resource manual* (4th ed.). Clifton Park, NY: Delmar Learning.

Simser, J., & Estabrooks, W. (2001). What is the hand cue? What is acoustic highlighting? In W. Estabrooks (Ed.), *50 Frequently asked questions about auditory-verbal therapy* (pp. 104–106). Toronto, Canada: Learning to Listen Foundation.

The Individuals with Disabilities Education Improvement Act of 2004, 20 U.S.C. § 1400 et seq. (2004). Retrieved from http://idea.ed .gov/download/statute.html

Tobin, K. (1987). The role of wait time in higher cognitive level learning. *Review of Educational Research, 57,* 69–95.

Trelease, J. (2006). *The read-aloud handbook* (6th ed.). New York, NY: Penguin Books.

Tur-Kaspa, H., & Dromi, E. (1999). Spoken and written language assessment of orally trained children with hearing loss: Syntactic structures and deviations. *The Volta Review, 100*(3), 186–199.

Walker, B., & Wilson, K. (2011 January/February). *It's too late baby now, it's too late—or is it?* [PowerPoint slides]. Presentation for the South Carolina School for the Deaf and Blind Hearing Outreach Program, Columbia, SC.

Waterman, B. B. (1994). Assessing children for the presence of a disability. *National Dissemination Center for Children with Disabilities News Digest, 4*(1), 1–27. Retrieved from http://nichcy.org/ wp-content/uploads/docs/nd23.pdf

Weaver, B. (n.d.). *Formal vs. informal assessments.* Retrieved from http://www.scholastic .com/teachers/article/formal-versus-informal-assessments

Williams, K. T. (2007). *Expressive Vocabulary Test* (2nd ed.). Toronto, Canada: Pearson.

Zimmerman, I., Steiner, V., & Pond, R. (2011) *Preschool Language Scales* (5th ed.). Bloomington, MN: Pearson.

CHAPTER 7

Psychoeducational Assessment

Susan Randich

- Psychoeducational evaluation of children with hearing loss can be used to assess cognitive, language, and academic skills as well as to diagnose secondary challenges including learning disabilities, intellectual disabilities, and behavioral issues. Evaluation provides an understanding of the child as an individual and a learner in order to better support the child in the educational setting.

- An effective psychoeducational evaluation integrates formal test results with the child's history, previous evaluations, behavioral observations, and parent and teacher experience with the child in order to provide a better awareness of a child's functioning across multiple dimensions—cognitive, linguistic, academic, and/or emotional/behavioral—that affect ability to access curriculum and learn in school.

- Although standard intellectual, academic, and behavioral instruments can be used successfully to assess children with hearing loss, the choice,

administration, and interpretation of tests are all dictated by the child's level of hearing loss and language proficiency. For this reason the clinician performing the evaluation should have experience with the evaluation of children with hearing loss who use listening and spoken language to communicate. The psychologist must be knowledgeable in choosing and interpreting tests with children with hearing loss.

- Use of inappropriate instruments and uninformed interpretation of tests with children with hearing loss can result in erroneous conclusions and diagnoses. The central challenge for the psychologist in performing psychoeducational evaluation for this population lies in determining to what degree the child's struggles reflect language delay secondary to the hearing loss, and to what degree the problems may reflect comorbid disorders.

- In order to be useful, the results of the evaluation must be communicated to a diverse audience that includes parents, teachers, other clinicians, and the student. The clinician needs to be aware of the varied needs of all these individuals in report-writing as well as face-to-face communication.

INTRODUCTION: WHAT IS PSYCHOEDUCATIONAL ASSESSMENT?

This chapter discusses the psychoeducational evaluation of children with hearing loss who use listening and spoken language (LSL) as their method of communication. There are a number of guides for the psychoeducational assessment of children with hearing loss (Braden, 2005; Metz, Miller, & Thomas-Presswood, 2010; Sattler & Hardy-Braz, 2002), but although these resources mention children who communicate orally, the emphasis is on children who use some form of sign language as their primary method of communication. There is limited information available on the assessment of children who use LSL to communicate and learn.

When children with hearing loss are identified early, fitted with appropriate hearing technology, and provided with family-centered early intervention services from properly trained professionals, most are able to progress at age-appropriate rates (Kennedy et al., 2006; Moeller, 2000; Yoshinaga-Itano, Sedey, Coutler, & Mehl, 1998), and require fewer special education services by the time they enter elementary school. Many positive outcomes are associated with early identification and intervention, including better language, speech, and social-emotional development, than later-identified children; more typical rates of cognitive development; and lower paren-

tal stress as the child acquires language and increases communication (Dornan, Hickson, Murdoch, Houston, & Constantinescu, 2010; Geers, 2006; Niparko et al., 2010; Yoshinaga-Itano & Gravel, 2001).

Likewise, children who receive cochlear implants early and receive high quality early childhood services often develop similarly to typical peers (Geers & Hayes, 2011; Geers & Sedey, 2011) and may never be referred for psychoeducational evaluation. As Edwards (2007) notes, however, children with hearing loss and other comorbid diagnoses are increasingly receiving cochlear implants, and additional problems may become apparent after a child is implanted. Often, there is a question of differential diagnosis of intellectual disability, a language disorder in addition to the hearing loss, attentional issues, or specific learning disorder. Psychoeducational evaluation has a role in the assessment and diagnosis of all of these conditions.

Psychoeducational evaluation is often identified as "testing." It is better defined, however, as the process of using a combination of tests, measurements, and observations to develop a better understanding of a child's functioning across multiple dimensions—cognitive, linguistic, academic, and/or emotional/behavioral—that affect ability to access curriculum and learn in school (Pohlman, 2008). Psychoeducational evaluation typically includes some measure of general cognitive potential as an anchor to help determine what expectations may be appropriate for a child's academic and/or linguistic functioning. Cognitive processing, including memory, visual or auditory processing, or visual-motor ability may also be assessed. Evaluation usually addresses academic skill development in the areas of reading, written expression, and mathematics. For children with hearing loss, language proficiency is addressed, from basic interpersonal communication to higher-level oral and written discourse skills. Finally, the evaluation may include an assessment of behavior, including adaptive behavior skills, social-emotional functioning, activity level, attention, and executive skills.

Psychoeducational assessment is different from both classroom assessment and group-administered standardized assessment. Unlike classroom evaluation (i.e., quizzes, chapter tests, etc.), psychoeducational testing is standardized. Standardization in test procedure and the availability of norms allows comparisons both with other children and with other tests taken by a specific child. (See Chapter 2.) The student can be compared to typical children of the same age or grade level to determine whether skills and abilities are at expected levels of development. It is also possible to compare the student's abilities across various skill areas. Finally, standard scores allow an assessment of the child's growth and development over time (Table 7–1).

Unlike group standardized testing, psychoeducational assessment is conducted in a one-on-one setting with the student, so that the clinician is able to make observations about the child's behavior and functioning that may help to pinpoint areas of specific strength and weakness in cognitive and academic skills.

In the public setting, psychoeducational evaluation is an important tool in determining the child's eligibility for a range of special education services. Besides assisting with educational diagnosis, psychoeducational evaluation may suggest appropriate therapeutic interventions such as speech therapy or occupational therapy. In both public and private

Table 7–1. Using Standard Scores

	Comparisons	Examples
Across children	Comparisons with hearing peers	• Is the child intellectually gifted? • How similar are the child's language skills to those of his or her hearing peers? • Is this child's activity level typical for children of the same age and sex? • Is the child ready to transition into a general education setting?
Within the child	Comparisons across skill areas	• Is the child's memory as strong as would be expected given his or her cognitive ability? • Is the child's language ability commensurate with his or her intelligence? • What are the child's areas of academic strength and weakness?
	Comparisons across time	• Is the child making progress toward "closing the gap" with hearing peers in language? • Has the child made expected growth in reading skills over the past year?

school contexts, evaluation also provides a better understanding of the child as a learner and communicator and allows teaching to be individualized to the needs of the child. It can also monitor the progress of the child in language acquisition and academic skills development, and can be a useful tool in assessing when or the degree to which a child is ready to transition into a general education setting.

ISSUES AND CONSIDERATIONS IN CONDUCTING PSYCHOEDUCATIONAL EVALUATION WITH CHILDREN WITH HEARING LOSS

Limitations of Tests and the Necessity of Multiple Sources of Information

In interpreting psychoeducational tests, it is important to remember that tests are powerful but imperfect tools. Every test incorporates some level of measurement error, so that formal tests scores are best considered an estimate of the child's true abilities. The observations and judgment of the clinician are crucial in interpreting the meaning of test scores.

Ethics require that a diagnosis is never made on the basis of a single test (American Psychological Association, 2010). A good psychoeducational evaluation uses and integrates multiple sources of data, including not only current test results, but also behavioral observations, parent and teacher reports, and results of previous testing. Because the assessment of children with hearing loss can be especially challenging, the evaluator may elect to use a battery that will include selected subtests or portions of several different tests.

Evaluator Qualifications

Psychoeducational assessment of a child with a hearing loss is a complex process that requires an understanding of the dynamics of hearing loss and amplification, a familiarity with language and academic skills development in children with hearing loss, and an awareness of how these issues impact evaluation results. The clinician should have experience with the evaluation of children with hearing loss and in particular should have experience in working with children with cochlear implants. The psychologist should also be knowledgeable in choosing and interpreting tests with children with hearing loss. In the absence of this expertise, the evaluator would benefit from consultation with an expert or working under the supervision of a knowledgeable practitioner (Krouse & Braden, 2011).

Planning the Evaluation

The assessment of the child begins with a clear definition of the referral question. Referral may originate with a therapist, an educator, or a parent, and may result from disappointing progress in the child's development of language and/or academic skills or concerns about the appropriateness of the child's current educational placement and/or services. Parents or educators may be seeking an assessment for Attention-Deficit/Hyperactivity Disorder (ADHD) or a specific learning disability. There may be explicit or unspoken questions about whether the child has an intellectual disability or is exhibiting symptoms of an autism spectrum disorder. It is important to spend adequate time with parents and teachers or therapists in order to fully understand their concerns about the child and what questions are to be addressed by the evaluation.

The second step in preparing for the evaluation is the review of records (Table 7–2). It is important to review the child's birth history, the cause of hearing loss if known, and the age at diagnosis. Knowledge of the child's history with amplification—for example, when amplified or implanted and how consistently the device was or is worn—is essential in assessing whether a language delay is attributable to lack of access to sound or to processing deficits intrinsic to the child. Similarly, it is crucial to know the child's history of therapeutic intervention and education. The difficulties of a child who was implanted early and had consistent LSL services since implantation would be interpreted very differently from a child who was implanted late, has been taught using Total Communication, or has had minimal intervention after implantation. Finally, the psychologist should examine any previous evaluation records, including psychoeducational reports and speech and language evaluations.

In evaluating a child with hearing loss, it is vital that the clinician understand the level of the child's current auditory ability. Children with hearing loss vary widely in their unaided loss, method of amplification, aided detection, and ability to use hearing to comprehend speech. Some children with cochlear implants are able to function quite well using audition alone, but other children may need to use speechreading to supplement listening to a greater or lesser extent. In evaluating a child with hearing loss, the evaluator will need to ensure that the child's equipment is working properly and to be aware of the degree to which the child depends on speechreading. A quiet room with good lighting is also essential.

Some prior knowledge of the child's language competence is also necessary for planning the evaluation, choosing a test battery, and interpreting tests. For a child with communication competence close to that of hearing peers, a standard test battery and standard administration is generally possible. For a child with significantly delayed or impaired language, however, both test administration and interpretation will be affected, with concerns raised about the child's ability to understand instructions and comprehend test items as well as ability to adequately demonstrate the skills or knowledge he or she possesses.

Table 7–2. Case History Review

Review of History
• Prenatal and birth history
• Presence of any illnesses or additional disabilities
• Attainment of major developmental milestones
• Cause of hearing loss
• Age of diagnosis of hearing loss
• History of amplification
• Type of current amplification
• Consistency of use of amplification
• Educational/therapeutic history
• Previous psychoeducational evaluations
• Previous language evaluations

Use of Accommodations and Modifications in Testing

To obtain an accurate assessment of the student's abilities and skills, the clinician may sometimes elect to make changes to the test format, administration, or content. The term **accommodation** is used to describe an alteration of environment, format, or equipment that allows an individual with a disability to gain access to content. A key principle is that accommodations should affect features of the test that are related to the disability but should not change the construct being measured. The term **modification** is used to describe a change in the administration or actual content of the test made in such a way that both students with disabilities and typical students would potentially benefit (Case, 2008). In practice, it can be difficult to differentiate between accommodations and modifications when testing children with hearing loss. For example, in a test of math reasoning in which word problems are administered orally, providing items in print is an accommodation aimed at decreasing the degree to which the auditory comprehension of a child with hearing loss affects the result. However, this accommodation also provides the stimulus to the student for a longer period of time, making fewer demands on the child's working memory as well as compensating for processing slowness, changes that might also improve the performance of a typical child being administered the test. Accommodations by definition alter standardized testing procedures, and there is usually no way of knowing exactly how or to what degree they affect the validity of the resulting scores (Sattler & Dumont, 2004).

In spite of these concerns, accommodations can provide important diagnostic information, particularly for children with complex needs and/or serious language delays (Sattler & Dumont, 2004). They should, however, be used as infrequently as possible and only to the degree necessary. Case (2008) provides a summary of possible accommodations, with an anal-ysis of the degree to which each accommodation would be likely to change the construct measured. If the clinician elects to use accommodations, he or she will need to record and justify the use in the evaluation report and interpret the resulting scores in light of the accommodations. If accommodations are used, the resulting score should be interpreted with caution, as a rough estimate of the student's true ability in the construct being measured. The more that the clinician deviates from standardized procedure, the more likely it is that scores obtained may be inflated.

Behavioral Observations

Observations of the child are a fundamental aspect of the psychoeducational evaluation, providing information about the child that is not available from test scores. Through observation and interaction with the child, the psychologist will gain important information about the child's speech and language skills (Table 7–3). The clinician can also develop a sense of the child's ability to interact with an adult in a cooperative fashion, motivation to perform well, and ability to engage with a cognitive task: Does the child enjoy problem-solving? Is the child self-confident or a "discouraged learner"? By observing the child as he or she engages in various kinds of problem-solving and academic tasks, the psychologist can observe the student's level of organization, how the student approaches tasks, and whether the student uses any kind of compensatory strategies.

It is also important to observe the child's activity level, attention, and task focus during testing, both within and between tasks. The child's level of atten-

Table 7–3. Behavioral Observations

Interpersonal skills	• Eye contact • Cooperation with an adult • Affect and emotional responsiveness • Self-confidence • Sense of humor
Language and audition	• Ability to use listening to understand speech • Accommodations necessary for comprehension (speechreading, print) • Speech intelligibility • Language comprehension • Expressive abilities • Conversational skills • Language pragmatics
Cognition	• Ability to engage with a cognitive task • Level of organization • Perseverance and frustration tolerance • Use of compensatory strategies
Attention and task–focus	• Activity level • Visual vs. aural distractibility • Daydreaming • Need for cues or redirection

tion during various activities can be diagnostic. Sometimes children will be particularly restless or inattentive when the area of deficit is being assessed; behavior may regress during tasks that are challenging because the student has learned that difficult tasks can be avoided by oppositional behavior or emotional outbursts. Finally, careful observation can discern strengths of the child, such as sense of humor, intellectual curiosity, interpersonal skills, perseverance, or frustration tolerance, which can be used to offset or compensate for areas of weakness. All of the above are qualities that can only be assessed by observation, rather than by formal test results.

COGNITIVE ASSESSMENT

Formal testing in a psychoeducational evaluation generally begins with an intelligence test that will provide a measure of the child's general nonverbal intellectual potential. Intellectual testing provides information about the child's cognitive strengths and weaknesses and assesses for the presence of processing deficits that can affect learning. This score will also act as an anchor that will offer the evaluator some sense of where the student should be functioning linguistically and academically.

The cognitive assessment of children with hearing loss has historically been controversial. Individuals with hearing loss tend to score similarly to hearing peers on nonverbal IQ measures. For example, a review of 324 studies of intelligence scores of individuals with hearing loss found a mean nonverbal IQ of 97.14, very close to the mean of 100 (Sattler & Hardy-Braz, 2002). Individuals with hearing loss, however, even when educated orally, often score significantly below average on verbal intelligence measures, typically greater than 15 points or one standard deviation below the mean (Braden, 2005; Krouse & Braden, 2011). Administration of the verbal sections of intelligence tests has been seen as unfair for individuals with hearing loss, and the recommendation has sometimes been that the verbal subtests not be administered. Yet, modern conceptualizations of intelligence posit that verbal ability is a key component of general intelligence, and verbal skills are seen as being integral to higher-order thinking (Horn & Cattell, 1966; Krouse & Braden, 2011). Success in school tends to be much more closely correlated with verbal IQ scores than with nonverbal IQ scores, and children with hearing loss have historically had low reading scores and poorer academic outcomes (Sattler & Hardy-Braz, 2002).

The above issues indicate that both verbal and nonverbal portions of intelligence tests provide valuable information and should be administered to children with hearing loss, but that the two domains be interpreted differently. In general, it is recommended that the nonverbal portions of intelligence tests be interpreted as the best estimate of general intelligence, and that the verbal score be interpreted as a measure of acquired language (Akamatsu, Mayer, & Hardy-Braz, 2008; Braden, 2005; Simeonsson, Wax, & White, 2001). Since verbal and nonverbal scores are seen as assessing different domains in children with hearing loss, a "Total IQ" that combines the two is not considered an unitary ability and should not interpreted as such (Flanagan & Kaufman, 2009).

Measures of Intelligence

Most modern intelligence tests are based on the Horn-Cattell-Carroll (CHC) model of intelligence (McGrew, 2005). With the use of this model, the verbal subtests are seen as tapping **crystallized intelligence**, defined as the individual's store of acquired knowledge and ability to reason and communicate verbally. The nonverbal abilities include **fluid reasoning,** defined as the ability to recognize patterns and use inductive and deductive reasoning to solve novel problems not taught in school,

and **visual-spatial processing**, defined as the ability to perceive, analyze, and think with visual patterns, including the ability to mentally manipulate, store, and recall visual representations. Two other key cognitive abilities tapped by modern intelligence tests are **short-term/working memory**, the ability to hold information in mind while using it to solve problems, and **processing speed,** the ability to perform simple cognitive tasks quickly and accurately, requiring focused attention and concentration.

In the assessment of the nonverbal skills of a child with hearing loss, administration of the nonverbal subtests of one of the comprehensive intelligence tests usually provides adequate measures of nonverbal fluid reasoning, visual-spatial reasoning, and processing speed. However, for a child with minimal language skills, behavioral issues, suspected intellectual disability, motor limitations, or other complex issues, a specialized nonverbal cognitive test may be used by itself or to supplement the standard intelligence test.

The Wechsler family of intelligence tests, including the Wechsler Preschool and Primary Scale of Intelligence, 4th Edition (WPPSI-IV; Wechsler, 2013), normed for children ages 3 through 7;11; the Wechsler Intelligence Scale for Children, 4th Edition (WISC-IV; Wechsler, 2003a), normed for ages 6 through 16;11, and the Wechsler Adult Intelligence Scale, 4th Edition (WAIS-IV; Wechsler, 2008), normed for individuals 16 and older, are the most widely researched and commonly used tests for evaluating individuals with hearing loss (Braden, 2005). Each of the Wechsler scales provides a verbal score as well as scores for working memory and processing speed. The WISC-IV and the WAIS-IV provide a Perceptual Reasoning Index that incorporates both fluid reasoning and visual-spatial ability, while the WPPSI-IV provides separate index scores for fluid reasoning and visual-spatial reasoning. Krause and Braden (2011) provide evidence for the reliability, as well as preliminary evidence for the validity, of the WISC-IV with students with hearing loss.

The Stanford-Binet, 5th Edition (SB-5; Roid, 2003) is an intellectual measure normed for individuals age 2 years through adulthood. It includes measures of fluid reasoning, knowledge, quantitative reasoning, visual-spatial processing, and working memory, with each domain measured with both verbal and nonverbal subtests. The nonverbal general intelligence scale thus represents all of the primary areas of the CHC model. It is notable that the SB-5 is one of the only intelligence tests that includes a nonverbal measure of crystallized intelligence (Braden & Athonasiou, 2005; Roid & Pomplun, 2005).

The Woodcock-Johnson, 3rd Edition (WJ-3; Woodcock, McGrew, & Mather, 2001) is a set of tests, normed for individuals aged 3 years through adulthood, which assesses general intellectual ability, specific cognitive abilities, oral language, and academic achievement. The intellectual battery includes a "low verbal" scale of general intelligence. A drawback for use with students with hearing loss is that, while it is possible to obtain a score for visual-spatial processing with nonverbal subtests, the fluid reasoning scale includes both verbal and nonverbal subtests (Schrank, 2005).

The Kaufman Assessment Battery for Children, 2nd Edition (KABC-II; Kaufman & Kaufman, 2004) is grounded in dual theoretical foundations, the CHC model as well as the neuropsychological model that includes sequential and simultaneous processing, learning, and planning (Kaufman, Kaufman, Kaufman-Singer, & Kaufman, 2005). Similar to the WJ III, the KABC-II includes a nonverbal general intelligence score, but the structure of the composite scores does not afford an easy assessment of verbal versus nonverbal abilities.

Accurate assessment of a child with a hearing loss may necessitate the use of a nonverbal intellectual test. Available tests include the Leiter-III (Roid, Pomplun, & Koch, 2013), the Wechsler Nonverbal (WNV; Wechsler & Naglieri, 2006), the Universal Nonverbal Intelligence Test (UNIT; Bracken & McCallum, 1998), and the Comprehensive Test of Nonverbal Intelligence, 2nd Edition (CTONI-2; Hammill, Pearson, & Wiederholt, 2009). Each of these tests is designed to be culturally neutral and nonlanguage dependent in both instructions and content. In addition, some of these tests are designed to have reduced motor demands, making them useful with children who have cerebral palsy or other motor impairments.

In addition to comprehensive cognitive tests, it may be useful to assess the child's skills in specific processing areas. Visual-motor integration is a key skill for learning to print and write and is often assessed using The Beery-Buktenica Developmental Test of Visual-Motor Integration, 6th Edition (Beery, Buktenica, & Beery, 2010). The psychologist may also elect to administer a memory scale, such as the Children's Memory Scale (CMS; Cohen, 1997). The CMS provides an assessment of the child's abilities in auditory/verbal versus visual memory, as well as short-term versus long-term memory. However, this test is not designed to be administered to individuals with hearing loss, and interpretation of the auditory/verbal memory tasks is problematic with children who have hearing loss and/or language delay. The psychologist will need to interpret results tentatively, especially in the auditory/verbal areas, in light of the student's ability to hear and understand the stimuli. Finally, a test of phonological processing such as the Comprehensive Test of Phonological Processing, 2nd Edition (CTOPP-2; Wagner, Torgesen, Rachotte, & Pearson, 1999), may be helpful in assessing children suspected of having dyslexia. Again, this test does not have data to support use with children with hearing loss and the experienced clinician will need to rely on clinical judgment in interpreting the results of the test.

Practical Considerations in Cognitive Testing

Sattler and Dumont (2004) provide extensive instructions for administering the WISC-IV and WPPSI-III Perceptual Organization (nonverbal) scales to children with hearing loss, including written task instruction, instructions for pantomiming directions, and examples for extra practice. In my experience of administering the Wechsler tests to students with hearing loss who use LSL, however, this author has found that significant modifications or accommodations are not typically necessary for the nonverbal portions. On occasion, extra practice items may be effective in helping students learn the task. For older children, this can often be accomplished by dropping back and administering earlier items normed for younger children. The Digits Backwards (repeating strings of digits in reverse) subtest can sometimes be difficult to explain to young children with limited language who may not understand the word "backward." In this case it can be helpful to use print to explain the task.

Interpreting Cognitive Test Results

In interpreting intelligence test results, the nonverbal composite score is considered to be the best estimate of the child's general intellectual potential, as discussed in an earlier section. In general, the more consistent the scores are across nonverbal subtests, the more confidence the evaluator can place in the resulting composite score as a valid measure of the child's intellectual potential (Flanagan & Kaufman, 2009). When subtest scores are significantly different from one another, the profile may reflect the presence of processing weaknesses, and the nonverbal composite score may not be an adequate measure of the child's potential. Additionally, although the subtests measuring working memory and processing speed provide important information, it is important to remember that scores on these subtests are often depressed in children with a variety of problems, including ADHD, learning and memory problems, and hearing loss (Pisoni et al., 2008). These scores should not be considered a measure of general intelligence for children with hearing loss.

LANGUAGE ASSESSMENT

Although an in-depth assessment of a child's language skills is typically undertaken by the speech-language pathologist, a standard psychoeducational battery provides a great deal of data about a child's language proficiency that may not be tapped in standard language tests such as the Clinical Evaluation of Language Fundamentals, 5th Edition (CELF-V). Specifically, the verbal scales of the standard intelligence tests provide information about the child's complex language and discourse skills. The student's ability to comprehend and respond to questions of increasing length and complexity, store of verbal knowledge, and ability to express ideas and complex thoughts in words are crucial to functioning in an academic environment.

An understanding of the historically poor academic outcomes for children with hearing loss may be provided in the concepts of basic interpersonal communication skills (BICS) and cognitive-academic language proficiency (CALP; Cummins, 2008). BICS refers to primary, face-to-face language interaction that occurs in home or social settings. This language is typically about the here-and-now and uses basic, high frequency vocabulary, and relatively simple sentence structures. In contrast, CALP is the language that allows individuals to communicate about topics that are distant in time and space. It uses low frequency, abstract, and often technical vocabulary as well as complex sentence structures. Academic areas including math, science, and social studies require skills such as conceptual and categorical thinking, consideration of evidence, manipulation of information, and logical argument that necessitate CALP. Although BICS can be used to read and write about familiar topics, as a child progresses through school CALP is increasingly required to discuss, read, and write about academic content. While children with hearing loss, especially children with good access to sound using cochlear implants or hearing aids, typically have adequate BICS, they are often weak in CALP, explaining the common experience of disappointing academic progress (Akamatsu et al., 2008).

Assessing Academic Language Skills

Akamatsu and colleagues (2008) argue that verbal portions of published intelligence tests are generally a good measure of CALP, and that while general intelligence in individuals with hearing loss is best estimated by a nonverbal measure, the verbal scores provide an important measure of the student's academic language, including the ability to comprehend increasingly complex sentence and question forms, the ability to express complex thoughts and ideas in words, verbal knowledge, vocabulary, and verbal reasoning skills.

For children with hearing loss, the difference between the child's nonverbal and verbal scores on an intelligence test has traditionally been seen as a useful index of the gap between the student's intellectual potential and the level of his or her language development. Ideally, we would like to see the verbal and nonverbal scores of children with hearing loss as small as possible. For comparison purposes, in typical hearing children the difference between the WISC-IV Perceptual Organization (nonverbal) Index and Verbal Comprehension (verbal) Index is generally less than 10 points. A difference of 10 to 12 points, depending on the age of the child, would be considered statistically significant, and differences of 20 or more points would be seen in less than about 6% of children (Wechsler, 2003b).

In addition to the information about language skills provided by the verbal portions of intelligence tests, commonly used academic achievement tests such as the Wechsler Individual Achievement Test, 3rd Edition (WIAT-III) and the Woodcock-Johnson III Tests of Achievement (WJ III) include measures of receptive and expressive language, which may be helpful in assessing the child's language skills as applied in a classroom situation. At the same time, some of these may be redundant with similar tasks on language tests such as the CELF-5 (Semel, Wiig, & Secord, 2013). For example, many of the WIAT-III Oral Language tasks, such as repeating oral sentences, are shorter versions of CELF-5 subtests. If the child is being administered a language test as part of the assessment battery, administration of these language portions of the achievement test may be unnecessary.

Practical Considerations

For children with receptive language weaknesses but some reading ability, comprehension of verbal items on intelligence tests can be improved by providing the test items in print as well as orally. This accommodation provides a visual stimulus and makes the stimulus available to the student for a longer period of time, but the child still must comprehend the question, have the necessary information, and express the knowledge in words. Provision of items in print is best accomplished by presenting each test item on a separate index card (Sattler & Dumont, 2004). In certain cases, it may be helpful to test limits on verbal items by simplifying the wording of questions, although this is a modification that clearly changes the content of the test. Because the above practices deviate from standardization procedures, the validity of the obtained score will be affected to a greater or lesser degree. If the clinician is trying to gain an accurate comparison of the verbal abilities of the student with those of hearing peers (for example, to determine the child's readi-

ness to transition into a general education setting), standardized procedures must be followed. For a student with delayed language, however, these adaptations can provide some discrimination of whether the child's poor performance reflects language comprehension deficits versus deficits in acquired knowledge. They can also result in useful information about what kinds of accommodations (such as use of print) may be helpful to the child in the classroom.

ASSESSMENT OF ACADEMIC SKILLS

Individually-administered academic achievement tests allow an in-depth assessment of a student's acquired academic skills and abilities. Comprehensive academic achievement tests are typically organized around the domains delineated in the Individuals with Disabilities Education Act (IDEA): basic reading (word recognition and decoding), reading comprehension, math reasoning, math computation, written expression, and oral language. The most commonly used tests are conormed with cognitive tests (for example, the WIAT-III with the WISC-IV). This means that the intelligence test and the achievement test are normed on the same sample of test-takers, facilitating comparison of scores across the two measures.

Use of academic achievement tests allows a comparison of the child with hearing students of the same age or grade. Because the tests are individually administered, the evaluator is able to observe the child engaged in a variety of academic tasks, providing an assessment of key academic subskills, as described in Table 7–4. The clinician can also discern the impact

Table 7–4. Academic Subskills

Reading	Math	Written Expression
Phonemic awareness	Number sense	Sound–symbol association
Sound–symbol association	Quantitative reasoning	Graphomotor ability (printing/writing)
Decoding	Math facts	
Fluency	Math procedures	Spelling
Reading vocabulary	Math concepts	Capitalization and punctuation
Factual comprehension	Word problems	Written language structure
Inferential comprehension		Ideas and content

of language delay versus processing deficits, as well as the effects of attention, motivation, persistence, and so forth, on the child's performance. This deeper and more nuanced assessment of the child's reading, writing, and math skills can be used to pinpoint areas of specific deficit and allow an individualized and targeted approach to remediating specific skill deficits.

The choice of an academic achievement battery will depend on the referral question as well as the language proficiency of the child. In general, the closer the student is to being at age- and grade-expectation, the more standard the battery can be. For example, a student who is in a full-time LSL day program and is being considered for mainstreaming should be administered the achievement test conormed with the cognitive test used, without modifications or accommodations, in order to obtain a clear assessment of how this child's abilities compare with typical peers in a general education setting. On the other hand, students with language delays or who are suspected of having learning disabilities may require a more complex, cross-battery assessment in order to tease out issues of language

proficiency as well as academic strengths and weaknesses.

A central issue for clinicians in choosing appropriate tests for children with hearing loss is that of the item format of the test (Overton, 2006). Published tests use various formats for assessing skills and knowledge. Input format refers to the way the child is presented with the items. The input format may be visual (print and/or pictures) or auditory (the examiner asks a question or presents a verbal stimulus). Output format refers to the way the child is asked to respond. The child may be allowed to give a nonverbal response, such as pointing to a picture or word in print, or may be required to write or verbalize a response. The response may be a forced choice within a closed set of responses, or it may be open-ended. The student may be able to respond in one or a few words, or may be required to provide longer response. Test instructions themselves may contain complex language, or may use simple language and afford visual demonstration. For a child with a serious language delay, tests that are heavily language-loaded may not actually tap the skill or knowledge that the instrument is designed to test (i.e., memory, reading skill, math competence), but may rather primarily reflect the level of the child's acquired language.

For children whose delayed language affects reading and writing skills, the use of a diagnostic reading or written expression tests incorporated into one of the newer language tests such as the OWLS-II (Carrow-Woolfolk, 2012) or the CELF-5 (Semel et al., 2013) can be useful. These tests target the lexical/semantic, syntactic, supra-linguistic, and pragmatic aspects of reading and written expression and allow an analysis of how deficits in specific language areas are affecting literacy.

BEHAVIORAL ASSESSMENT

A complete understanding of a child with hearing loss often requires the use of one or more behavioral measures. Behavioral measures fall into three general categories: tests assessing general emotional and behavioral functioning; tests tapping attention, task focus, and executive functioning; and tests that assess adaptive skills. There is overlap, however, among the tests.

Behavioral tests are generally in the form of questionnaires designed to be completed by the child's teachers and parents. Self-report forms are available for children who have adequate reading skills, generally upper elementary and high school age. Potential problems with the use of behavioral inventories include inter-rater reliability and possible response bias (Reynolds, Livingston, & Willson, 2006). A well-developed test will include scales that assess whether the rater tended to either exaggerate or deny problems in the child, or was inconsistent in responding, indicating possible problems with the rater's comprehension of items. Best practices across all of these measures call for the tests to be completed by multiple observers in multiple settings (Barkley & Edwards, 2006; Reynolds et al., 2006). Thus, the child's behavior should be rated in the home as well as by several raters in the school environment, if possible. The clinician can have greater confidence in the results of testing when two or more sources of information are available and provide generally consistent ratings. When the use of multiple raters results in conflicting data, it is useful to resolve the differences, possibly by interviewing the raters. Questioning the informant about specific items can help determine whether differences are due to confusion or misunderstanding by the rater, to biased responding, or to a true difference in the child's behavior from one environment to another (Harrison & Oakland, 2003b).

Measures of General Behavior

General or "omnibus" behavior rating scales tap a broad range of emotional and behavior symptoms. They are sensitive to both internalizing problems such as anxiety and depression and externalizing problems such as hyperactivity and oppositional or aggressive behavior. Behavior rating scales are commonly used for clinical diagnosis and educational classification (Reynolds et al., 2006). However, they can also be useful in better understanding and managing behavioral issues in the classroom. For example, a child who presents with aggressive or oppositional behavior may be found to have underlying depression or anxiety.

The Behavior Assessment System for Children, 2nd Edition (BASC-2; Reynolds & Kamphaus, 2004) is a multimethod, multidimensional instrument used to evaluate behavior and self-perceptions of children and young adults ages 2 through 25 years. It includes parent and teacher rating scales, a self-report scale for older children and adolescents, a structured developmental history form, and a form for recording and classifying directly observed classroom behaviors. The BASC-2 includes items that tap both positive, adaptive behaviors and negative, problematic, or clinical behaviors. It yields quantitative composite scales, including adaptive skills, internalizing problems, externalizing problems, and school problems. The BASC-2 Manual states that it can be used to assess behavioral and emotional issues in children with sensory impairments such as hearing loss, but also asserts that the interpretation of test scores for these children requires specialized training and expertise.

The Achenbach System of Empirically Based Assessment (ASEBA; Achenbach, 2009) is a comprehensive system that assesses competencies, adaptive functioning, and behavioral, emotional, and social problems in individuals ages 1½ years through adulthood. There are forms for parents, caregivers, and teachers as well as a self-report form. The ASEBA is administered as paper-and-pencil behavioral inventories that yield quantitative scores. It also includes open-ended questions that offer opportunities for respondents to document their own concerns about the child as well as their perceptions of the child's strengths and weaknesses, providing information that may not be captured by quantitative scores alone. The ASEBA has been used in a number of clinical studies that involve children with hearing loss (see, for example, Barker et al., 2009; Vostanis, Hayes, Du Feu, & Warren, 1997).

Measures of Activity Level, Attention, and Executive Ability

Although general behavioral tests include scales that tap hyperactivity, impulsivity, and attention, tests that specifically assess for hyperactivity and attention deficit are often helpful in evaluating children for ADHD. The Conners 3rd Edition (Conners, 2008) is an assessment system that includes long and short forms for parents, teachers, and self-report. An early childhood version is also available. The Conners-3 includes quantitative scales that tap activity level, inattention, impulsivity, and executive function. There are also scales tapping associated problems such as family and peer relations, as well as scales tapping common comorbid disorders, including conduct disorder and oppositional defiant disorder.

Increasingly seen as associated with ADHD, executive skills are defined as those abilities that allow people to regulate behavior in order to solve problems and complete tasks, including planning, organization, time management, working memory, and metacognition (Dawson & Guare, 2010). These skills are typically impaired in individuals with ADHD, although some research has found that children with hearing loss also tend to be delayed in developing executive skills (Hauser, Lukomski, & Hillman, 2008). The Behavior Rating Inventory of Executive Function (BRIEF; Gioia, Isquith, & Kenworthy, 2000) is a behavioral inventory that taps executive skills, including behavioral regulation skills (such as emotional control and inhibition) and metacognitive skills (i.e., planning and organization, organization of materials, task initiation, working memory, and self-monitoring). Forms are available for parents and teachers, and there is a preschool version.

Measures of Adaptive Behavior

Adaptive behavior is defined as those age-appropriate skills necessary for people to live independently and to function safely and appropriately in daily life. Adaptive behavior assessed by common tests include practical and self-help skills; ability to follow home and school rules and routines; behaviors affecting health and safety; communication and social skills; and self-direction, including emotional self-regulation and ability to engage in goal-directed behavior. At younger ages, motor skills may be tapped; for adolescents and adults, work-related skills are assessed. Children with sensory impairments, language and learning impairments, ADHD, and intellectual disabilities may all demonstrate some degree of impairment in adaptive behavior skills (Harrison & Oakland, 2003b). Adaptive behavior scales can be used for diagnosis, for assessment of strengths and limitations, and to document and monitor an individual's progress over time.

In assessing the adaptive behavior of children with hearing loss, it is important to determine the degree to which items are influenced by the language proficiency of the child. While adaptive behavior scales typically include subtests that specifically tap communication skills, some items in other scales may also require language ability. For example, an item under "com-munity use" may ask if the child can provide his or her address or follow directions to a nearby place. An item under "social skills" may ask if the child can name three classmates, state whether he or she is happy or sad, or apologize when he or she has hurt someone. Thus, for a child with limited language, a low score in one of these domains may reflect the language delay rather than a true weakness in the named domain. When a child with hearing loss receives low scores on an adaptive behavior scale, the clinician is encouraged to examine the individual items, following up with the rater if necessary, in order to determine to what degree the low score reflects language delay versus true limitations in a given domain.

The Adaptive Behavior Assessment System, 2nd Edition (ABAS-II; Harrison & Oakland, 2003a) is a comprehensive, multi-informant, norm-referenced assessment of adaptive skills for individuals ages birth through 89 years. The ABAS-II is a behavioral inventory with forms for parents, teachers, and adults. Some preliminary data exists regarding use with children with hearing loss. The performance of a sample of 19 deaf and hard of hearing children was compared with a matched control (Harrison & Oakland, 2003b). The authors draw the conclusion that children with hearing loss do not demonstrate major deficits in adaptive behavior as measured by the ABAS-II, but they may exhibit slightly lower adaptive functioning as well as deficits in specific skill areas such as communication.

The Vineland Adaptive Behavior Scales, 2nd Edition (Vineland-II; Sparrow, Ciccheti, & Balla, 2005) is a multimodal and multi-informant, norm-referenced assessment of adaptive behavior. While the Vineland-II, like the earlier editions, includes survey and expanded interview forms that are administered in a semistructured interview format with a parent or caregiver, it also includes parent/caregiver and teacher rating forms.

SPECIFIC DIAGNOSTIC ISSUES

Intellectual Disability

Diagnosis of intellectual disability in children with hearing loss can be a challenging task, particularly when the child is preschool age. In order to be diagnosed with an intellectual disability, a child must exhibit very significant deficits (greater than two standard deviations below the mean) in cognitive functioning, as well as significant deficits in two or more areas of adaptive behavior (American Psychiatric Association, 2013; Schalock, Borthwick-Duffy, Buntinx, Coulter, & Craig, 2010). For the child with a hearing loss, inappropriate interpretation of intelligence test scores, in particular using IQ scores that incorporate verbal skills, can result in erroneous diagnoses. In addition, even when the verbal score is discounted as a measure of intelligence, a child's nonverbal cognitive score can be depressed by a number of factors, including fine motor weakness, specific visual processing deficits, slow processing, and deficits in attention and task focus. These factors can be more pronounced in very young children who may have limited exposure to school-like tasks, immature self-regulation skills, and delayed communication skills.

For the above reasons, cognitive assessment of a child with hearing loss suspected of intellectual disability should include multiple cognitive measures, including a nonverbal intelligence test. A full scale IQ that includes verbal subtests should never be used as a measure of intellectual ability. It is important that the test used have an adequate "floor," that is, a sufficient number of items at the lower levels of the test such that a reliable discrimination can be made. When clinicians are using the Wechsler tests, children ages 6;0 to 7;11 who are suspected of having cognitive limitations should be administered the WPPSI-IV rather than the WISC-IV. As noted in a previous section, scores on adaptive behavior tests require careful interpretation in order to ensure the child's observed adaptive deficits are not primarily reflective of language delay.

In general, functioning across areas tends to be fairly uniformly depressed in children with intellectual disabilities (Flanagan & Kaufman, 2009), while a pattern of inter-subtest scatter, with some scores at or near age-expectancy and other scores well below expectation, will throw a diagnosis of intellectual deficiency into doubt. Consistent test results across multiple measures as well as across time lend confidence to obtained scores.

Learning Disability

The diagnosis of learning disabilities in children with hearing loss is a complex topic that is beyond the scope of the present chapter, but some comments may be helpful. Flanagan and Mascolo (2005) state best practice for all children in the diagnosis of learning disabilities currently involves the use of both Response to Intervention (RTI) and the Pattern of Strengths and Weaknesses Model (PSW). The older Discrepancy Model, however, is still sometimes used. The Discrepancy Model compares a student's cognitive ability as measured by the full scale IQ score to the student's skills in a specific academic area (for example, mathematics) as measured by an academic test. If the student's achievement test score is lower than the full scale IQ score by a predetermined number, usually one to 1½ standard deviations, the student can be diagnosed with a learning disability in that area. The Discrepancy Model, however, is difficult to apply with children with hearing loss because the full scale IQ cannot be considered an accurate measure of the student's cognitive potential. Furthermore, the nonverbal IQ score for a child with a processing deficit in a given area, such as visual-spatial reasoning, may also be compromised. For example, a child who has difficulty in math may also earn a lower nonverbal IQ score due to weakness in visual-spatial skills, resulting in a minimal ability-achievement discrepancy that might erroneously be interpreted as a lack of evidence for a learning disability.

Some score profiles commonly seen in children with hearing loss can be diagnostic. A child who has a language delay attributable to hearing loss but no other processing issues will, in an appropriate education setting, typically be able to acquire the mechanics of academic skills but will struggle in academic areas that require language. Thus, the student will demonstrate adequate skills in the areas of phonics and word recognition, math computation, and written language mechanics such as letter formation, capitalization, and punctuation. However, reading vocabulary may be limited and the student will struggle with literal and especially inferential comprehension. In math, he or she is likely to have difficulty with math concepts and especially word

problems. In writing, the student will exhibit problems with syntax and grammar as well as poor elaboration (Geers & Hayes, 2011). In contrast, a child with hearing loss who also has processing deficits or learning disabilities is likely to exhibit deficits in mechanics that are not attributable to language delay, such as sound-symbol association, grapho-motor skills, math computation, and retention and recall of previously learned skills and information.

Error analysis can be an important tool in interpreting the results of academic testing. The evaluator examines the incorrect responses of the student in an effort to determine where the breakdown occurred: Did the child appear to have the requisite information but have difficulty expressing the information coherently? Did the child's math errors reflect a lack of automaticity with math facts, a tendency to make careless errors, or with lack of acquisition of procedures such as regrouping? Table 7–5 demonstrates how analysis of students' spelling errors may lead to hypotheses about the nature of their difficulties.

COMMUNICATING RESULTS

The psychoeducational report is an essential vehicle for documenting and communicating the results of a psychoeducational evaluation. The task of the psychologist in writing the document is complex, as readers are likely to be diverse, including other psychologists, clinicians such as physicians or speech-language pathologists, teachers, and parents, who all have differing degrees of sophistication and knowledge. A comprehensive psy-

Table 7–5. Analysis of Spelling Errors

Type of Error	Example	Possible Interpretation
"Typical" errors	"ruff" for rough	Child is spelling word phonetically, shows adequate phonetic knowledge
	"rideing" for riding	Child is not applying spelling rule
Errors indicating possible processing weakness	"bog" for dog	Possible orthographic error—child reverses d and b
	"guass" for guess	Possible phonics error; child may have inadequate sound-symbol association
Errors specific to hearing loss	"sharsh" for charge	Possible auditory discrimination error; child may not be hearing word adequately
	"chart" for charge	Possible lexical/semantic error; child may be unfamiliar with the word and substituting a similar, familiar word

choeducational report will summarize background information as well as any previous test results. It should provide behavioral observations and a description of any adaptations or modifications in standardized test administration. It is helpful to provide results in both a tabular summary of test scores, which may be useful to other clinicians, and a narrative interpretation of scores that is understandable to nonprofessionals. A discussion of how the child's hearing loss and language delay, if any, affects the results is particularly useful for educating professionals who may not be familiar with this population. The conclusions section should integrate current and past results, discuss the child's strengths as well as areas of concern, and provide diagnostic impressions, if applicable. A useful report offers broad recommendations for further evaluation and/or services, as well as specific practical recommendations for therapists and teachers.

In addition to a written report, the psychologist generally provides verbal feedback to parents. This is a valuable opportunity to further interpret and clar-ify evaluation results, resolve misunderstanding, and answer questions. Tact and sensitivity are required when there is the possibility of a new diagnosis in addition to the hearing loss. Some parents may suspect their child is struggling with additional issues and welcome confirmation of their suspicions. For other parents, however, the diagnosis of a second problem is a significant emotional blow that may be challenging to accept (Edwards, 2007). Parents may react with denial, anger, or anxiety, and unresolved mourning issues around the original hearing loss may present themselves. The clinician must be ready to respond with patience, empathy, and understanding in order to assist the parents in the process of accepting the additional diagnosis and acting to meet the needs of their child.

Although psychologists less frequently provide feedback directly to students, a discussion of the evaluation results can be a valuable experience for the child who has adequate communication skills. Talking with students about their strengths and weaknesses can actually normalize and destigmatize areas of struggle, putting borders around the areas of difficulty. Students with greater self-knowledge have improved ability to advocate for themselves (Pohlman, 2008). With students with hearing loss, it can be useful to employ visuals and print in this process. Rather than attempting to provide an exhaustive account of the evaluation, it can be more effective to focus on a few key points that are easily understandable to the student, keeping the explanation simple and clear and checking frequently for comprehension.

SUMMARY

This chapter explained the process of psychoeducational evaluation of children with hearing loss, with an emphasis on children who use LSL as their method of communication. Although issues related to the use of sign language are not relevant for this population as they may be with other students with hearing loss, language proficiency is still a crucial focus in evaluating these students. The central challenge for the psychologist in performing psychoeducational evaluation for this population lies in determining to what degree the child's struggles reflect language delay secondary to the hearing loss, and to what degree the problems may reflect comorbid disorders. This question will affect choice of tests, test administration, and interpretation of results. With an adequate grasp of the issues involved in hearing loss, cochlear implants, and language acquisition, as well as an understanding of how these interact with other processing and behavioral issues, the psychologist will be able to provide assessments that are useful in

understanding the child as an individual and a learner, supporting the child in the educational setting, and helping the child to be successful.

CASE STUDIES

Kris (Intellectual Disability)

Kris was born 6 weeks premature and experienced severe neonatal complications. She spent one month in the newborn intensive care unit, during which time she was on a respirator and received ototoxic medication. Kris has cerebral palsy. She did not walk until she was 3 years old and continues to demonstrate gross and fine motor weakness. At 3 months of age she was diagnosed with a profound hearing loss and was fitted with hearing aids. She received a cochlear implant when she was 5 years old. Although Kris initially received early childhood services through an LSL early childhood program, after the age of 3 years, she attended rural public schools, with inconsistent services and communication modalities.

Kris was administered a psychoeducational battery in her home school when she was 6 years old. Administration of the WISC-IV resulted in a nonverbal score in the borderline range, with reported verbal and full scale scores in the severely delayed range, below the 1st percentile. An adaptive behavior measure yielded similar scores, and Kris' academic skills were found to be at or below the kindergarten level. Based on the Full Scale WISC-IV and adaptive behavior scores, Kris was given a diagnosis of multiple disabilities, including hearing loss and intellectual disability. Her home school recommended placement at the State School for the Deaf, where she would learn American Sign Language (ASL). However, Kris' parents did not agree that Kris was intellectually limited and they requested an independent evaluation.

When Kris was seen for the independent evaluation, she presented as a friendly, spunky little girl with an engaging sense of humor. Testing with the WISC-IV was seen as inappropriate due to the motor demands and timed nature of some of the subtests. Evaluation with a nonverbal intelligence test with minimal motor demands resulted in a measured IQ in the low average range, which was seen as a more accurate and appropriate estimate of Kris' intellectual potential than the previous WISC-IV Full Scale IQ. Administration of an adaptive behavior measure resulted in a low score in the area of conceptual abilities, reflecting language and academic delays, but Kris' practical and social skills scored at the lower limits of the average range. Kris' academic delays were seen as reflecting, to a large degree, lack of access to instruction due to her language delay.

Kris was enrolled in a full-time LSL day program. With consistent and intensive speech and listening services, she began making steady growth in audition and language acquisition. Oral motor weakness has limited her speech, but her receptive language skills are relatively well developed. Intensive teaching of academics in a small-group setting helped her to develop literacy and math skills. Although both Kris' language and academic skills continue to be delayed when she is compared with typical peers, she is expected to transition into a mainstream school with resource room assistance for middle school.

Tracy (Language Weakness in a Mainstreamed Student)

Tracy was initially seen for evaluation when she was 10 years old. Tracy has a progressive hearing loss and used hearing aids until she was 5½ years old, when she received a cochlear implant. She had consistent LSL early childhood services, attended a self-contained hearing-impaired classroom in kindergarten, and was mainstreamed in first grade. She began to struggle in the mainstream in 3rd grade, repeated 4th grade, and at the time of the evaluation had services that included a teacher's aide in the classroom, regular sessions with an itinerant teacher of the hearing impaired, twice weekly speech/language therapy, and academic tutoring, but was still struggling. Tracy's mother described her as being "burned out and frustrated" in school.

Tracy presented as an attractive, sociable youngster who demonstrated intelligible speech and good conversational skills. Evaluation indicated she was functioning in the average to above-average range of nonverbal intellectual functioning. There was no evidence of processing deficits in memory, visual functioning, or attention and task focus. Tracy demonstrated a strong language base and good basic communication skills. However, her academic language skills scored significantly lower than her nonverbal ability, and she was found to be weak in vocabulary, receptive and expressive discourse, and the ability to use higher level conjunctions. Her academic mechanics—reading decoding, math computation, spelling—were well-developed, but her reading comprehension was weak and she had difficulty with word problems in math. She performed poorly on classroom tests, and her written expression tended to be simple and limited in content. The assessment team concluded that Tracy's language skills were not adequate to access curriculum in a general education setting as she moved into the middle grades.

Tracy attended an LSL day school for 3 years, with an intensive focus on developing vocabulary, higher-level oral language, reading comprehension, and oral and written discourse. At the end of the third year, psychoeducational evaluation indicated that Tracy's academic language skills and vocabulary were now at or close to age-expectancy. All of her academic skills, including reading comprehension, written expression, and math reasoning, scored within normal limits for her grade level, and she had developed greater self-confidence and poise. Tracy was able to successfully transition back into her home school district with minimal support. She is currently attending college.

Mack (ADHD and Behavior)

Mack is a funny, animated 9-year-old boy with red hair and freckles. He was born 5 weeks premature but did not experience any severe neonatal complications. Mack was diagnosed with a profound hearing loss at 11 months, was fitted with hearing aids, and received a cochlear implant shortly thereafter. He received LSL early child services but transitioned into a public school early childhood special education program at age three. Mack's parents felt that his progress slowed after he was placed in the cross-categorical classroom, and they sought placement in an LSL day program when he was 5 years old. In the LSL program, Mack was described as a cheerful and sociable little boy, but he also displayed very frequent explosive

and disruptive behavior in the classroom that affected his availability for learning. He also exhibited a high activity level, impulsivity, and difficulty staying on task. Psychoeducational evaluation indicated that Mack's nonverbal intellectual ability was in the average range. He was a talkative child who demonstrated good pragmatic language and conversational skills, but it was discovered that his language skills were not as well developed as casual interaction would suggest. Behavioral evaluation indicated the presence of ADHD. Mack was also found to have significant deficits in visual-motor integration and graphomotor skills. His emotional breakdowns in the classroom were seen as reflecting impulsivity and deficits in self-regulation, as well as having the function of avoidance of frustrating activities such as writing. Mack was diagnosed with ADHD by his pediatrician and began taking stimulant medication with good benefit. Strategies to address his behavioral problems as well as to improve his attentional skills were implemented in the classroom. Mack's language and academic skills have shown excellent growth over time, and he has developed a strong interest in music and a real talent in dramatic performance.

Jeremy (Learning Disability)

Jeremy is a 7-year-old boy whose hearing loss was discovered in a newborn screening. He received his first cochlear implant at 15 months and a second, bilateral implant 2 years later. Jeremy received early childhood services in an LSL program and transitioned into a kindergarten program in his neighborhood public school, while continuing to receive speech and language therapy outside the school day. Jeremy's teacher and speech therapist reported that Jeremy was a motivated child who worked hard and was eager to participate in the classroom and in individual therapy sessions. Even so, Jeremy's progress in acquiring academic skills was slow, and he was functioning far below grade level in reading, writing, and math. Evaluation was sought to determine the cause of his delays.

Results of psychoeducational evaluation indicated that Jeremy was a child of average intellectual potential who was able to use thinking skills to solve visually presented problems. His language skills were seen as adequate to support him in the general education classroom. However, Jeremy demonstrated processing deficits that were seen as having a negative impact on his ability to acquire academic skills. Jeremy was found to have very significant weakness in working memory. He had difficulty holding information in mind, storing it in long-term memory, and retrieving it. Jeremy's visual-spatial skills were also found to be weak. He demonstrated problems with the integration and synthesis of part-whole relationships as well as directionality. These weaknesses resulted in Jeremy struggling to perceive, learn, and reproduce visual symbols such as letters, numerals, and mathematical symbols. The combination of limitations in both visual-spatial processing and working memory were seen as affecting phonemic awareness and sound-symbol association in reading.

The psychoeducational evaluation recommended that Jeremy receive special education services through his public school to address his weaknesses in early reading and math skills. Specific recommendations were made for helping his teacher address Jeremy's learning issues in the mainstream classroom. In addition, his parents elected to pursue private tutoring with a reading specialist. With these interventions, Jeremy is making rapid progress in developing reading and math skills.

REFERENCES

Achenbach, T. M. (2009). *The Achenbach System of Empirically Based Assessment (ASEBA): Development, findings, theory, and applications*. Burlington, VT: University of Vermont Research Center for Children, Youth, and Families.

Akamatsu, C. T., Mayer, C., & Hardy-Braz, S. (2008). Why considerations of verbal aptitude are important in educating deaf and hard-of-hearing students. In M. Marschark & P. C. Hauser (Eds.), *Deaf cognition: Foundations and outcomes* (pp. 131–169). New York, NY: Oxford University Press.

American Psychiatric Association. (2013). *Diagnostic and statistical manual of mental disorders* (5th ed.). Washington, DC: Author.

American Psychological Association. (2010). *Ethical principles of psychologists and code of conduct*. Retrieved November 26, 2013, from http://www.apa.org/ethics/code/index.aspx

Barker, D. H., Quittner, A. L., Fink, N. E., Eisenberg, L. S., Tobey, E. A., & Niparko, J. K. (2009). Predicting behavior problems in deaf and hearing children: The influences of language, attention, and parent-child communication. *Development and Psychopathology, 21*(2), 373–392. doi:10.1017/S0954579409000212

Barkley, R. A., & Edwards, G. (2006). Diagnostic interview, behavior rating scales, and the medical examination. In R. A. Barkley (Ed.), *Attention-deficit hyperactivity disorder: A handbook for diagnosis and treatment* (3rd ed.). New York, NY: Guilford Press.

Beery, K. E., Buktenica, N. A., & Beery, N. (2010). *Beery-Buktenika test of visual-motor integration* (6th ed.). San Antonio, TX: Pearson Education.

Bracken, B. A., & McCallum, R. S. (1998). *Universal test of nonverbal intelligence*. Rolling Meadows, IL: Riverside.

Braden, J. P. (2005). Hard of hearing and deaf clients: Using the WISC-IV with clients who are hard of hearing or deaf. In A. Prifitera, D.

H. Saklofske, & L. G. Weiss (Eds.), *WISC-IV: Clinical use and interpretation, scientist-practitioner perspectives* (pp. 351–380). London, UK: Elsevier Press.

Braden, J. P., & Athonasiou, M. S. (2005). A comparative review of nonverbal measures of intelligence. In D. P. Flanagan & P. L. Harrison (Eds.), *Contemporary intellectual assessment: Theories, tests, and issues*. New York, NY: Guilford Press.

Carrow-Woolfolk, E. (2012). *Oral and Written Language Scales* (2nd ed.). Austin, TX: Pro-Ed.

Case, B. J. (2008). *Policy report: Accommodations to improve instruction and assessment of students who are deaf or hard of hearing* [Policy report]. San Antonio, TX: Pearson Education. Retrieved from http://images.pearsonassessments.com/images/tmrs/tmrs_rg/Deaf.pdf?WT.mc_id=TMRS_Accommodations_for_the_Deaf

Cohen, M. (1997). *Children's Memory Scale*. San Antonio, TX: Pearson Education.

Conners, C. K. (2008). *Conners 3rd Edition*. North Tonawanda, NY: Multi-Health Systems.

Cummins, J. (2008). BICS and CALP: Empirical and theoretical status of the distinction. In N. H. Hornberger (Ed.), *Encyclopedia of language and education* (pp. 487–499). New York, NY: Springer. Retrieved from http://link.springer.com/referenceworkentry/10.1007/978-0-387-30424-3_36

Dawson, P., & Guare, R. (2010). *Executive skills in children and adolescents: A practical guide to assessment and intervention*. New York, NY: Guilford Press.

Dornan, D., Hickson, L., Murdoch, B., Houston, T., & Constantinescu, G. (2010). Is auditory-verbal therapy effective for children with hearing loss? *Volta Review, 110*(3), 361–387.

Edwards, L. C. (2007). Children with cochlear implants and complex needs: A review of outcome research and psychological practice. *Journal of Deaf Studies and Deaf Education, 12*(3), 258–268. doi:10.1093/deafed/enm007

Flanagan, D. P., & Kaufman, A. S. (2009). *Essentials of WISC-IV assessment* (2nd ed.). Hoboken, NJ: John Wiley and Sons.

Flanagan, D. P., & Mascolo, J. T. (2005). Psychoeducational assessment and learning disability diagnosis. In D. P. Flanagan & P. L. Harrison (Eds.), *Contemporary intellectual assessment: Theories, tests, and issues* (pp. 521–544). New York, NY: Guilford Press.

Geers, A. (2006). Factors influencing spoken language outcomes in children following early cochlear implantation. *Advanced Otorhinolaryngology, 64*, 50–65.

Geers, A. E., & Hayes, H. (2011). Reading, writing, and phonological processing skills of adolescents with 10 or more years of cochlear implant experience. *Ear and Hearing, 32*(Suppl. 1), 49S–59S. doi:10.1097/AUD.0b013e3181fa41fa

Geers, A. E., & Sedey, A. L. (2011). Language and verbal reasoning skills in adolescents with 10 or more years of cochlear implant experience. *Ear and Hearing, 32*(Suppl. 1), 39S–48S. doi:10.1097/AUD.0b013e3181fa41dc

Gioia, G., Isquith, P., & Kenworthy, L. (2000). *Behavior rating inventory of executive function*. Lutz, FL: Psychological Assessment Resources.

Hammill, D. D., Pearson, N. A., & Wiederholt, J. L. (2009). *Comprehensive Test of Nonverbal Intelligence* (2nd ed.). Austin, TX: Pro-Ed.

Harrison, P. L., & Oakland, T. (2003a). *Adaptive Behavior System* (2nd ed.). San Antonio, TX: Harcourt Assessment.

Harrison, P. L., & Oakland, T. (2003b). *Manual for the adaptive behavior system* (2nd ed.). San Antonio, TX: Harcourt Assessment.

Hauser, P. C., Lukomski, J., & Hillman, T. (2008). Development of deaf and hard of hearing students' executive function. In M. Marschark & P. C. Hauser (Eds.), *Deaf cognition: Foundations and outcomes* (pp. 286–307). New York, NY: Oxford University Press.

Horn, J. L., & Cattell, R. B. (1966). Refinement and test of the theory of fluid and crystallized general intelligences. *Journal of Educational Psychology, 57*(5), 253–270. doi:10.1037/h0023816

Kaufman, A. S., & Kaufman, N. L. (2004). *Kaufman Assessment Battery for Children* (2nd ed.). Circle Pines, MN: AGS.

Kaufman, J. C., Kaufman, A. S., Kaufman-Singer, J., & Kaufman, N. L. (2005). The Kaufman Assessment Battery for Children (2nd ed.) and the Kaufman Adolescent and Adult Intelligence Scale. In D. P. Flanagan & P. L. Harrison (Eds.), *Contemporary intellectual assessment: Theories, rests, and issues* (2nd ed.). New York, NY: Guilford Press.

Kennedy, C. R., McCann, D. C., Campbell, M. J., Law, C. M., Mullee, M., Petrou, S., . . . Stevenson, J. (2006). Language ability after early detection of permanent childhood hearing impairment. *New England Journal of Medicine, 354*(20), 2131–2141.

Krouse, H. E., & Braden, J. P. (2011). The reliability and validity of WISC-IV scores with deaf and hard-of-hearing children. *Journal of Psychoeducational Assessment, 29*(3), 238–248. doi:10.1177/0734282910383646

McGrew, K. S. (2005). The Cattell-Horn-Carrol Theory of Cognitive Abilities: Past, present, and future. In D. P. Flanagan & P. L. Harrison (Eds.), *Contemporary intellectual assessment: Theories, tests, and issues* (2nd ed.). New York, NY: Guilford Press.

Metz, K., Miller, M., & Thomas-Presswood, T. N. (2010). Assessing children who are deaf or hard of hearing. In D. C. Miller (Ed.), *Best practices in school neuropsychology: Guidelines for effective practice, assessment, and evidence-based intervention.* New York, NY: John Wiley and Sons.

Moeller, M. P. (2000). Early intervention and language development in children who are deaf and hard of hearing. *Pediatrics, 106,* E43.

Niparko, J. K., Tobey, E. A., Thal, D. J., Eisenberg, L. S., Nae-Yuh, W., Quittner, A. L., & Fink, N. E. (2010). Spoken language development in children following cochlear implantation. *Journal of the American Medical Association, 303*(15), 1498–1506.

Overton, T. (2006). *Assessing learners with special needs: An applied approach* (5th ed.). Upper Saddle River, NJ: Pearson Education.

Pisoni, D. B., Conway, C. M., Kronenberger, W. G., Horn, D. L., Kapicke, J., & Henning, S. C. (2008). Efficacy and effectiveness of cochlear implants in deaf children. In M. Marschark & P. C. Hauser (Eds.), *Deaf cognition: Foundations and outcomes* (pp. 52–101). New York, NY: Oxford University Press.

Pohlman, C. (2008). *Revealing minds: Assessing to understand and support struggling learners.* San Francisco, CA: Jossey Bass.

Reynolds, C. R., & Kamphaus, R. W. (2004). *Behavior assessment system for children* (2nd ed.). Circle Pines, MN: AGS.

Reynolds, C. R., Livingston, R. B., & Willson, V. (2006). *Measurement and assessment in education.* Boston, MA: Pearson Education.

Roid, G. H. (2003). *Stanford-Binet Intelligence Scales* (5th ed.). Itasca, IL: Riverside.

Roid, G. H., & Pomplun, M. (2005). Interpreting the Stanford-Binet Intelligence Scales, 5th ed. In D. P. Flanagan & P. L. Harrison (Eds.), *Con-*

temporary intellectual assessment: Theories, tests, and issues (2nd ed.). New York, NY: Guilford Press.

Roid, G. H., Pomplun, M., & Koch, C. (2013). *Leiter-International Performance Scale* (3rd ed.). Wood Dale, IL: Stoelting.

Sattler, J. M., & Dumont, R. (2004). *Assessment of children: WISC-IV and WPPSI-III supplement.* La Mesa, CA: Jerome M. Sattler.

Sattler, J. M., & Hardy-Braz, S. (2002). Hearing impairments. In J. M. Sattler (Ed.), *Assessment of children: Behavioral and clinical applications* (4th ed., pp. 377–389). La Mesa, CA: Jerome M. Sattler.

Schalock, R. L., Borthwick-Duffy, S. A., Buntinx, W. H. E., Coulter, D. L., & Craig, E. M. (2010). *Intellectual disability: Definition, classification, and systems of support* (11th ed.). Washington, DC: American Association on Intellectual and Developmental Disabilities.

Schrank, F. A. (2005). Woodcock-Johnson III Tests of Cognitive Ability. In D. P. Flanagan & P. L. Harrison (Eds.), *Contemporary intellectual assessment: Theories, tests, and issues* (2nd ed.). New York, NY: Guilford Press.

Semel, E., Wiig, E. H., & Secord, W. (2013). *Clinical Evaluation of Language Fundamentals* (5th ed.). San Antonio. TX: Pearson.

Simeonsson, R. J., Wax, T. M., & White, K. (2001). Assessment of children who are deaf or hard of hearing. In R. J. Simeonsson & S. L. Rosenthal (Eds.), *Psychological and developmental assessment: Children with disabilities and chronic conditions* (pp. 248–266). New York, NY: Guilford Press.

Sparrow, S. S., Ciccheti, D. V., & Balla, D.A. (2005). *Vineland Adaptive Behavior Scales* (2nd ed.). Circle Pines, MN: AGS.

Vostanis, P., Hayes, M., Du Feu, M., & Warren, J. (1997). Detection of behavioural and emotional problems in deaf children and adolescents: Comparison of two rating scales. *Child: Care, Health and Development, 23*(3), 233–246. doi:10.1111/j.1365-2214.1997.tb00966.x

Wagner, R., Torgesen, J., Rachotte, C., & Pearson, N. (1999). *Comprehensive Test of Phonological Processing.* Austin, TX: Pro-Ed.

Wechsler, D. (2003a). *Wechsler Intelligence Scale for Children* (4th ed.). San Antonio, TX: Pearson.

Wechsler, D. (2003b). *Wechsler Intelligence Scale for Children, 4th Edition: Administration and scoring manual.* San Antonio, TX: Pearson.

Wechsler, D. (2008). *Wechsler Adult Intelligence Scale* (4th ed.). San Antonio, TX: Pearson.

Wechsler, D. (2013). *Wechsler Preschool and Primary Scale of Intelligence* (4th ed.). San Antonio, TX: Pearson.

Wechsler, D., & Naglieri, J. A. (2006). *Wechsler Nonverbal Scale of Intelligence*. San Antonio, TX: Pearson Education.

Woodcock, R. W., McGrew, K. S., & Mather, N. (2001). *Woodcock-Johnson* (3rd ed.). Itasca, IL: Riverside.

Yoshinaga-Itano, C., & Gravel, J. S. (2001). The evidence for universal hearing screening. *American Journal of Audiology, 10*(2), 62–63.

Yoshinaga-Itano, C., Sedey, A. L., Coutler, D. K., & Mehl, A. L. (1998). Language of early- and later-identified children with hearing loss. *Pediatrics, 102,* 1161–1171.

CHAPTER 8

Literacy Assessment

Krystal L. Werfel

KEY POINTS

- Literacy outcomes for children with hearing loss as a group continue to lag behind peers with normal hearing, despite advances in amplification technology.
- Literacy consists of emergent literacy, word-level literacy, and text-level literacy skills.
- Literacy deficits can be seen in individuals or across domains of literacy.
- A problem-solving approach to literacy assessment provides detailed information about an individual's needs for literacy interventions, effectiveness of specific literacy interventions, and impacts of interventions on general literacy skills.
- Literacy assessment should include both normative comparisons and progress monitoring.

INTRODUCTION

Children with hearing loss have notoriously poor literacy achievement. Although there is wide individual variability in reading and writing outcomes in the population, the average reading level for 18-year-olds with hearing loss is roughly 3rd grade, and this achievement level has been remarkably consistent since the 1970s (Qi & Mitchell, 2012). This finding is particularly alarming in light of technological advances in amplification, including digital hearing aids and cochlear implants. Although a small group of children who received cochlear implants prior to age 2 have demonstrated reading outcomes that fall within the range of normal, professionals have noted that access to sound at an early age does not guarantee successful literacy development (Geers & Hayes, 2011). Given such poor average outcomes for children with hearing loss, it is vital to appropriately assess literacy, as well as emergent literacy skills, including both normative comparisons and progress monitoring. This chapter details a problem-solving approach to literacy assessment for children with hearing loss.

LITERACY ACHIEVEMENT

Attaining proficient literacy achievement requires one to use a complex system of knowledge and skills across a variety of linguistic domains. Skilled reading involves fluent word recognition and comprehension of text meaning (Scarborough, 2001), and skilled writing involves sufficient planning, fluent transcription of ideas to text, and adequate reviewing of the written product (Flower & Hayes, 1981). Scarborough (2001) presented a model that includes many linguistic skills, including vocabulary, syntax, phonological awareness, and others, intertwined to support skilled reading. Likewise, Flower and Hayes' (1981) model of skilled writing includes many linguistic (e.g., syntax, spelling) as well as cognitive (e.g., organizing, self-monitoring) processes. Indeed, research over the past several decades has supported the linguistic basis of literacy (e.g., Apel, Fowler-Wilson, Brimo, & Perrin, 2012; Carlisle, 2000; Catts, Fey, Zhang, & Tomblin, 1999; NELP, 2008).

Clearly, children do not simply enter formal schooling and immediately learn to read. Instead the process of attaining proficient literacy achievement extends over the schooling years and beyond. To effectively select literacy assessments that are developmentally appropriate for individual children, it is necessary to understand the levels of literacy achievement. These levels of literacy knowledge do not represent a stage model of literacy acquisition, in which children master skills in a lower level before moving to the next. Rather, the levels represent specific literacy tasks. Table 8–1 displays descriptions and examples of each level.

Emergent Literacy

Emergent literacy widely is thought of as the body of knowledge and skills that are precursors to later reading and writing (Whitehurst & Lonigan, 1998). Emergent literacy consists of three broad categories: **oral language** (e.g., vocabulary, morphology, syntax), **phonological processing** (e.g., phonological awareness, **phonological memory,** and **phonological recoding**), and **print knowledge** (e.g., alphabet knowledge, print concepts, written word concepts; Snow, Burns, & Griffin, 1998). As such, most have assigned emergent literacy to the preschool years, when one

Table 8–1. Levels of Literacy Achievement

Level	Description	Examples of Skills to Assess
Emergent	Language skills that are foundational to reading and writing	Vocabulary Syntax Phonological awareness Letter Names/Sounds Print Concepts
Word-Level	Literacy skills involving single words	Automatic Word Recognition Decoding Spelling
Text-Level	Literacy skills involving connected text	Reading Fluency Reading Comprehension Written Expression

is developing oral language, phonological awareness, and foundational print knowledge that will support word-level literacy in the early grades, and text-level literacy achievement during later school years. Emergent literacy indeed does encompass the majority of literacy achievement during the preschool years; however, these emergent literacy skills (that is, oral language, phonological processing, and print knowledge) continue to support reading and writing throughout the process of literacy acquisition (e.g., Apel et al., 2012; Berninger et al., 1992; Werfel, 2012). Figure 8–1 illustrates these differing approaches to thinking about the role of emergent literacy in literacy acquisition.

In terms of assessment, we must put aside the notion that emergent literacy skills lessen in importance after the onset of formal literacy instruction. We must continue to identify, develop, and

use assessments of these foundational literacy skills that are developmentally appropriate for school-age children and adolescents. There is much evidence in reading and growing evidence in writing that emergent literacy skills underlie literacy achievement throughout acquisition (Apel et al., 2012; Berninger, Mizokawa, & Bragg, 1991; Carlisle, 2000; Catts et al., 1999; Werfel, 2012). To provide the most effective instruction and intervention, it is extremely important to continue assessing emergent literacy skills with literacy in mind beyond preschool.

Children with hearing loss, including those who are developing spoken language, exhibit difficulties across many emergent literacy skills. (For a detailed review, see Moeller, Tomblin, Yoshinaga-Itano, Connor, & Jerger, 2007.) Oral language skills for children with hearing loss are poorer than their peers with normal

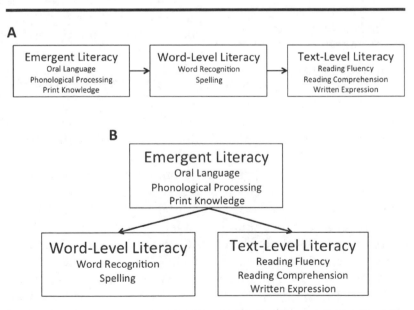

Figure 8–1. Differing views of the role of emergent literacy. **A.** Emergent literacy skills are precursors to later word- and text-level literacy. **B.** Emergent literacy skills are foundational to word- and text-level literacy throughout acquisition.

hearing in vocabulary (Pittman, Lewis, Hoover, & Stelmachowicz, 2005; Wake, Poulakis, Hughes, Carey-Sargeant, & Rickards, 2005), morphology (McGuckian & Henry, 2007), and syntax (Elfenbein, Hardin-Jones, & Davis, 1994). Likewise, phonological processing deficits abound (Ambrose, Fey, & Eisenberg, 2012; Easterbrooks et al., 2007; Harris & Beech, 1998). Within print knowledge, alphabet knowledge appears to be relatively intact in children with hearing loss (Easterbrooks et al., 2007; Werfel, Lund, & Schuele, 2014); however, conceptual print knowledge is impaired (Werfel et al., 2014). Monitoring performance relative to same-age peers with normal hearing as well as growth relative to an individual's previous performance for each of the emergent literacy skills throughout schooling for children with hearing loss can inform areas that should be targeted in instruction and intervention.

Word–Level Literacy

Word-level literacy consists of word recognition (reading) and spelling (writing). Ample evidence exists to confirm the language basis (e.g., emergent literacy skills) of both word recognition and spelling (Apel et al., 2012; Catts et al., 1999). Word-level literacy, spanning both word recognition and spelling, is predicted by linguistic knowledge such as phonological processing, morphological knowledge, print knowledge, orthographic knowledge, and vocabulary knowledge (Apel et al., 2012; Carlisle, 2000; Catts et al., 1999; Mattingly, 1972; NELP, 2008; Scarborough, 1998; Stahl & Murray, 1994; Walker & Hauerwas, 2006; Werfel, 2012).

For many children with hearing loss, deficits are apparent in both areas of word-level literacy (Bess, Dodd-Murphy, & Parker, 1998; Geers & Hayes, 2011; Wake et al., 2005). Some studies, however, have reported that word recognition of real words for children with hearing loss as a group does not differ from children with normal hearing (e.g., Briscoe, Bishop, & Norbury, 2001). In terms of spelling, children with hearing loss are less likely than children with normal hearing to make phonologically accurate errors, but they do not appear to use a visual memorization strategy (Hayes, Kessler, & Treiman, 2011). Such findings suggest that linguistic knowledge underlies literacy skills for children with hearing loss; however, it is possible that the relation of linguistic knowledge and literacy differs for children with hearing loss. As with emergent literacy skills, it is important to monitor children's word-level literacy both in comparison to normative standards and progress monitoring compared to their individual previous performance.

Text–Level Literacy

Text-level literacy consists of reading fluency and comprehension, as well as written expression. As with word recognition, language skills predict children's outcomes in text-level literacy (Cutting & Scarborough, 2006). The types of knowledge, however, that predict word-level literacy and text-level literacy differ somewhat (Apel et al., 2012).

Apel et al. (2012) reported that vocabulary and morphological awareness were related to reading comprehension, whereas **orthographic** awareness, phonological encoding, and morphological awareness were related to word recognition. In a study of 2nd grade students, the contribution of oral language, as measured by vocabulary and syntax, was higher than phonological processing for reading comprehension; additionally, the contribution of oral language was higher for reading comprehension than word recognition (Catts et al., 1999). Importantly, linguistic skills such as vocabulary and syntax predict reading comprehension even after word recognition skills are accounted for.

Likewise, Berninger et al. (1992) reported that the language skills that underlie spelling and written expression also differ somewhat. For example, verbal IQ was a contributor to quality of compositions but not spelling for elementary school children. In addition, one important predictor of written expression that is generally not needed in spelling is syntactic knowledge. McCutchen (1986) reported that mastery of syntactic structures is an important underlying component of high quality text composition. Spelling in word-level contexts generally does not require the use of syntactic structure knowledge.

Literacy deficits at the text level seem to be particularly prevalent in children with hearing loss. Children with hearing loss exhibit deficits in both reading comprehension (Qi & Mitchell, 2012) and written expression (Antia, Reed, & Kreimeyer, 2005). Recall that the average reading comprehension level for 18-year-olds with hearing loss is only 3rd grade (Qi & Mitchell, 2012). Additionally, over 50% of children with hearing loss in grades 3 through 12 scored below average on a measure of written expression (Antia et al., 2005). As with other types of literacy skills, it is important to monitor children's text-level literacy both in comparison to

normative standards and progress monitoring compared to their previous individual performance.

Clearly, children with hearing loss are at high risk for poor literacy achievement. To provide effective literacy instruction and intervention to this population, it is vital to identify specific literacy deficits for individual children. Therefore, the next section of this chapter highlights the types of literacy impairments children may exhibit.

TYPES OF LITERACY IMPAIRMENT

When we categorize literacy impairments, emergent literacy traditionally doesn't have a seat at the table. However, as previously discussed, deficits in those emergent literacy skills differentially underlie traditional categories of literacy impairment.

Reading

Gough and Tunmer (1986) detailed three categories of reading impairment: inadequate word recognition skills, inadequate comprehension skills, or both. Inadequate decoding skills leads to dyslexia, inadequate comprehensions skills to poor comprehension, and inadequate word recognition and comprehension leads to garden variety poor reading (Figure 8–2).

Dyslexia

Dyslexia is characterized by difficulties in accurate and/or fluent word recognition (Lyon, Shaywitz, & Shaywitz, 2003). Recall that word recognition consists of both explicit decoding (e.g., sounding out

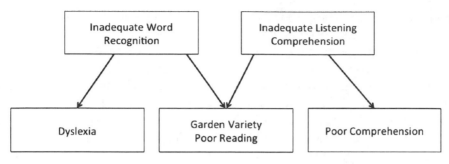

Figure 8–2. Reading impairments.

words) and automatic recognition of written words (e.g., sight-word naming), and both should be assessed. The overwhelming deficit in emergent literacy skills for individuals with dyslexia is phonological awareness, not general weakness in oral language (Catts, Adlof, Hogan, & Ellis Weismer, 2005; Stanovich, 1988).

Dyslexia is the most common of literacy impairments among children with normal hearing. The prevalence of dyslexia in the United States is estimated to be between 5% and 17% of school-age children with normal hearing (Shaywitz & Shaywitz, 2003). In a recent study of 3rd and 4th graders in a rural United States school district, however, we found that approximately 30% of students met the diagnostic criteria for dyslexia (Werfel, Crowe, & Schuele, 2012). Prevalence estimates for children with communication disorders are even higher. For example, reports of the prevalence of dyslexia in children with specific language impairment range from approximately 25% (Catts et al., 2005) to 50% (McArthur, Hogben, Edwards, Heath, & Mengler, 2000). Prevalence estimates of dyslexia in children with hearing loss are not currently available. Given the frequency of general oral language deficits in children

with hearing loss, it may be likely that few would meet diagnostic criteria for dyslexia but instead exhibit word recognition and reading comprehension deficits (discussed below in "garden variety poor reading"). When assessing reading, it is important to measure both word recognition and reading comprehension to create a complete picture of an individual child's strengths and weaknesses.

Poor Comprehension

Poor comprehension is characterized by poor reading comprehension in spite of adequate word recognition skills (Nation, Clarke, Marshall, & Durand, 2004). In contrast to children with dyslexia, in poor comprehenders phonological processing skills in the school years appear to be intact (Catts, Adlof, & Ellis Weismer, 2006; Nation et al., 2004). However, poor comprehenders as a group score lower on measures of oral language such as vocabulary, morphosyntax, figurative language, and grammatical understanding than children with typical reading achievement (Catts et al., 2006; Nation et al., 2004; Nation, Cocksey, Taylor, & Bishop, 2010).

Researchers in the UK report that the prevalence of poor comprehension is between 10% and 20% of school-age children with normal hearing (Nation & Snowling, 1997; Yuill & Oakhill, 1991). Prevalence estimates of poor comprehension are not readily available for U.S. students. In our screening of 3rd and 4th graders in a rural U.S. school district, approximately 6% met the diagnostic criteria for poor comprehension (Werfel et al., 2012). As with dyslexia, prevalence estimates of poor comprehension in children with hearing loss are not currently available.

Garden Variety Poor Reading

It is possible for children to exhibit deficits in either word recognition or reading comprehension. However, particularly for children with hearing loss, it is likely that deficits are present across these skills. Gough and Tunmer (1986) called readers who struggle with word recognition and comprehension **garden variety poor readers**. Because children with hearing loss tend to have language deficits across domains, including phonological processing, semantics, and syntax, assessing both levels of reading skills, along with the emergent literacy skills that are foundational to each, is vital for this population.

Writing

As with reading, writing deficits can vary across component domains (Berninger & Hart, 1993; Figure 8–3). Writing outcomes, however, are widely overlooked in the learning disability literature (Mayes & Calhoun, 2006). As a result, much less is known about writing impairments than reading impairments. The Nation's Report Cards in Reading and Writing (NCES, 2011a, 2011b) suggest that children struggle more to develop adequate writing skills as opposed to reading skills. Therefore, it is important to include writing skills in literacy assessments for children with hearing loss.

Dysgraphia

Writing's counterpart to word recognition is single-word spelling. Although word recognition and spelling rely on the same types of underlying word knowledge (e.g., sounds, letters, morphemes of words; Zutell & Rasinski, 1989), it is possible for individuals to exhibit deficits only in spelling (Frith, 1980). Spelling impairment, or **dysgraphia**, has not been as widely studied as dyslexia. There is some evidence that the spelling of individuals

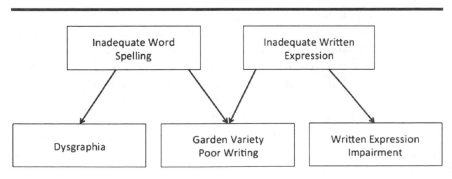

Figure 8–3. Writing impairments.

who have spelling deficits in the absence of word recognition deficits differ from those who have deficits in both (Nelson & Warrington, 1974).

In recent work in my lab, approximately 22% of 2nd through 4th grade children with typical language scored below the average range on single-word spelling. For same-age children with specific language impairment, the rate of spelling impairment was 63% (Werfel, 2013). The prevalence of spelling impairment in children with hearing loss is unknown, but as with other components of literacy, it is reasonable to assume that it is closer to the rate for children with specific language impairment than children with normal hearing and typical language.

Written Expression Impairment

The writing counterpart to poor comprehension, **written expression impairment,** involves deficits in planning, translating, and/or reviewing a written composition in the absence of word-level spelling deficits. Written expression deficits can be driven by impairments in linguistic and cognitive skills, including working memory, syntax, and vocabulary, among others (Berninger et al., 1991).

Prevalence estimates of written expression impairment are rare. However, the Nation's Report Card in Writing (NCES, 2011b) reported that only 27% of 8th and 11th grade students produced written compositions that were scored "proficient" or higher. For students with clinical diagnoses, Mayes and Calhoun (2006) reported higher levels of impairment in written expression than any other literacy skill. As with other types of literacy skills, the prevalence of written expression impairments in children with hearing loss is unknown.

Garden Variety Poor Writing

Similar to the case of garden variety poor reading, it is likely that children with hearing loss who struggle with writing will exhibit deficits across both spelling and written expression. Such students can be considered to be **garden variety poor writers**, to parallel Gough and Tunmer's (1986) terminology for reading impairments. Children with hearing loss often exhibit deficits across language domains; therefore, it is necessary to assess writing skills broadly and thoroughly, along with linguistic skills known to underlie writing, to identify areas in need of intervention.

PRINCIPLES OF ASSESSMENT

When considering what types of assessments to administer to an individual child with hearing loss, it is important to first determine the purpose of assessing him or her. Possible purposes for assessment include identifying impairments, qualifying for services, and evaluating the effects of instruction or intervention. Depending on your purpose for assessing, you should select appropriate types of tests that allow you to fulfill that purpose. For example, if your purpose in assessment is to qualify an individual for services, you will select tests that evaluate an individual's performance compared to a normative group. In contrast, if you want to evaluate the effects of an intervention, you should choose an assessment that allows you to measure performance before beginning the intervention and then monitor growth in the target skill throughout teaching. Such assessments are called curriculum-based measures.

For children with hearing loss, using a problem-solving approach to literacy assessment is suggested. Bransford and Stein (1984) proposed a model of effective problem solving, and Deno (2005) adapted their model to fit specifically educational problems. Such a problem-solving approach involves five steps, and each step involves specific types of assessment (Figure 8–4). First, the problem must be identified. Next, the specifics of the problem should be defined. Once the problem has been identified and defined, one should explore possible solutions. When a viable solution has been selected and implemented, the progress in solving the problem (i.e., improving the skill) should be monitored. Finally, at the conclusion of intervention, the effectiveness of the solution should be evaluated. Each step in this model is explained in detail

below, and suggestions for measures at each point in the problem-solving process are provided.

Identify the Problem

If you are reading this chapter, chances are you have already identified the problem of interest here: literacy achievement in children with hearing loss. As discussed above, literacy outcomes are generally quite poor for this population. However, we would be remiss to skip this particular step of the problem-solving model of assessment with any individual child. When considering literacy assessment in light of the problem-solving model, the "Identify the Problem" step is analogous

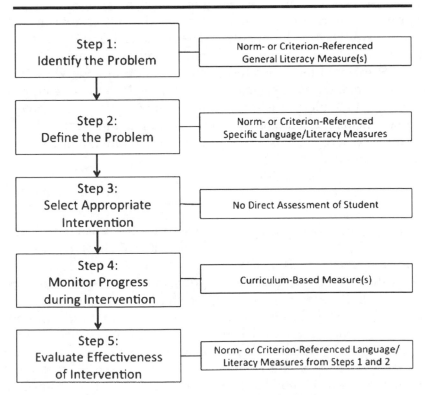

Figure 8–4. A problem–solving model of literacy assessment.

with norm-referenced assessment that is already standard practice.

The purpose of norm-referenced assessment is to compare an individual's performance to a normative sample of their same-age peers. Limitations of norm-referenced clinical and educational assessment have been discussed elsewhere (e.g., Brown-Chidsey, 2005; McCauley & Swisher, 1984) and are not repeated here. Despite those limitations, there are compelling reasons to use norm-referenced literacy assessment during the problem identification stage. Norm-referenced assessment is used to qualify students for intervention services in school systems and for third-party payment, as well as quantify the severity of the problem (i.e., how far below peers an individual's performance falls).

In the problem identification step in the problem-solving model of assessment, the primary goal is to determine if the literacy skills of an individual child with hearing loss are low enough to indicate a need for intervention. Therefore, choosing a norm-referenced assessment that broadly measures literacy is essential. Such assessments are often referred to omnibus and measure a range of reading and/or writing skills and can provide a general estimate of the magnitude of an individual's literacy deficit.

Omnibus Emergent Literacy Assessments

Several norm-referenced measures exist that provide estimates of emergent literacy skills as a whole. For example, the Test of Preschool Early Literacy (TOPEL; Lonigan, Wagner, Torgesen, & Rashotte, 2007) measures phonological awareness, print knowledge, and vocabulary and can be used through age 5 year, 11 months. The

Test of Early Reading Ability-3 (TERA-3; Reid, Hresko, & Hammill, 2001) measures alphabet knowledge, print knowledge, and meaning and can be used through 8 years, 6 months. Administering one of these omnibus emergent literacy measures can provide evidence that emergent literacy is or is not an area of deficit for an individual child with hearing loss.

Omnibus Literacy Assessments

The Woodcock-Johnson Tests of Achievement III (WJ III; Woodcock, McGrew, & Mather, 2001) and the written language portion of the Oral and Written Language Scales-II (OWLS-II; Carrow-Woolfolk, 2011) are two examples of omnibus literacy assessments. Subtests of the WJ III cover the full range of literacy skills, including word recognition, reading fluency, reading comprehension, spelling, writing fluency, and written expression. The Reading Comprehension and Written Expression subtests of the OWLS-II can provide an overview of students' literacy skills. As with emergent literacy, these omnibus measures can provide evidence that require further detailed testing is needed for an individual child.

Define the Problem

Once a problem has been identified, the second step of the problem-solving model of assessment is to further define that problem. In the case of literacy assessment for children with hearing loss, defining the problem means determining exactly which areas of literacy are impaired, as well as the emergent literacy skill deficits that underlie the literacy impairments. This step is much more complicated than simply identifying the presence of a problem, and as such, requires a more complicated approach to assessment. To define the problem, a combination of norm-referenced and criterion-referenced assessments should be used. Criterion-referenced assessments differ from norm-referenced assessments because instead of comparing an individual's performance to his or her same-age peers, they compare his or her performance to a specified benchmark in performance. (See Chapter 2 for more information.) Using both types of assessments provides a more complete picture of an individual's skills than using either in isolation.

First, the goal of defining the problem in literacy assessment is to determine which areas of literacy are impaired. The broad literacy assessments used to identify the problem can be used as a guide for further exploration. Select follow-up assessments to explore in more detail an individual's performance on specific literacy skills, such as word recognition or written expression.

Emergent Literacy Assessments

As previously emphasized, assessment of emergent literacy skills should begin in the preschool years and continue throughout formal schooling, as appropriate. To fully understand literacy impairments and design and/or select effective intervention strategies, a comprehensive picture of a child's underlying deficits is essential. During the preschool and early elementary school years, assessment in the area of emergent literacy should be comprehensive. Identifying any such deficits early in development allows prediction of later difficulties, as well as initiation of appropriate instruction and

intervention in a timely manner. During the later school years, assessment in these foundational areas should focus on those (a) known to be previously impaired in an individual and (b) known to underlie literacy skills of interest for that individual.

One good place to begin after identifying a deficit in emergent literacy is to administer a criterion-referenced measure that taps multiple areas of emergent literacy skills. The University of Minnesota developed the Individual Growth & Development Indicators (myIGDIs) for measuring emergent literacy skills in 4- and 5-year-olds, which include measures of phonological awareness, alphabet knowledge, vocabulary, and comprehension (McConnell, Bradfield, & Wackerle-Hollman, 2013). The Phonological Awareness Literacy Screenings (PALS; Invernizzi, Juel, Swank, & Meier, 2004; Invernizzi, Meier, & Juel, 2003; Invernizzi, Sullivan, Meier, & Swank, 2004) assess a range of emergent literacy skills, including alphabet knowledge, print concept knowledge, phonological awareness, word recognition, and spelling, and can be used from preschool to 3rd grade. These broad measures can provide further guidance in choosing specific areas of emergent literacy that need comprehensive assessment.

Oral Language

For many children with hearing loss, assessment of oral language skills begins soon after identification. For very young children, parent reports of vocabulary, such as the MacArthur-Bates Communicative Development Inventories (CDI; Fenson et al., 2007), characterize early oral language assessment. The CDI norms begin at 8 months and continue through 37 months; it is also appropriate for older children with developmental delays. In addition to parent report, two normative pairs of vocabulary assessments are available. The Peabody Picture Vocabulary Test–4 (PPVT–4; Dunn & Dunn, 2007) assesses receptive vocabulary; the Expressive Vocabulary Test–2 (EVT–2; Williams, 2007) is its expressive vocabulary counterpart. The PPVT–4 and EVT–2 have normative data available from age 2:6 to 90+ years. The Receptive One Word Picture Vocabulary Test (ROWPVT; Brownell, 2000b) and the Expressive One Word Picture Vocabulary Test (EOWPVT; Brownell, 2000a) are also available, with normative data available from age 2 to 80+ years. For clinicians who work with children with hearing loss who are Spanish–English bilingual, Spanish-bilingual normative data for children ages 4 to 12 years is available for the ROWPVT and EOWPVT.

As children's vocabularies expand, oral language assessment should include assessment of morphological skills as well as syntax. The Rice/Wexler Test of Early Grammatical Impairment (TEGI; Rice & Wexler, 2001) assesses morphosyntactic grammatical deficits in children ages 3 to 8 years. The Structured Photographic Expressive Language Test–Preschool 2 (SPELT-P2; Dawson et al., 2004) measures morphology and syntax in children ages 3 to 5;11 years; the Structured Photographic Expressive Language Test–3 (SPELT–3; Dawson, Stout, & Eyer, 2005) has normative data for children ages 4 to 9;11 years. For older children, the Test of Morphological Structure (Carlisle, 2000) can be used to measure knowledge of derivational morphology. Language sample analysis is also a viable method of assessing expressive use of vocabulary, morphology, and syntax. Hadley (1998) provides guidance in eliciting spoken language samples, and Barako Arndt and Schuele (2013) provide guidance in coding.

Phonological Processing

Overwhelmingly, phonological awareness is the primary component of phonological processing measured in children with hearing loss. Many standardized measures of phonological awareness are available. However, it is important to be cautious when interpreting tests in which the phonological awareness composite includes print knowledge subtests (e.g., alphabet knowledge, print concept knowledge). Such composite scores likely will not yield an accurate reflection of an individual's ability to analyze speech sounds separate from letters. It is also important when assessing phonological processing in children with hearing loss to keep in mind that speech perception and speech production deficits may be confounding factors in interpreting errors. It may be useful to administer measures of speech perception and speech production to alleviate such concerns.

The Comprehensive Test of Phonological Processing–2 (Wagner, Torgesen, Rashotte, & Pearson, 2013) measures each type of phonological processing—awareness, memory, and recoding—and provides composites for each. In addition, it has normative data from ages 6 to 24. Therefore, its use is recommended for measuring phonological processing skills relative to an individual's same-age peers. It is also important to measure phonological processing skills relative to a benchmark. The PALS has subtests appropriate for such assessment in preschool through third grade.

Print Knowledge

In comparison to oral language and phonological processing, there are relatively few measures of print knowledge. Several published assessments contain subtests that tap print knowledge (e.g., TOPEL, PALS). In addition, the Preschool Word and Print Awareness (PWPA) is available as an appendix of Justice and Ezell (2001). The PWPA is a measure that was adapted from Clay's (1979) Concepts about Print Test to be more appropriate for preschoolers who are not yet reading. It measures print and word concept knowledge in the context of an adult–child shared reading experience. Justice, Bowles, and Skibbe (2006) provide print concept knowledge estimates for the PWPA for preschoolers as a group (ages 3 to 5). Clay's (1979) Concepts about Print Test can be used to measure print concept knowledge in school-age children.

Word Recognition

In terms of word recognition, there are two general types of measures: untimed word recognition and timed word recognition. The WJ III and the Woodcock Reading Mastery Test (WRMT-III; Woodcock, 2011) both contain subtests that tap untimed word recognition. These normative assessments measure untimed word recognition of both real words and nonwords. The Test of Word Reading Efficiency (Torgesen, Wagner, & Rashotte, 2012) measures timed word reading. Similar to the WJ III and WRMT-III, the TOWRE-2 measures timed word recognition of both real words and nonwords. In addition to these normative assessments, criterion-referenced assessments such as the DIBELS (http://dibels.uoregon.edu) are also available to measure word recognition.

For children with hearing loss, it is important to consider certain testing accommodations when administering word recognition tests (similar to those needed for phonological processing assessment). For example, it is important to determine if errors reflect a deficit in word recognition skills or are simply the result of speech sound production errors, particularly in the case of nonwords. To tease out the source of errors in this case it may be helpful to administer a measure of speech sound production, particularly if you are an unfamiliar listener of the child being assessed.

Spelling

Relatively fewer measures of word-level spelling exist. The most widely used measures include the Test of Written Spelling (Larsen, Hammill, & Moats, 2013) and the WJ III Spelling subtest. The TWS-5 measures dictated spelling of single words. The WJ III Spelling subtest actually measures spelling recognition, which is not recommended as an estimate of spelling production. In addition to these normative assessments, the Words Their Way spelling inventories (Bear, Invernizzi, Templeton, & Johnston, 2011) can be used to identify appropriate spelling intervention targets for children. Masterson and Apel (2010) detailed a spelling scoring system that can be used to characterize students' spelling errors based on linguistic features and monitor developmental change during intervention. This scoring system may be particularly useful in identifying specific areas to target in intervention.

Reading Comprehension

Reading comprehension can be measured in a number of ways. The Gray Oral Reading Tests (Wiederholt & Bryant, 2012) measure students' ability to answer multiple choice questions about a passage after reading it aloud. The WRMT-III measures students' ability to fill in a missing word from a sentence or passage when reading silently, as well as knowledge of antonyms, synonyms, and the ability to complete analogies. The Test of Reading Comprehension (Brown, Wiederholt, & Hammill, 2008) uses a variety of silent reading comprehension tasks, including sentence completion, relational vocabulary, ordering sentences of a passage, and contextual fluency. Reading comprehension assessments should be selected based on the need for information about an individual child's skills.

Written Expression

As with spelling, there are fewer published measures of written expression than reading comprehension. The Test of Written Language (Hammill & Larsen, 2009) measures a variety of written expression tasks, including story composition, contextual conventions, and writing sentences to dictation. Written samples can also be analyzed for use of correct spelling and punctuation, types of syntactic structures, story/argument organization, vocabulary, and other linguistic features of interest.

Explore Solutions to the Problem

After defining the specific literacy deficits of an individual with hearing loss,

the third step in the problem-solving model is to select or design an appropriate intervention approach to address the problem. During this stage, there is no new assessment of a child's skills. Rather, the assessment from the previous step is used to guide intervention decisions. For example, if the problem definition assessment revealed impairments in spelling and phonological processing, an appropriate intervention design would address phonological processing with spelling outcomes in mind.

Assess Progress During Solution Implementation

When an intervention plan is in place, a vital (and often overlooked) component is progress monitoring. In general, norm-referenced assessments should not be used for progress monitoring. Instead, **curriculum-based measurement** has emerged as an alternative to continuously monitor the effects of intervention on a child's performance. Curriculum-based measures should be developed based on the specific intervention that a child receives. For example, in the above example of a child with deficits in spelling and phonological processing, assessments that tap the specific targets of the intervention should be created. Let's say that the focus of intervention is segmentation of the initial and final sounds of words and spelling CVC (consonant-vowel-consonant) words with short vowels. In this case, three curriculum-based measures would be appropriate: initial sound segmentation, final sound segmentation, and CVC spelling.

Deno (1985) described several necessary components of curriculum-based measures. First, they should be developed based on the intervention that the child receives. It is vital that these measures assess the specific skills that the child should gain as a direct of the intervention. Second, there should be multiple forms of the measure that are of the same difficulty level. Having multiple forms of equivalent difficulty ensures that the child's improved performance is a result of increased skill and not simply familiarity with the test items (a problem of using norm-referenced and criterion-referenced assessments to monitor progress). Third, the measure should be efficient for frequent administration. Progress monitoring assessment should take place at the beginning of each intervention session. Clearly, this requires curriculum-based measures to be easy and fast to administer.

Administering curriculum-based measures during intervention is a method of closely monitoring the effectiveness of the chosen intervention. In contrast to traditional practice, in which an intervention is selected and the effectiveness is measured with a pretest/post-test comparison, utilizing progress monitoring throughout the intervention provides immediate feedback on its effectiveness. Because of this feature of curriculum-based measures, an ineffective intervention can be altered immediately rather than after weeks or months of wasted time. Curriculum-based measures must not be neglected in literacy assessment for children with hearing loss.

Evaluate the Effectiveness of the Solution

When conducting literacy interventions, it is imperative to measure the effects of intervention on students' general literacy skills in addition to monitoring their progress on the specifically targeted skills. Indeed, general improvement in literacy skills is the ultimate goal of any specific literacy intervention. To measure the effects of an intervention on general literacy skills, it is important to readminister the same standardized assessments from steps one and two upon completion of the intervention. The nature of norm-referenced standardized assessments makes them quite difficult to be useful in measuring progress and you are likely to see little improvement on these types of assessments, particularly for short interventions (i.e., six months or less). Most norm-referenced tests can be administered only one or two times per year; always check individual test manuals for guidelines on how frequently it can be administered. Therefore, in most cases, criterion-referenced assessments (remember, these compare an individual's knowledge to specific benchmarks for his or her age) will be most useful in measuring general literacy outcomes after specific interventions.

SUMMARY

Children with hearing loss remain at high risk to experience poor literacy achievement despite advances in amplification technology. Therefore, a focus on literacy assessment even before formal literacy instruction begins is needed. Assessment should be individualized for a particular child's needs and should be continued throughout intervention. Using a problem-solving model of literacy assessment for children with hearing loss can inform intervention strategies and convey effectiveness of our chosen approaches more quickly than an annual or semiannual testing. Children with hearing loss are likely to experience difficulty across areas of emergent literacy and literacy, and our assessment should include at least broad testing of each type and level of literacy skills. Early assessment and identification of literacy difficulties for children with hearing loss will allow us to begin intervention early and provide more support for these children to achieve proficiency in literacy skills.

REFERENCES

Ambrose, S., Fey, M., & Eisenberg, L. (2012). Phonological awareness and print knowledge of preschool children with cochlear implants. *Journal of Speech, Language, and Hearing Research, 55,* 811–823.

Antia, S., Reed, S., & Kreimeyer, K. (2005). Written language of deaf and hard-of-hearing students in public schools. *Journal of Deaf Studies and Deaf Education, 10,* 244–255.

Apel, K., Fowler-Wilson, E., Brimo, D., & Perrin, N. (2012). Metalinguistic contributions to reading and spelling in second and third grade students. *Reading and Writing, 25,* 1283–1305.

Barako Arndt, K., & Schuele, C. M. (2013). Multiclausal utterances aren't just for big kids: A framework for analysis of complex syntax in spoken language production of preschool- and early school-age children. *Topics in Language Disorders, 33,* 125–139.

Bear, D., Invernizzi, M., Templeton, S., & Johnston, F. (2011). *Words their way: Word study for phonics, vocabulary, and spelling instruction* (5th ed.). Upper Saddle River, NJ: Pearson.

Berninger, V., & Hart, T. (1993). From research to clinical assessment of reading and writing disorders: The unit of analysis problem. In R. M. Joshi & C. K. Leong (Eds.), *Reading disabilities: Diagnosis and component processes* (Vol. 74, pp. 33–61). Dordrecht, The Netherlands: Kluwer.

Berninger, V., Mizokawa, D., & Bragg, R. (1991). Theory-based diagnosis and remediation of writing disabilities. *Journal of School Psychology, 29,* 57–79.

Berninger, V., Yates, C., Cartwright, A., Rutberg, J., Remy, E., & Abbott, R. (1992). Lower-level developmental skills in beginning writing. *Reading and Writing: An Interdisciplinary Journal, 4,* 257–280.

Bess, F., Dodd-Murphy, J., & Parker, R. (1998). Children with minimal sensorineural hearing loss: Prevalence, educational performance, and functional status. *Ear and Hearing, 19,* 339–354.

Bransford, J., & Stein, B. (1984). *The IDEAL problem solver.* New York, NY: W. H. Freeman.

Briscoe, J., Bishop, D., & Norbury, C. (2001). Phonological processing, language, and literacy: A comparison of children with mild-to-moderate sensorineural hearing loss and those with specific language impairment. *Journal of Child Psychology and Psychiatry, 42,* 329–340.

Brown, V., Wiederholt, J., & Hammill, D. (2008). *Test of Reading Comprehension* (4th ed.). Austin, TX: Pro-Ed.

Brown-Chidsey, R. (2005). The role of published norm-referenced tests in problem-solving based assessment. In R. Brown-Chidsey (Ed.), *Assessment for intervention: A problem-solving approach.* New York, NY: Guilford Press.

Brownell, R. (2000a). *Expressive One-Word Picture Vocabulary Test.* Novato, CA: Academic Therapy.

Brownell, R. (2000b). *Receptive One-Word Picture Vocabulary Test.* Novato, CA: Academic Therapy.

Carlisle, J. (2000). Awareness of the structure and meaning of morphologically complex words: Impact on reading. *Reading and Writing: An Interdisciplinary Journal, 12,* 169–190.

Carrow-Woolfolk, E. (2011). *Oral and Written Language Scales* (2nd ed.). Torrance, CA: Western Psychological Services.

Catts, H., Adlof, S., & Ellis Weismer, S. (2006). Language deficits in poor comprehenders: A case for the simple view of reading. *Journal of Speech, Language, and Hearing Research, 49,* 278–293.

Catts, H., Adlof, S., Hogan, T., & Ellis Weismer, S. (2005). Are specific language impairment and dyslexia distinct disorders? *Journal of Speech, Language, and Hearing Research, 48,* 1378–1396. doi:1092-4388/05/4806-1378

Catts, H., Fey, M., Zhang, X., & Tomblin, J. B. (1999). Language basis of reading and reading disabilities: Evidence from a longitudinal investigation. *Scientific Studies of Reading, 3,* 331–361.

Clay, M. (1979). *The early detection of reading difficulties: A diagnostic survey with recovery procedures.* Portsmouth, NH: Heinemann.

Cutting, L., & Scarborough, H. (2006). Prediction of reading comprehension: Relative contributions of word recognition, language proficiency, and other cognitive skills can depend on how comprehension is measured. *Scientific Studies of Reading, 10,* 277–299.

Dawson, J., Stout, C., & Eyer, J. (2005). *Structured Photographic Expressive Language Test* (3rd ed.). DeKalb, IL: Janelle.

Dawson, J., Stout, C., Eyer, J., Tattersall, P., Fonkalsrud, J., & Crowley, K. (2004). *Structured Photographic Expressive Language Test–Preschool* (2nd ed.). DeKalb, IL: Janelle.

Deno, S. (1985). Curriculum-based measurement: The emerging alternative. *Exceptional Children, 52,* 219–232.

Deno, S. (2005). Problem-solving assessment. In R. Brown-Chidsey (Ed.), *Assessment for intervention: A problem-solving approach.* New York, NY: Guilford Press.

Dunn, L., & Dunn, D. (2007). *Peabody Picture Vocabulary Test* (4th ed.). San Antonio, TX: Pearson.

Easterbrooks, S., Lederberg, A., Miller, E., Bergeron, J., & Connor, C. M. (2007). Emergent literacy skills during early childhood in children with hearing loss: Strengths and weaknesses. *The Volta Review, 108,* 91–114.

Elfenbein, J., Hardin-Jones, M., & Davis, J. (1994). Oral communication skills of children who are hard of hearing. *Journal of Speech, Language, and Hearing Research, 37,* 216–226.

Fenson, L., Marchman, V., Dale, P., Reznick, J., Thal, D., & Bates, E. (2007). *MacArthur-Bates Communicative Development Inventories* (2nd ed.). Baltimore, MD: Brookes.

Flower, L., & Hayes, J. (1981). A cognitive process theory of writing. *College Composition and Communication, 32,* 365–387.

Frith, U. (1980). Unexpected spelling problems. In U. Frith (Ed.), *Cognitive processes in spelling.* London, UK: Academic Press.

Geers, A., & Hayes, H. (2011). Reading, writing, and phonological processing skills of adolescents with 10 or more years of cochlear implant experience. *Ear & Hearing, 32,* 49S–59S.

Gough, P., & Tunmer, W. (1986). Decoding, reading, and reading disability. *Remedial and Special Education, 7,* 6–10.

Hadley, P. (1998). Language sampling protocols for eliciting text-level discourse. *Language, Speech, and Hearing Services in Schools, 29,* 132–147.

Hammill, D., & Larsen, S. (2009). *Test of Written Language* (4th ed.). Austin, TX: Pro-Ed.

Harris, M., & Beech, J. (1998). Implicit phonological awareness and early reading development in prelingually deaf children. *Journal of Deaf Studies and Deaf Education, 3,* 205–216.

Hayes, H., Kessler, B., & Treiman, R. (2011). Spelling of deaf children who use cochlear implants. *Scientific Studies of Reading, 15,* 522–540.

Invernizzi, M., Juel, C., Swank, L., & Meier, J. (2004). *Phonological Awareness Literacy Screening–K.* Charlottesville, VA: University of Virginia.

Invernizzi, M., Meier, J., & Juel, C. (2003). *Phonological Awareness Literacy Screening 1–3.* Charlottesville, VA: University of Virginia.

Invernizzi, M., Sullivan, A., Meier, J., & Swank, L. (2004). *Phonological Awareness Literacy Screening–PreK.* Charlottesville, VA: University of Virginia.

Justice, L., Bowles, R., & Skibbe, L. (2006). Measuring preschool attainment of print-concept knowledge: A study of typical and at-risk 3- to 5-year-old children using item response theory. *Language, Speech, and Hearing Services in Schools, 37,* 224–235.

Justice, L., & Ezell, H. (2001). Word and print awareness in 4-year-old children. *Child Language Teaching and Therapy, 17,* 207–225.

Larsen, S., Hammill, D., & Moats, L. (2013). *Test of Written Spelling* (5th ed.). Austin, TX: Pro-Ed.

Lonigan, C., Wagner, R., Torgesen, J., & Rashotte, C. (2007). *Test of Preschool Early Literacy.* Austin, TX: Pro-Ed.

Lyon, G. R., Shaywitz, B., & Shaywitz, S. (2003). A definition of dyslexia. *Annals of Dyslexia, 53,* 1–14.

Masterson, J., & Apel, K. (2010). The spelling sensitivity score: Noting developmental changes in spelling knowledge. *Assessment for Effective Intervention, 36,* 35–45. doi:10.1177/1534508410380039

Mattingly, I. (1972). Reading, the linguistic process, and linguistic awareness. In J. Kavanagh & I. Mattingly (Eds.), *Language by ear and by eye: The relationships between speech and reading* (pp. 133–147). Cambridge, MA: MIT Press.

Mayes, S., & Calhoun, S. (2006). Frequency of reading, math, and writing disabilities in children with clinical disorders. *Learning and Individual Differences, 16,* 145–157.

McArthur, G., Hogben, J., Edwards, V., Heath, S., & Mengler, E. (2000). On the "specifics" of specific reading disability and specific language impairment. *Journal of Child Psychology and Psychiatry, 41,* 869–874. doi:0021-9630/00

McCauley, R. & Swisher, L. (1984). Use and misuse of norm-referenced tests in clinical assessment: A hypothetical case. *Journal of Speech and Hearing Disorders, 49,* 338–348.

McConnell, S., Bradfield, T., & Wackerle-Hollman, A. (2013). *Individual growth and development indicators of early literacy* (2nd ed.). St. Paul, MN: Early Learning Labs.

McCutchen, D. (1986). Domain knowledge and linguistic knowledge in the development of writing ability. *Journal of Memory and Language, 25,* 431–444.

McGuckian, M., & Henry, A. (2007). The grammatical morpheme deficit in moderate hearing impairment. *International Journal of Language and Communication Disorders, 42*(S1), 17–36.

Moeller, M. P., Tomblin, J. B., Yoshinaga-Itano, C., Connor, C. sM., & Jerger, S. (2007). Current state of knowledge: Language and literacy of children with hearing impairment. *Ear and Hearing, 28,* 740–753.

Nation, K., Clarke, P., Marshall, C., & Durand, M. (2004). Hidden language impairments in children: Parallels between poor reading comprehension and specific language impairment? *Journal of Speech, Language, and Hearing Research, 47,* 199–211. doi:1092-4388/04/4701-0199

Nation, K., Cocksey, J., Taylor, J., & Bishop, D. (2010). A longitudinal investigation of early reading and language skills in children with poor reading comprehension. *Journal of Child Psychology and Psychiatry, 51,* 1031–1039.

Nation, K., & Snowling, M. (1997). Assessing reading difficulties: The validity and utility of current measures of reading skill. *British Journal of Educational Psychology, 67,* 359–370.

NCES. (2011a). *The nation's report card: Reading 2011 (NCES 2012-457).* Washington, DC: Institute of Education Sciences, U.S. Department of Education.

NCES. (2011b). *The nation's report card: Writing 2011 (NCES 2012-470).* Washington, DC: Institute of Education Sciences, U.S. Department of Education.

NELP. (2008). *Developing early literacy: Report of the National Early Literacy Panel.* Washingtion, DC: National Institute for Literacy.

Nelson, H., & Warrington, E. (1974). Developmental spelling retardation and its relation to other cognitive abilities. *British Journal of Psychology, 65,* 265–274.

Pittman, A., Lewis, D., Hoover, B., & Stelmachowicz, P. (2005). Rapid word-learning in normal-hearing and hearing-impaired children: Effects of age, receptive vocabulary, and high-frequency amplification. *Ear and Hearing, 26,* 619–629.

Qi, S., & Mitchell, R. (2012). Large-scale academic achievement testing of deaf and hard-of-hearing students: Past, present, and future. *Journal of Deaf Studies and Deaf Education, 17,* 1–18.

Reid, D., Hresko, W., & Hammill, D. (2001). *Test of Early Reading Ability* (3rd ed.). Austin, TX: Pro-Ed.

Rice, M., & Wexler, K. (2001). *Rice/Wexler Test of Early Grammatical Impairment.* San Antonio, TX: The Psychological Corporation.

Scarborough, H. (1998). Predicting the future achievement of second graders with reading disabilities: Contributions of phonemic awareness, verbal memory, rapid naming, and IQ. *Annals of Dyslexia, 48,* 115–136.

Scarborough, H. (2001). Connecting early language and literacy to later reading (dis)abilities: Evidence, theory, and practice. In S. Neuman & D. Dickinson (Eds.), *Handbook for research in early literacy.* New York, NY: Guilford Press.

Shaywitz, S., & Shaywitz, B. (2003). Dyslexia (specific reading disability). *Pediatrics in Review, 24,* 147–152.

Snow, C., Burns, M., & Griffin, P. (1998). *Preventing reading difficulties in young children.* Washington, DC: National Academy Press.

Stahl, S., & Murray, B. (1994). Defining phonological awareness and its relationship to early reading. *Journal of Educational Psychology, 86,* 221–234.

Stanovich, K. (1988). Explaining the differences between the dyslexic and the garden-variety poor reader: The phonological-core variable-difference model. *Journal of Learning Disabilities, 21,* 590–604.

Torgesen, J., Wagner, R., & Rashotte, C. (2012). *Test of Word Reading Efficiency* (2nd ed.). Austin, TX: Pro-Ed.

Wagner, R., Torgesen, J., Rashotte, C., & Pearson, N. (2013). *Comprehensive Test of Phonological Processing* (2nd ed.). Austin, TX: Pro-Ed.

Wake, M., Poulakis, Z., Hughes, E., Carey-Sargeant, C., & Rickards, F. (2005). Hearing impairment: A population study of age at diagnosis, severity, and language outcomes at 7–8 years. *Archives of Disease in Childhood, 90,* 238–244.

Walker, J., & Hauerwas, L. (2006). Development of phonological, morphological, and orthographic knowledge in young spellers: The case of inflected verbs. *Reading and Writing, 19,* 819–843.

Werfel, K. (2012). *Contributions of linguistic knowledge to spelling performance in elementary school children with and without language impairment* (Unpublished doctoral dissertation). Vanderbilt University, Nashville, TN.

Werfel, K. (2013). *Spelling in children with and without language impairment.* Unpublished data.

Werfel, K., Crowe, C., & Schuele, C. M. (2012, November). *Prevalence of poor comprehenders in a rural U.S. school district.* Paper presented at the Annual Convention of the American-Speech-Language-Hearing Association, Atlanta, GA.

Werfel, K., Lund, E., & Schuele, C. M. (2014). Print knowledge of preschool children with hearing loss. *Communication Disorders Quarterly.* Advance online publication. doi: 10.1177/1525740114539002

Whitehurst, G., & Lonigan, C. (1998). Child development and emergent literacy. *Child Development, 69,* 848–872.

Wiederholt, J., & Bryant, B. (2012). *Gray Oral Reading Tests* (5th ed.). Austin, TX: Pro-Ed.

Williams, K. (2007). *Expressive Vocabulary Test* (2nd ed.). San Antonio, TX: Pearson.

Woodcock, R. (2011). *Woodcock Reading Mastery Tests* (3rd ed.). San Antonio, TX: Pearson.

Woodcock, R., McGrew, K., & Mather, N. (2001). *Woodcock-Johnson III Tests of Achievement.* Rolling Meadows, IL: Riverside.

Yuill, N., & Oakhill, J. (1991). *Children's problems in text comprehension: An experimental investigation.* New York, NY: Cambridge University Press.

Zutell, J., & Rasinski, T. (1989). Reading and spelling connections in third and fifth grade students. *Reading Psychology, 10,* 137–155.

CHAPTER 9

Assessment of the Listening Environment

Carrie Spangler and Carol Flexer

- Every sound has to pass through an environment before it reaches the child's hearing technology and then on to the child's brain; therefore, acoustic access must be made available to the child in all life settings—home, school and playground, car, and after-school activities.
- A construct of a *"listening map"* illustrates the complexity of a child's acoustic navigational demands inside and outside of school. These demands escalate as a child advances from grade to grade and require careful, thoughtful management of a child's acoustic accessibility.
- The child's amplification technologies need to be effectively connected to the many changing educational technologies (e.g., computers, tablets, smartphones) that are used in today's fast paced, dynamic classrooms.
- High performance in the Common Core Standards of Speaking and Listening is expected throughout the child's educational life span.
- One possible yearly acoustic accessibility assessment protocol may include: home and school environmental noise measurements using smartphone and tablet computer apps; classroom observation; teacher, parent, and student interviews; collaboration with a clinical/educational audiologist in managing **Hearing Assistance Technologies (HAT)**; and administering the *Functional Listening Evaluation* (FLE) in the classroom.
- An implementation plan for managing the child's acoustic accessibility in home and school environments could include: report or summary of the results of the assessment protocol for parents and school team members; team meeting, including parents and audiologist, to review the report or summary and to write Individualized Educational Plan (IEP) goals and accommodations for acoustic accessibility; staff in-services

about acoustic accessibility goals and accommodations; and ongoing follow-up conversations with parents, child, and staff to ensure sustainable implementation of acoustic accessibility technologies and accommodations.

WHY IS ACOUSTIC ACCESSIBILITY IMPORTANT— WHAT IS THE PROBLEM?

Children are dynamic beings—constantly moving from one setting to the next in their daily home, school, and community environments. Every location has an acoustic footprint that changes minute by minute, and a child is expected to learn and interact in all of these environments. How do practitioners make that acoustic interaction possible?

Let's examine a typical day in the life of a kindergartner from an acoustic accessibility perspective, distinguishing the multitude of acoustic transitions the child must navigate across numerous environments. This flow chart of acoustic navigational demands can be called the child's **Listening Map** (Figure 9–1).

The child's listening map becomes more challenging, complex, and dynamic each year. For example, by 3rd grade, the child's listening map includes class changes, numerous teachers, increasing numbers of classmates, a variety of classrooms with unique demands in each classroom, more technology-based learning, grouping of children according to academic levels, multiple small-groups interacting within a single space, and peer collaboration. Our job as listening and spoken language specialists is more

critical than it has ever been because hearing technology changes quickly, becoming more advanced and complicated each year. In addition, today's classrooms are different learning environments from the past. Ninety-two percent of children with permanent hearing loss are born to two hearing parents and 96% of children with permanent hearing loss are born to one hearing parent and one parent with hearing loss (Mitchell & Karchmer, 2004). Furthermore, 90% of children with hearing loss are using listening and spoken language; thus, children with hearing loss are most likely to be mainstreamed (Cole & Flexer, 2011). Therefore, the acoustics of the entire school must be considered, not just the child's classroom(s).

This chapter offers information and suggest tools that can be used to continually distinguish and assess a child's **acoustic accessibility**. No matter how amazing the instruction is in a setting, if that information does not reach the child's brain due to acoustic barriers, learning will not occur. The purpose of this chapter is to understand and manage acoustic accessibility in all of the child's learning environments inside and outside of school. To that end, the following topics are covered: acoustic and **educational accessibility**, classroom and personal amplification technologies used by children with hearing loss, educational technologies and their impact on acoustic accessibility, assessment protocols for understanding and managing acoustic accessibility in all of a child's environments, parent and teacher collaboration, accessibility goals for Evaluation Team Report (ETR) and Individualized Education Plan (IEP) and 504 Plans, and possible modifications to the listening environments in school and at home.

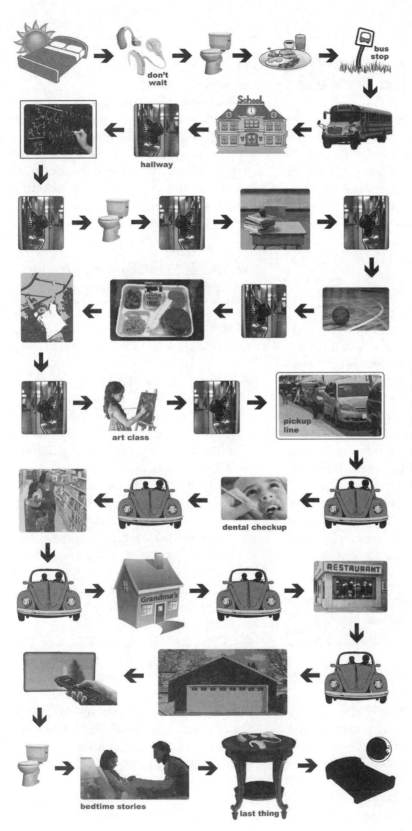

Figure 9–1. This flow chart, referred to as the child's *Listening Map*, depicts a portion of the multiple and complex acoustic navigational demands experienced by a kindergartner on a typical day.

WHAT IS ACOUSTIC ACCESSIBILITY?

Acoustic accessibility deals with the behavior of sound in a room (any room—home, school, or community-based), its impact on children, and its effect on the ability of a child to extract meaning from sound. The behavior of sound is influenced by room variables such as noise, reverberation, and distance from the speaker; these concepts are discussed later in the chapter.

The classroom is one of the most challenging learning domains for all children, who spend much of their time in noisy classroom environments where teachers demand constant, detailed listening to critical, often fast-paced instruction that is spoken at a distance from them. The major factors that affect auditory learning in the classroom (or in any room, inside or outside of school) include the hearing and attention capabilities of the child and the actual classroom environment (e.g., noise, reverberation, and distance from the speaker). Additional variables include the speech of the teacher and of pupils, and their relative positions in the room.

WHAT IS EDUCATIONAL ACCESSIBILITY?

Educational accessibility means access to curriculum and instruction in the classroom at the same level and rate as typically hearing peers—not a simple task because today's children face enormous challenges in the classroom (Anderson & Arnoldi, 2011). Over 90% of children with hearing loss will be in general education; they will be held to the same learning and performance standards as their peers (Cole & Flexer, 2011).

Below are some examples of Common Core Standards in the area of Speaking and Listening for Kindergartners—standards that have been adopted by 45 states to date (National Governors Association, 2010). Note the complexity of listening and spoken language expectations in the classroom, even for kindergartners.

Sample of Speaking and Listening Standards for Kindergarten

Used with permission from: http://www.corestandards.org/ELA-Literacy/SL/K

- CCSS.ELA-Literacy.SL.K.1: Participate in collaborative conversations with diverse partners about *kindergarten topics and texts* with peers and adults in small and larger groups.
  - CCSS.ELA-Literacy.SL.K.1a: Follow agreed-upon rules for discussions (e.g., listening to others and taking turns speaking about the topics and texts under discussion).
  - CCSS.ELA-Literacy.SL.K.1b: Continue a conversation through multiple exchanges.
- CCSS.ELA-Literacy.SL.K.2: Confirm understanding of a text read aloud or information presented orally or through other media by asking and answering questions about key details and requesting clarification if something is not understood.
  - CCSS.ELA-Literacy.SL.K.3: Ask and answer questions in order to seek help, get information, or clarify something that is not understood.

Common core standards do not stop in kindergarten; they continue and escalate all the way through high school. For example, the College and Readiness Standards for Speaking and Listening mandates: "To build a foundation for college and career readiness, students must have ample opportunities to take part in a variety of rich, structured conversations—as part of a whole class, in small groups, and with a partner. Being productive members of these conversations requires that students contribute accurate, relevant information; respond to and develop what others have said; make comparisons and contrasts; and analyze and synthesize a multitude of ideas in various domains"(National Governors Association, 2010).

The point is, there is a great deal at stake in managing acoustic accessibility for the purpose of ensuring the child has educational accessibility throughout his or her school experience. Each year brings escalating learning challenges and those challenges demand that children have acoustic access to teachers, peers, and to their own spoken communication. The child's academic trajectory needs to be sustained by thoughtful management of the child's acoustic and educational demands, first by parents and teachers, and ultimately by the child him- or herself.

WHAT IS THE SCIENCE INVOLVED IN UNDERSTANDING AND MANAGING THE LISTENING ENVIRONMENT?

There are several features that must be understood and managed for children to have acoustic accessibility: noise, **rever-beration**, and distance from the desired sound source.

Noise: Signal-To-Noise Ratio (SNR)

A child's speech recognition is reduced by background noise that covers up or masks important acoustic/linguistic cues in the message. This masking is especially problematic for consonants because they carry most of the intelligibility of speech necessary for accurate perception. Background noise in a room tends to mask the weaker consonant phonemes significantly more than the louder vowel phonemes.

Signal-to-noise ratio (SNR) is the relationship between a primary signal such as the teacher's or parent's speech, and background noise. Noise is anything and everything that conflicts with the desired auditory signal and may include others talking, noise from heating or cooling systems, classroom or hall noise, playground sounds, computer noise, and wind, among others (Nelson & Blaeser, 2010). The quieter the room and the more favorable the SNR, the clearer the auditory signal will be for the child's brain. The noisier the environment, the poorer the SNR and the more garbled the signal will be for the brain. The dominant source of noise in a room is the children in the room and the number of acoustic events that are co-occurring.

Adults with normal hearing and intact listening skills require a consistent SNR of approximately +6 dB for the reception of intelligible speech (Kramer, 2014). Children need a much more favorable SNR because their neurological immaturity and lack of life and language experiences reduce their ability to perform auditory/cognitive closure (Chermak, Bellis, & Musiek, 2014). Moreover, all children and especially children with hearing loss require the signal to be about 10 times louder than competing sounds. Interestingly, children with sensorineural hearing loss have a spatial processing disorder, a particular type of auditory processing disorder that makes them less able to attend to target sounds coming from one direction by suppressing sounds coming from other directions (Ching, van Wanrooy, Dillon, & Carter, 2011). Therefore, children with sensorineural hearing loss require a SNR higher than required by their normally hearing peers in the classroom if they are to equally understand speech when there is background noise. Due to noise, reverberation, and variations in teacher position, the SNR in a typical classroom is unstable and averages out to only about +4 dB and may be as low as 0 dB, often less than ideal even for adults with normal hearing and normal auditory processing capabilities (Smaldino, 2011).

Reverberation

Reverberation, specifically reverberation time (RT) refers to the amount of time it takes for a steady state sound to decrease 60 dB from its peak amplitude. In a room with much reverberation, speech is reflected from various hard room surfaces (such as floors, walls, and windows), so that some of the speech elements are delayed in reaching the ear of the listener. The reflected speech thus overlaps with the direct speech signal and covers up or masks critical acoustic phonemic elements, especially the weaker consonant sounds that carry the vast majority of the acoustic information important for speech recognition (Smaldino, 2011). Speech recognition, therefore, tends to worsen with increases in reverberation time.

Distance

Speech sounds lose 6 dB of amplitude for every doubling of distance as they travel away from the talker. In a landmark study, Leavitt and Flexer (1991) reported an example of the interplay between classroom acoustics, distance from the sound source, and speech. Using the Rapid Speech Transmission Index (RASTI), they demonstrated that only 83% of the speech energy delivered in the front of a classroom was actually available to a listener seated in the front row of a typical classroom-sized environment. Moreover, in the back row of the same classroom, only approximately 50% of the speech energy was available. RASTI is a measure of speech energy as it traverses a room, and is an index of the amount of energy available to be perceived when influenced by SNR and RT, not the amount actually perceived by the listener. Even less of the signal would be available if the listener has a hearing loss, and/or reduced auditory or language processing. These factors would interfere with the student's actual perception of the available speech energy. That is, add the impact of the classroom acoustical environment to the distortion imposed by a damaged auditory or linguistic system and it becomes apparent why simply using a hearing aid is not likely to result in satisfactory communication in the classroom.

ANSI Standards for Classroom Noise and Reverberation

Undesirable acoustics (noise and reverberation) can be a barrier to listening and learning in the classroom. Therefore, a working group composed of a wide variety of stakeholders produced the first American standard, which was published in 2002: *Acoustical Performance Criteria, Design Requirements, and Guidelines for Schools* (ANSI/ASA S12.60-2002). A second review of the standard resulted in some minor modifications and a separate part devoted to issues unique to portable classrooms.

The first part of the revised standard, *American National Standard Acoustical Performance Criteria, Design Requirements, and Guidelines for Schools, Part 1: Permanent Schools* (ANSI/ASA S12.60-2010) is a refined version of the 2002 standard. Theprimary performance requirement for furnished but unoccupied classrooms is basically unchanged from the 2002 standard. Specifically, the one-hour average A-weighted background noise level (A-weighting is based on the equal loudness contour for human hearing—attenuating low frequencies) cannot exceed 35 dB (55 dB if C-weighting is used—C-weighting does not attenuate low frequencies) and for averaged sized classrooms the reverberation time (RT60) cannot exceed 0.6 seconds (35/55 dBA/C and 0.7 seconds if the volume is greater than 10,000 but less than or equal to 20,000 cubic feet). Among other changes are improvements in the requirements for exterior walls and roofs in noisy areas, consideration of activities close to classrooms, clarification of the definition of a core learning space" addition of the limit of 45 dBA for sound in hallways, clarification and simplification of measurement procedures, and addition of the requirement that if a **classroom audio distribution system (CADS)** is believed appropriate it should provide even coverage and be adjustable so as not to disturb adjacent classes (Smaldino, 2011).

WHAT HEARING ASSISTANCE TECHNOLOGIES (HATS) ARE USED IN THE CLASSROOM BY CHILDREN WITH HEARING LOSS?

The purpose of all amplifications technologies is to channel the clearest and most complete speech information to the child's brain during every waking moment. The child's brain growth can be influenced only by sounds that actually reach and stimulate neural pathways.

While primary technologies—hearing aids, bone anchored hearing devices (BAHD) and cochlear implants (CI) (covered in Chapters 10 and 11 of this text)—allow auditory brain access in quiet, close situations, any noisy situation requires a remote microphone to overcome unfavorable environments and channel intelligible speech directly to neural centers (Dillon, 2012).

Personal–Worn FM System

Frequency modulation (FM) and other types of wireless systems improve signal quality and intelligibility far more than any signal processing scheme, such as noise reduction and directional microphones, located entirely within the hearing aid (Dillon, Ching & Golding, 2014). A **personal-worn FM system** is a wireless personal listening device that includes a remote microphone placed near the desired sound source, usually the speaker's mouth, and a receiver for the listener who can be positioned anywhere within approximately 50 feet of the person talking. Because the unit is really a small FM radio that transmits and receives on a single frequency, no wires are required to connect the talker and listener. The talker wears the remote microphone within 6 inches of his or her mouth, causing the personal FM unit to create a listening situation that is comparable to a parent or teacher being within 6 inches of the child's ear at all times, thereby allowing a positive and constant SNR (Nguyen & Bentler, 2011). The amount of SNR benefit will vary depending on a number of factors such as FM ratio (the relationship of the loudness of the FM signal compared to the loudness of the CI or hearing aid microphone signal), whether or not the hearing aid or CI microphone is activated, how well the personal technology is programmed, how appropriately the FM microphone is physically placed on the talker, and how effectively the talker uses the FM transmitter. SNR improvement using the FM microphone can be as much as 20 dB (HAT, 2008, retrieved from http://www.audiology.org/resources/document library/Documents/HATGuideline.pdf).

Personal FM systems, historically, have employed an analog frequency modulated (FM) radio frequency (RF) signal to transmit the desired signal. Currently, manufacturers have started introducing digitally-modulated RF systems, which are similar to Bluetooth® technologies often used in recreational and business products. **Digital RF systems** (also called DM, digital modulation systems) are able to provide a higher level of analysis and control over the signal received by the microphone and then delivered to the listener. Furthermore, these DM systems typically use a carrier frequency that "hops" from frequency to frequency hundreds of times per second, a feature that makes these systems less susceptible to interference from nearby RF devices (Wolfe et al., 2013). Studies have shown that hearing aid and cochlear implant users receive great benefit from dynamic

digital RF systems when compared to traditional/classic and dynamic FM systems, especially in higher levels of background noise (Thibodeau, 2013; Wolfe et al., 2013).

Personal FM/DM Use in School

Personal FM units are essential for a child with any type and degree of hearing loss, from minimal to profound, who is in any classroom or group learning situation (Anderson, Goldstein, Colodzin, & Inglehart, 2005; ASHA, 2000; Flynn, Flynn, & Gregory, 2005). Listening in a classroom is difficult, even for a child with a mild hearing loss. Parents often report that children with hearing loss arrive home exhausted, because even if the child appears to be doing relatively well in school, listening requires a great deal of work. An FM system significantly reduces the level of effort the child expends just receiving instructional information, leaving the child with more cognitive capacity for thinking about the new concepts offered by the teacher (Anderson, 2004). The most common styles of personal FM technology currently used include one in which the FM receiver is integrated into the ear-level hearing aid case and another in which a small FM receiver boot or audioshoe is attached directly to the bottom of the ear-level hearing aid, or to a cochlear implant speech processor.

Personal FM/DM Use Outside of School

The value of FM systems and remote microphones in classrooms is well documented. Very little has been written about FM use outside of school settings, but clinicians who have used them in other settings have reported very positive results. Acoustic accessibility is critical in all of a child's environments. That is, auditory information must reach the child's brain in all situations for psychosocial as well as academic neural development to occur. A personal worn FM/DM is therefore critical outside of school, too.

The work of Hart and Risley (1999) has clearly demonstrated that the number of words children speak is directly related to the number of words spoken to the child. For a child with hearing loss, hearing enough words is clearly an issue. When the primary speaker is not in close proximity to the child, the child hears fewer words. Parents report that wearing the microphone is a reminder for them to speak more, so an FM system can significantly increase the number of words actually heard by a child with hearing loss (Moeller, Donaghy, Beauchaine, Lewis, & Stelmachowicz, 1996). They also reported that children felt an increased sense of security when they could hear their parents from a distance.

FM use in the car or on the playground or in difficult communication situations provides additional listening time. Nguyen and Bentler (2011) found that children are more likely to practice their emerging spoken language with caregivers when using an FM system, and when the infant or preschooler is not close by, parents still can communicate easily. Parents uniformly report that the systems are easy to manage and that the children seem more attentive and more alert to sound when the FM is being used.

As children grow older and become involved in other activities, more opportunities for use develop. For example, children who play sports can have a great deal of difficulty hearing on a playing field. If the coach uses an FM system, the child will have good acoustic access to directions. Participating in family conversations at the dinner table and the kitchen also can be an acoustic challenge (Figure 9–2), and a FM system with conference microphone capabilities could be beneficial.

The transmitter will also be useful in ballet class, religious school, scouts, and on the playground. Friends, as well as adults, can learn to use the transmitter to assist in communication.

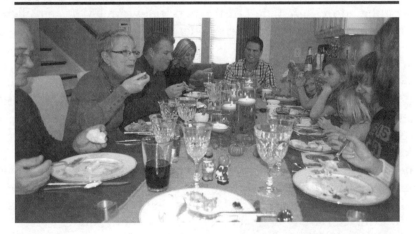

Figure 9–2. This family photo characterizes the listening challenges that can be present during family meals. These include acoustical barriers (hard floors, large table, noise of tableware) as well as conversational challenges.

Desktop Sound System

Desktop or totable sound field systems are an option for enhanced acoustic accessibility for individual students. A small loudspeaker is placed on a student's desk and the teacher wears a wireless FM microphone. Obviously not all students in the room benefit from this kind of system because it does not provide uniform amplification throughout the classroom. Anderson et al. (2005) found that desktop units and personal-worn FMs provide better speech perception scores than CADS for some children with hearing aids and cochlear implants by providing a more effective SNR.

Classroom Audio Distribution Systems (CADS)

Sound field technology, now often called CADS, is an effective educational tool that allows control of the acoustic environment in a classroom, thereby facilitating acoustic accessibility of teacher instruction for all children in the room (Smaldino & Flexer, 2012). A CADS looks like a wireless public address system, but it is designed specifically to ensure that the entire speech signal, including the weak high frequency consonants, reaches every child in the room. Through the use of this technology, an entire classroom can be amplified through the use of one, two, three, or four wall-or ceiling-mounted loudspeakers, or in some instances, a stand-alone loudspeaker array.

Using an FM or infrared signal, CADS facilitates the reception of consistently more intact signals than those received in an unamplified classroom, but signals are not as complete as those provided by using a personal FM unit (Smaldino & Flexer, 2012). In addition, the equipment, especially the loudspeakers, must be installed appropriately, and teachers must receive in-service training about the rationale and effective use of the technology.

A primary value of CADS is that it can focus the pupils and facilitate attention to relevant information. To that end, the effective use of the CADS microphone can be a powerful teaching tool. Teachers need to be shown how to use the microphone to create a listening attitude in the room; the purpose of the microphone is for quieting and focusing the room, not for exciting or distracting the children.

CADS and Personal FM Together

In many instances, the best listening and learning environment can be created by using both a CADS infrared (IR) and a personal-worn FM system at the same time. The CADS IR unit, appropriately installed and used in a mainstreamed classroom, improves acoustic access for all pupils and creates a listening environment in the room. The individual personal-worn FM system allows the particular child with hearing loss to have the most favorable SNR within that environment. So, the CADS focuses and quiets all students in the classroom while allowing the teacher to control and modulate her voice, and the personal FM provides the best SNR directly to the ear of the child. In addition, most CADS have two microphones—a teacher mic and a pass-around mic—which allow the child with hearing loss better acoustic accessibility of both the teacher and student voices.

Due to the continuous advancements in hearing assistance technologies (HAT), it is advisable to consult with the educational/clinical audiologist to determine how the child's personal FM unit and the CADS best can be used together. That is, it would appear that the simplest solution would to be to couple the child's personal FM transmitter to the designated FM port of the CADS, using an appropriate patch cord. In this instance, the teacher need wear only the microphone of the CADS and his or her voice will be transmitted to both the child's personal FM receiver and the classroom loudspeakers. Unfortunately, for some technologies, this coupling causes a poorer signal to be transmitted to the child's personal FM. Therefore, in the absence of data to the contrary, it is advisable for the teacher to wear two microphones; one for the personal FM and one for the CADS; electroacoustic verification of personal FM benefit should be performed for each arrangement according to HAT guidelines (HAT Guidelines, p. 10). Figure 9–3 shows pictures of a wrong way (Figure 9–3A) and a right way (Figure 9–3B) for the teacher to wear both the FM and CADS microphones at the same time.

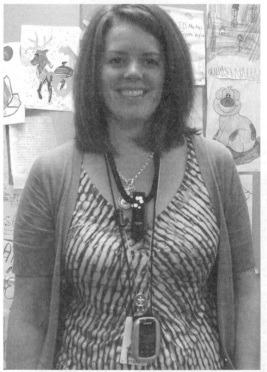 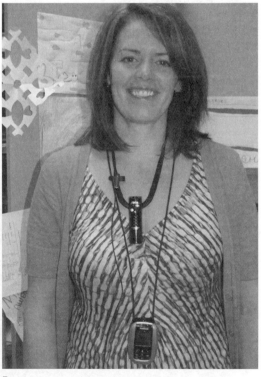

A   B

Figure 9–3. A. Pictured is an incorrect placement of a teacher wearing two microphone transmitters. Note that the microphone placements for the personal microphone and CADS are too low, and the teacher is wearing jewelry which causes unwanted noise to the listeners. **B.** Pictured is a correct placement of a teacher wearing two microphone transmitters. Note that the teacher has moved both the personal and CADS microphones closer to her mouth and has removed jewelry. Even though the personal FM transmitter is not close to her mouth, the microphone of the personal FM is now clipped high on a soft lavalier cord closer to her mouth.

HOW DOES EDUCATIONAL TECHNOLOGY IMPACT ACOUSTIC ACCESSIBILITY?

There are many educational technologies used in today's classrooms, for example:

- Tablets
- iPods
- Smartboards
- eLearning
- eBooks
- computers
- laptops
- streaming of videos
- YouTube videos
- Apps for educational learning
- Standardized tests on computers

Educational technology certainly enhances the learning environment, but for a student with hearing loss, these technologies can present challenges in their implementation and utilization. Professionals and students need to realize that in today's fast-paced classrooms, there is not a once and done solution to managing challenges posed by ever-changing educational technologies, challenges such as connectivity, streaming, and electromagnetic interference.

Connectivity Issues

Every kind of technology will have different **connectivity** issues and problems. Connectivity, in this instance means, how we couple or connect the child's personal HAT to the various educational technologies. Connectivity problems involve finding the appropriate connecting cords (Figure 9–4), ensuring adequate volume and quality of sound for each device when coupled to an educational device,

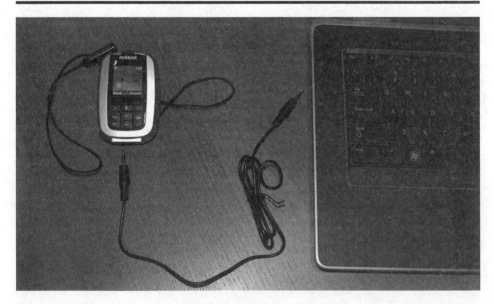

Figure 9–4. Pictured is a laptop computer that is one type of educational technology used in the classroom. The picture displays the setup of a personal FM transmitter with the audio input cord needed to connect the FM transmitter to the headphone jack of the computer.

eliminating distortion of the sound signal, and ensuring teacher knowledge of connectivity issues and troubleshooting strategies when connectivity is problematic. See box below.

Educational Streaming

Educational streaming refers to the mode of delivery of videos from YouTube, websites, and other online educational programming to the child's and/or classroom's computer system. Streaming allows transmission of audio, video, and other multimedia over the internet. Specifically, streaming media services deliver audio and video programs and information without making the viewer wait and endure the tedium of actually downloading large files. An issue is created, for example, when teachers stream YouTube segments that have poor audio quality and no captioning. Good connectivity of the child's FM to the child's computer will not overcome a video that is streamed

---

Here is a case example of managing connectivity (acoustic accessibility) of sound from a laptop, computer, or an iPad to the child's FM unit and hearing aids.

A fully mainstreamed 5th grade student with a moderate to moderately severe hearing loss uses an FM system appropriately fitted to bilateral ear level hearing aids. In school, the child is expected to complete independent learning activities as well as take standardized tests using his school laptop/tablet. Using a standard headphone attached to the computer and worn over the student's ears with or without hearing aids does not give the student adequate access to the computer's sound. In order to ensure the child has acoustic accessibility to computer-based learning and test taking, the following has to happen:

1. Involve an educational audiologist in the child's educational plan.
2. Obtain the appropriate audio input cord from the FM manufacturer, a cord that matches both the headphone jack of the child's computer, and the child's FM transmitter.

3. Ensure that the student's personal hearing aids are functioning, using both a biologic and functional listening check.
4. Ensure that the student's personal FM system is functioning, using both a biologic and functional listening check.
5. Locate the audio input jack on the child's FM transmitter, and the audio headphone jack on the personal computer or tablet. (See Figure 9–4.)
6. Listen to the sound quality of the computer signal through the connected hearing aid and FM transmitter using a listening stethoset.
7. Ensure that the volume on the computer is set to a comfortable listening level for the student.
8. Investigate whether captioning is available for the selected computer program, and if so, turn it on.
9. Monitor the student's comprehension closely because even though this arrangement provides an improved listening experience for the student, the student may still miss auditory information that is presented through the computer.

with poor audio quality. One solution might be for the teacher to include only closed-captioned YouTube video options when searching a topic.

Electromagnetic Interference

Electromagnetic interference is disturbance that affects an electrical circuit. Sources of electromagnetic interference in any of the child's environments include: fluorescent lights, computers, cell phone towers nearby, and hearing aid and cochlear implant telephone coil use for FM systems. Every room in a building may have different sources and problems with interference. Current amplification and FM technologies are designed to have fewer problems with interference, but interference still persists in various forms.

> WHAT ASSESSMENT PROTOCOLS CAN BE USED TO UNDERSTAND AND MANAGE ACOUSTIC ACCESSIBILITY IN ALL OF A CHILD'S ENVIRONMENTS?

There are many excellent direct and indirect protocols available for evaluating acoustic accessibility in home and school settings; indeed, there are so many tools that selection can be overwhelming (Anderson & Arnoldi, 2011; HATS, 2008; Johnson & Seaton, 2012; Madell & Flexer, 2014; Smaldino & Flexer, 2012). In an effort to streamline the selection of numerous available tools, the authors suggest a short list of assessments that can be used to begin the evaluation of home and school acoustic environments from preschool to high school. This list is far from exhaustive and the educational audiologist and

educational team may determine which of many available protocols are necessary to obtain all information relevant to a particular child's listening needs.

One possible acoustic accessibility assessment battery that can be repeated yearly, may include:

- Home and school environmental noise measurements using smartphone and tablet apps;
- Classroom observation using the Classroom Observation at a Glance Form (Johnson & Seaton, 2012, pp. 393 H–M) and a Classroom Observation Data Management Form (Appendix 9–A);
- Teacher, parent, and student interviews and checklists using the *LIFE-R* (Anderson, Smaldino, & Spangler, 2011);
- Use of *Guidelines for Remote Microphone Hearing Assistance Technologies for Children and Youth from Birth to 21 Years* (HAT, AAA, 2008) when collaborating with clinical/educational audiologists in managing FM and CADS; and
- Administer the Functional Listening Evaluation (FLE) in the classroom in order to collect evidence of the benefit of HAT and to identify the child's listening challenges (e.g., noise/distance/ visual) with and without the use of HATS (Johnson & Seaton, 2012, pp. 154–157).

Home and School Environmental Noise Measurements Using Smartphone and Tablet Apps

Because parents, teachers and practitioners who work with children with hearing loss are very focused on acoustic accessibility, all should have sound level meter apps on phones and tablets to obtain a general idea of the noise levels in all environments.

A recent search of sound level meter apps available for Apple and Android platforms identified several that could to be useful for the measurement of classroom acoustics. A few appeared to have been designed by audio professionals and could possibly be considered equivalent to stand-alone, Type II sound level meters (SLMs). The other apps seem to be designed more for estimation purposes, lacking features such as A-weighting, spectral analysis, and measures of reverberation time. While the options may be limited, the well-designed apps can be extremely functional and convenient (Smaldino, 2011; Smaldino & Ostergren, 2012).

Classroom Observation Protocol: Using the Classroom at a Glance Form and a Classroom Observation Data Collection Sheet

Before the classroom observation is conducted, the child's audiologist needs to verify and validate that the child's primary amplification provides access to the entire speech spectrum at soft levels (Madell, 2014). The audiologist also needs to verify hearing aid and FM coupling electroacoustically and also behaviorally in the sound booth in order to ensure transparency between both devices.

Before the Classroom Observation:

1. If the observer (Educational Audiologist, SLP, LSLS) is familiar with the child and his or her case history, proceed to step two. Some school districts

hire a consulting professional when faced with a student with hearing loss for the first time. If this is the case, it is important for the consulting professional to gain as much background information as possible about the child (ETR/IEP/case history information) before spending time in the school.

2. Contact the special education director, principal, or case manager to arrange a day to spend at the school. Explain that it is important to be able to spend the majority of the school day observing the child in order to analyze *all* acoustic environments in the student's "listening map." Avoid school days that deviate from a normal day (e.g., state testing day, day before a holiday, etc.).

3. Organize all of the assessment tools that will be used for the day (SLM app on the observer's smartphone or tablet, listening stethoscope, Classroom at a Glance form, Functional Listening Evaluation [FLE] form, Classroom Observation Data Management form, and Listening Inventory for Educational Risk-Revised [LIFE-R] forms).

4 Obtain a copy of the student's schedule and list of teachers ahead of time.

5. If possible, send an e-mail or other correspondence ahead of time, and ask the teacher to complete the LIFE-R in advance of your visit.

Day of the Observation:

1. On the day of and prior to the classroom observation, a biologic check of the child's hearing aid should be performed by the observer, using a listening stethoscope.

2. Next, the observer needs to verify that the child's personal FM is working

optimally and coupled appropriately to the child's personal technology and to the CADS if one is present in the classroom (American Academy of Audiology, 2008).

3. The Classroom at a Glance form should be completed according to the child's school schedule in each of his or her educational settings. The Classroom at a Glance form gives the observer the ability to look at different aspects of the educational situation that may affect a child's acoustic accessibility in various classroom environments, for example, physical characteristics of the room, teacher-student characteristics, classroom technology, amplification, and student participation/social aspects (Johnson & Seaton, 2012, pp. 393 H–M).

4. Use the Classroom Observation Data Management form (Appendix 9–B) to collect information about the child's performance on specific designated behaviors, for example, number of times in a 10-minute period that the child initiates interaction with peers in a collaborative activity, on- and off-task behavior.

Teacher, Parent, and Student Interviews Using the LIFE–R: A Series of Checklists for Verification of Acoustic Accessibility
(Anderson, Smaldino, & Spangler, 2011)

An understanding of the acoustic barriers to listening and learning in a classroom by the teacher and/or parents should not be assumed; data must be obtained. Checklists offer a way to obtain very useful information about how a child performs in a number of different situations. Some of these tools are designed to be completed by parents, some by students, and some by the professionals who work with the child; it can be very useful to have forms completed by a number of different people to obtain a broad picture. Results of rating scales are very helpful in counseling children, parents, and teachers about school concerns and in developing plans for acoustic accessibility, self-advocacy, and problem management. The LIFE-R (Listening Inventory for Education–Revised) is one such tool that offers a number of inventories and rating scales (for parents, teachers, and students) that are applicable across a wide range of ages and situations.

The LIFE-R

The LIFE-R has two main rating forms that can be used multiple times during the year to investigate the effect of changes in the child's technology or changes in the child's behavior:

1. The Teacher Life Inventory-Revised
2. Student Life Inventory-Revised

Both rating forms present with a variety of classroom listening situations and social listening/advocacy situations in school. For each of these questions, the student and teacher must judge the student's level of difficulty hearing and understanding.

The Student and Teacher LIFE-R also can be used as a pretest and post-test after a trial with hearing assistance technologies (HAT). Although use of HAT may improve the student's performance in some of the additional listening situations, it is likely that self-advocacy skills and other access activities may need to be used to show benefit in situations such as listening when others are talking, or teacher moving around the room. After completion of the rating forms, the LIFE-R provides a "listening difficulty summary" that allows the professional to identify the student's self-advocacy needs, develop appropriate goals, and track the student's progress over time.

Starting School LIFE-R

In addition to the Student and Teacher LIFE-R rating forms, there is another inventory called the Starting School LIFE. This tool usually focuses on the younger child, and is a framework for the school IEP team to use annually to gather information and observations from the family, child and educators in order to appropriately serve the whole child. The family is requested to complete the CHILD (Children's Home Inventory of Listening Difficulties) which the school team can consider as an indication of how the student performs at home compared to similar situations encountered in school. The family and school team impressions of communication mode for verbal instruction, educational program or setting, technology, accommodations, skill development, and social interactions are also taken into account. The following link allows access and free download of all components of LIFE-R and Starting School Life: http://successforkidswithhearingloss.com/tests/life-r

Collaborate With Clinical/Educational Audiologist in Managing FM and CADS Using the *Guidelines for Remote Microphone Hearing Assistance Technologies for Children and Youth from Birth to 21 Years* (HAT, AAA, 2008)

In order to ensure that the child's personal amplification devices and hearing assistance technologies (HAT) have been fitted and are functioning appropriately, the child's educational and clinical audiologists must collaborate. The American Academy of Audiology's *Clinical Practice Guidelines for Remote Microphone Hearing Assistance Technologies for Children and Youth from Birth to 21 Years* (2008) can be very helpful in the collaboration process. These guidelines provide a rationale and comprehensive protocol (selection, fitting, and management of HAT) for devices that use remote microphones such as personal-worn FMs, CADS and loop systems. The guidelines also discuss regulatory considerations and qualifications of personnel. Monitoring and managing equipment is discussed in detail, including procedures for checking systems to be sure they are working. Strategies for implementing guidelines in the schools are offered.

The following information in the HAT Guidelines is particularly useful:

a. HATS Table 5.3.3: Listening environment considerations/school (p. 14).
b. HATs Table 5.3.4: Listening considerations for home and community.
c. HATS Appendix B: Remote microphone HAT implementation worksheet; there is an in- school form and out-of-school form.
d. HATS Appendix D: Common functional outcome measures used to assess amplification benefit, pp. 44–46)

For Web access to the full document, please refer to American Academy of Audiology; 2008: http://www.audiology.org/resources/documentlibrary/Documents/HATGuideline.pdf

Administer the Functional Listening Evaluation (FLE) in the Classroom to Collect Evidence of the Benefit of HAT and to Identify the Child's Listening Challenges (e.g., noise/distance) With and Without the Use of HATS
(Johnson & Seaton, 2012, pp. 154–157)

The need to document a student's ability to hear in the school environment is evident. The functional listening evaluation (FLE) is designed to evaluate a student in his or her classroom, taking into account the classroom characteristics, using sound-level meters or sound measurement apps. A student's ability to listen in eight different environments is evaluated; four in quiet with close and distant proximities and auditory-only and auditory-visual access, and the same four conditions with background noise present. In addition, the FLE allows the examiner to compare how the student performs with no amplification, with personal amplification, and with HAT. The results of this test can help demonstrate the negative effects of distance and noise as well as enhance the team's understanding of the benefit of both HAT and acoustical modification in the classroom environment.

WHAT IS AN IMPLEMENTATION PLAN FOR MANAGING THE CHILD'S ACOUSTIC ACCESSIBILITY IN HOME AND SCHOOL ENVIRONMENTS?

After completing the acoustic accessibility assessment battery, an implementation plan must be devised. A possible implementation plan includes:

- *Detailed written report* of the acoustic accessibility assessment battery results sent to all team members.
- *Team meeting* to include parents and audiologist for reviewing results of the assessment protocol and writing Individualized Education Plan (IEP) goals and accommodations for acoustic accessibility.
- *Staff in-service training* about acoustic accessibility goals, management of HAT, and acoustic accessibility accommodations.
- *Ongoing follow-up* to ensure sustainable implementation of acoustic accessibility technologies and acoustic accessibility accommodations.

Team Meeting Including Parents and Audiologist to Review Results of the Assessment Protocol and to Summarize and Write IEP Goals and Accommodations for Acoustic Accessibility

The LIFE-R has a very helpful feature that generates a report for the particular student based on information obtained from the student appraisal form. (See Appendix 9–B for an example of this report.) This report can be extremely useful in writing IEP and 504 objectives specifying accommodations and self-advocacy, as shown in the following example:

Adam is 10 years old in the 5th grade with bilateral cochlear implants that he received at 2 years of age. He has been fully mainstreamed since kindergarten, with appropriate and thoughtful accommodations. Adam currently is performing at grade level. The Student LIFE-R, administered with assistance by the LSL specialist after 6 weeks of school (when the first report card was issued) generated a report in which one of many items on the report indicated the student "mostly has difficulty hearing and understanding when the teacher is walking around the room." Currently, the teacher reports that Adam is not displaying any advocacy strategies for his hearing and listening needs. Therefore, the information from the Teacher and Student LIFE-R report indicated that one of the goals the IEP team ought to consider specifying that the child will have access to instruction through appropriate modifications and accommodations.

Following is an example of one of several IEP goals for acoustic accessibility identified by information obtained from the LIFE-R Student Appraisal report. (This is a simple summary of one goal; please refer to other chapters in this book for additional details about IEP development and implementation): "The student will have auditory access to academic instruction in large, small, group settings and assemblies."

Objective 1: Child will determine appropriate strategic seating in the classroom, measured through classroom observation, in 3 out of 4 trial situations.

Objective 2: Child will identify a malfunctioning personal FM system (in a controlled sabotaged situation), and notify his teacher of the malfunction unit in 3 out of 4 trials.

Objective 3: Child will identify 3 communication barriers and implement 3 communication solutions in his classroom setting in 3 out of 4 trials.

Staff In-Service Training About Acoustic Accessibility Goals and Accommodations

A staff in-service training is a critical component of managing acoustic accessibility; the in-service training can include the following components:

- Be sure to include all staff members and school personnel who have contact with the child.
- Begin with "the brain talk"! Emphasize the importance of hearing and acoustic accessibility as the foundation of the child's auditory brain development—and auditory brain development is the basis of language, reading, and learning.
- Demonstrate use of the SLM app and make sure all staff members have an app on their smartphones or tablets. Have teachers practice making noise measurements.
- Play unfair spelling test or other recorded simulation of hearing loss; it is vital for teachers and others to hear how a hearing loss distorts the intelligibility of speech.
- Discuss and demonstrate the child's personal technologies, for example, HA, or CI, and show how to troubleshoot. Have the teacher practice.

- Emphasize factors that impact acoustic and educational access in the classroom (e.g., noise, reverberation, distance, visual distractions, attention, etc.).
- Illustrate how the classroom can be made more educationally and acoustically accessible by using environmental modifications (e.g., carpet, noise reduction, close hallway door, windows, monitor HVAC systems). Johnson and Seaton (2012) have developed a very useful checklist that can identify "Accommodations and Modifications for Students Who are Deaf or Hard of Hearing" (pp. 528–529 [13A]).
- Demonstrate the child's personal-worn FM system, and have the staff handle and listen to the technology.
- Show how to functionally validate and record that the equipment is working to ensure that the child has optimal acoustic accessibility each day.
- Arrange for follow-up conversations and coaching throughout the year for sustainable implementation of strategies.

What modifications can be made to the listening environments in school, at home, on the playground, and in the community to improve acoustic accessibility?

All sounds must pass through an environment before they arrive at the child's technology. Therefore, the first step in reaching the child's brain is managing the environment. Some noise sources can be controlled and others cannot. It is essential that we manage the controllable factors in order to provide children with appropriate listening and learning environments. The home environment is the primary concern for infants. For toddlers, concerns revolve around the home, playground, and possibly day care. As children get older, preschool, school, and after-school activities become added concerns.

Classroom Accommodations

- No child with hearing loss or other auditory disorders such as auditory processing should be placed in an open classroom. An open classroom is one where several classes are in one open space with dividers such as bookcases separating

---

Here is one strategy for promoting school/educational collaboration in identifying and solving acoustic accessibility problems in various school listening environments. This strategy can be used as part of an in-service training.

- Show pictures of a variety of classrooms and educational situations. Actual pictures of the child's listening environments make this activity personal.
- Using one picture at a time, ask

the audience to identify barriers to acoustic accessibility in that room.
- Ask the teachers to generate solutions to identified acoustic barriers.
- Then, list all solutions.
- Also, have students with hearing loss do the same exercise so they are aware of the educational and listening needs and barriers in specific educational settings. Start by taking a picture of their classroom and ask them to analyze acoustic accessibility, in an age-appropriate manner.

groups; because many children and activities share this large space, acoustic accessibility typically is horrible.

- The classroom selected for the child with hearing loss should be located away from particularly noisy areas such as the gym, lunchroom, bathrooms, playground, and noisy streets.
- Acoustic floor materials should be installed in classrooms and in hallways to reduce noise.
- Acoustic tiles should be placed on ceilings (and on walls, too, in some instances) to reduce reverberation.
- Tennis balls or "chair socks" should be placed on the feet of all movable chairs and tables to reduce the noise made as chairs scrape on the floor.
- Windows and doors should be tightly fitted and kept closed to reduce extraneous noise.
- Noise from the heating, ventilation, and air-conditioning systems should be monitored and reduced.
- Computers can also be noisy and also should be monitored.

Not Preferential Seating: Call It "Strategic Seating." The term preferential seating has been used for years and typically implies the child is seated at the front of the room, near the teacher. From that location, the assumption is that all information can be heard. Because the classroom is a dynamic environment, a fixed location at the front of the room may be too restrictive and isolating. A more descriptive term might be strategic seating, as described below:

- No matter how good the classroom accommodations, if a child is not seated close to the person talking, listening will be difficult.

Therefore, an FM system must be used and will permit the child to hear words spoken directly into the microphone/transmitter; however, listening to "nonmicrophone talkers" will continue to be difficult.

- Seating should be in the front third of the room, off to the side, with a full view of the classroom. This placement should permit the student to turn and face the group, monitor the activity occurring in the room, and both identify the talker and see the talker's face.
- The student should have permission to move about the classroom as needed to hear relevant activities. For example, if English is taught in the front of the room and math at the back, the student may need to move to hear the academic conversations.
- For small group work, the student with hearing loss should be assigned to a table that is at the side of the room and should be permitted to sit with his or her back to the wall to reduce the amount of noise swirling around.

Teaching Accommodations to Improve Listening. The following soft, common sense recommendations that are related specifically to acoustic accessibility can make the difference between a successful or a stressful school experience for children with hearing loss. Teachers should be coached and mentored in implementation.

- Teachers should be advised to try and keep the classroom quiet, encouraging students not to talk among themselves or chatter during desk work time, and not to call out answers.

- The teacher should be encouraged to use "clear speech," speak at a normal or slightly slower conversational rate with pauses, and at a normal pitch to facilitate listening and auditory processing. Most adults speak faster than most children can process.
- The teacher should be asked to face the student with hearing loss when speaking to him or her, and to call the student by name to be sure he or she knows he or she is being addressed.
- It is important the teacher verifies, by asking specific informational questions, that the child understands what is being said.
- Students should be encouraged to ask for clarification when they do not understand; they should be empowered to advocate for themselves.
- Implement strategies for note-taking, voice-to-text, and so forth as the child advances in grades.
- Receiving outlines, lesson plans, agendas, and so forth, in advance, all through school, will be very useful for pretutoring and studying, and can allow the child to predict upcoming words and concepts.
- Listening all day can be exhausting, and children with hearing loss expend a great deal of effort focusing in class; listening breaks could be scheduled throughout the day to allow the child to rest.
- The daily schedule should be organized so the child with hearing loss does not have difficult subjects back-to-back.

WHAT ONGOING FOLLOW–UP SHOULD BE PERFORMED TO ENSURE IMPLEMENTATION OF ACOUSTIC ACCESSIBILITY TECHNOLOGIES AND ACCOMMODATIONS?

The cornerstone of acoustic accessibility is the function and use of the child's technologies (HA, CI, BAHD and FM systems). Auditory information must reach the child's brain in order for neural connections to be generated. No strategies or instruction can compensate for technologies that are not in optimal condition and used every waking moment. So, there must be a specific amplification plan in place to monitor and fix the child's technologies.

That is:

- Who is to be notified if there is any suspicion of equipment malfunction? (e.g., the educational audiologist)
- Who is to notify the audiologist? (Anybody and everybody who notices a problem, e.g., the child, parent, teacher, bus driver, SLP, aide, lunchroom monitor, etc.)
- When is the audiologist to be notified? (Immediately!)
- What actions should be taken to resolve the problem? A plan of action should be specified.

In addition, there must be an organized in-service follow-up plan that includes teacher, parents, and other school staff. There is no such thing as an effective one-time meeting; communication must be ongoing, accommodations need to be monitored, and questions need to be answered. (Refer to Appendix 9–C for a sample amplification plan.)

SUMMARY

Assessment and management of the child's acoustic access is complex, and includes the child's entire day. Refer to Figure 9–1, the child's "listening map."

Auditory information must reach the brain in order for neural connections to develop. The purpose of all technologies is to direct sound to the child's brain for the development of listening, speaking, reading, learning, and psychosocial skills. The purpose of acoustic accessibility is to allow a pathway to the brain; all sounds must pass through an environment in order to reach the child's technologies. Even the best educational programming cannot substitute for poor acoustic access if listening and spoken language are the desired outcomes.

By using the assessment and follow-up strategies outlined in this chapter, professionals can generate a management plan for sustainable acoustic access in school and home environments for students who have hearing loss, which is foundational for student success.

REFERENCES

American Academy of Audiology. (2008). *Clinical practice guidelines for remote microphone hearing assistance technologies for children and youth from birth to 21 years.* Retrieved from http://www.audiology.org/resources/document library/documents/hatguideline.pdf

American National Standards Institute (ANSI). (2002). *ANSI/ASA S12.60-2002. American National Standard acoustical performance criteria, design requirements, and guidelines for schools.* Melville, NY: Acoustical Society of America.

American National Standards Institute (ANSI). (2010). *ANSI/ASA S12.60-2010 American National Standard acoustical performance criteria, design requirements, and guidelines for schools, Part 1: Permanent schools, and Part 2: Relocatable classrooms factors.* Melville, NY: Acoustical Society of America.

American Speech-Language-Hearing Association. (2000). *Guidelines for fitting and monitoring FM systems.* Retrieved from http://www.asha.org/members/deskref-journals/deskref/default

Anderson, K. (2004). The problem of classroom acoustics: The typical classroom soundscape is a barrier to learning. *Seminars in Hearing, 25*(2), 117–129.

Anderson, K. L., & Arnoldi, K. A. (2011). *Building skills for success in the fast-paced classroom: Optimizing achievement for students with hearing loss.* Hillsboro, OR: Butte.

Anderson, K. L., Goldstein, H., Colodzin, L., & Inglehart, F. (2005). Benefit of S/N enhancing devices to speech perception of children listening in a typical classroom with hearing aids or a cochlear implant. *Journal of Educational Audiology, 12*, 14–28.

Anderson, K. L, Smaldino, J. J., & Spangler, C. (2011). *LIFE-R.* Retrieved from http://success forkidswithhearingloss.com/tests/life-r

Chermak, G. D., Bellis, J. B., & Musiek, F. E. (2014). Neurobiology, cognitive science, and intervention. In G. D. Chermak & F. E. Musiek (Eds.), *Handbook of central auditory processing disorder: Comprehensive intervention, Volume II* (2nd ed., pp. 3–38). San Diego, CA: Plural.

Ching, T. Y., van Wanrooy, E., Dillon, H., & Carter, L. (2011). Spatial release from masking in normal-hearing children and children who use hearing aids. *Journal of the Acoustical Society of America, 129*(1), 368–375.

Cole, E., & Flexer, C. (2011). *Children with hearing loss: Developing listening and talking, birth to six* (2nd ed). San Diego, CA: Plural.

Dillon, H. (2012). *Hearing aids* (2nd ed). New York, NY: Thieme Medical.

Dillon, H., Ching, T., & Golding, M. (2014). Hearing aids for infants and children. In J. R. Madell & C. Flexer, *Pediatric audiology: Diagnosis, technology and management* (2nd ed., pp. 209–227). New York, NY: Thieme Medical.

Flynn, T. S., Flynn, M. C., & Gregory, M. (2005). The FM advantage in the real classroom. *Journal of Educational Audiology, 12*, 35–42.

Hart, B., & Risley, T. R. (1999). *The social world of children learning to talk.* Baltimore, MD: Brookes.

Johnson, C. D., & Seaton, J. B. (2012). *Educational audiology handbook* (2nd ed.). Clifton Park, NY: Delmar-Cengage Learning.

Kramer, S. (2014). *Audiology: Science to practice* (2nd ed.). San Diego, CA: Plural.

Leavitt, R. J., & Flexer, C. (1991). Speech degradation as measured by the rapid speech transmission index (RASTI). *Ear and Hearing, 12,* 115–118.

Madell, J. R. (2014). Evaluation of speech perception in infants and children. In J. R. Madell & C. Flexer, *Pediatric audiology: Diagnosis, technology and management* (2nd ed., pp. 103–120). New York, NY: Thieme Medical.

Madell, J. R., & Flexer C. (2014). *Pediatric audiology: Diagnosis, technology and management* (2nd ed.). New York, NY: Thieme Medical.

Mitchell, R. E., & Karchmer, M. A. (2004). Chasing the mythical ten percent: Parental hearing status of deaf and hard of hearing students in the United States. *Sign Language Studies, 4*(2), 138–163.

Moeller, M. P., Donaghy, K. F., Beauchaine, K. L., Lewis, D., & Stelmachowicz, P. G. (1996). Longitudinal study of FM system use in non-academic settings: Effects on language development. *Ear and Hearing, 17*(1), 28–41.

National Governors Association Center for Best Practices and Council of Chief State School Officers. (2010). *Common core core state standards.* Retrieved February 6, 2014, from http://www.corestandards.org/ELA-Literacy/CCRA/SL)

Nelson, P. B., & Blaeser, S. B. (2010). Classroom acoustics: What possibly could be new? *The ASHA Leader, 15*(11), 16–19.

Nguyen, H., & Bentler, R. (2011). Optimizing FM systems. *The ASHA Leader, 16*(12), 5–6.

Smaldino, J. (2011). New developments in classroom acoustics and amplification. *Audiology Today, 23*(1), 30–36.

Smaldino, J., & Flexer, C. (2012). *Handbook of acoustic accessibility: Best practices for listening, learning and literacy in the classroom.* New York, NY: Thieme.

Smaldino, J., & Ostergren, D. (2012). Classroom acoustic measurements. In, J. Smaldino & C. Flexer (Eds.), *Handbook of acoustic accessibility: Best practices for listening, learning and literacy in the classroom* (pp. 34–54). New York, NY: Thieme.

Thibodeau, L. (2013, December). *Results with devices that utilize DM technology.* Oral presentation at the Phonak Advances in Audiology Conference, Las Vegas, NV.

Wolfe, J., Morais, M., Schafer, E., Millis, E., Mulder, H. E., Goldbeck, F., . . . Lianos. L. (2013). Evaluation of speech recognition of cochlear implant recipients using a persona digital adaptive radio frequency system. *Journal of the American Academy of Audiology, 24*(8), 714–724.

Classroom Observation Form

Student: _____ Date: _____ Class: _____

School: _____ District: _____ Teacher: _____

Code: A = At task
T = Talking with another student
L = Looking around the room
P = Playing with objects at desk (toys, pencil, book)
Q = Asking questions about what is happening in class
S = Seeking information from other students
C = Making comments not pertaining to topic

Time:	Code:	Comments:
:	____	_____
:	____	_____
:	____	_____
:	____	_____
:	____	_____
:	____	_____
:	____	_____
:	____	_____
:	____	_____
:	____	_____
:	____	_____
:	____	_____
:	____	_____
:	____	_____
:	____	_____
:	____	_____
:	____	_____
:	____	_____

Adapted from: Dr. Jim Blair, Utah State University.   *continues*

Appendix 9–A. *continued*

Time:	Code:	Comments:
:	_____	_____
:	_____	_____
:	_____	_____
:	_____	_____
:	_____	_____
:	_____	_____
:	_____	_____
:	_____	_____
:	_____	_____
:	_____	_____
:	_____	_____
:	_____	_____
:	_____	_____
:	_____	_____
:	_____	_____
:	_____	_____
:	_____	_____
:	_____	_____
:	_____	_____
:	_____	_____
:	_____	_____
:	_____	_____
:	_____	_____
:	_____	_____
:	_____	_____

Summary of School Listening Challenges

Name: Test Student
Grade: 5
Date completed: Friday, December 20, 2013
Session ID: 1387546284
Teacher: Teacher
School: Hear and Learn

Hearing Aid: Left and Right
Cochlear Implant: None.
Bone Anchored Device: None.
Type of Classroom Hearing Technology: PersonalFM
Trial Period: None

Of the 15 Listening Inventory For Education questions, the following situations were rated Always Difficult (🍁🍁🍁), Mostly Difficult (🍁🍁), or Sometimes Difficult (🍁):

Test's most challenging listening situations:

🍁	Teacher talking in front of room
🍁🍁	Teacher talking with back turned
🍁🍁	Teacher talking while moving
🍁	Student answering during discussion
🍁🍁	Hearing and understanding directions
🍁	Other students making noise
🍁🍁🍁	Noise outside of the classroom
🍁🍁	Multimedia (video, computer)
🍁	Listening with fan noise on
🍁🍁	Simultaneous large and small group
🍁	Cooperative small group learning
🍁🍁	Announcements
🍁🍁	Listening in a large room (assembly)
🍁	Listening to others when outside
🍁🍁	Listening to students during informal social times

continues

TOP PRIORITIES

Student/teacher strategies should be implemented for the following school listening situations:

1. Noise outside of the classroom
2. Teacher talking with back turned
3. Teacher talking while moving
4. Hearing and understanding directions
5. Multimedia (video, computer)

Instructor Comments:

Amplification Plan

Student: _____ Teacher: _____

Audiologist: _____

Equipment: LE: _____

RE: _____

FM: _____

A daily listening check on the above equipment will be conducted by

_____. In the event that he or she is absent,

_____ will complete the daily listening check.

This will be documented by a daily check list/calendar.

If the child is using a personal FM system, it will be fit, programmed, and maintained

by _____ (Audiologist).

Teacher(s)/staff will be in-serviced on the child's hearing loss, use of equipment, and accommodations that are beneficial for students with hearing loss.

Date completed: _____ Initials: _____

In the event of equipment malfunction, the following actions will be taken:

1. Check settings (on/off).
2. Change battery.
3. Contact _____.
4. _____.
5. _____.
6. _____.

_____   _____
(Student)   (Parent)

_____   _____
(Teacher)   (Audiologist)

_____
(Speech-Language Pathologist)

CHAPTER 10

Hearing Aid Assessment

Ryan McCreery

KEY POINTS

- Amplification provides children with hearing loss auditory access and experiences they need to minimize developmental delays.
- The two primary goals of hearing aid assessment in children are to make speech audible across a range of everyday listening situations and to promote consistent hearing aid use.
- Selection of hearing aid features and signal processing strategies can help to maximize audibility.
- Consistent verification using probe microphone measures during childhood is crucial for maintaining audibility for speech as the child grows and develops.
- Monitoring outcomes is an important process for measuring the impacts of amplification the child's auditory skill development.

INTRODUCTION

The primary negative consequence of childhood hearing loss is impoverished access to the acoustic cues that are the basis of auditory-verbal communication. The long-term consequences of limited auditory access extend beyond delays in communication development to affect academic achievement, social opportunities, and quality of life (Calderon & Low, 1998; Wake et al., 2004). In the current era of universal newborn hearing screening (UNHS) and early diagnosis and intervention, positive outcomes can be supported through the provision of hearing aids and other auditory devices during the early stages of development (Tomblin et al., 2014). This chapter focuses on the provision of air conduction and bone conduction amplification for infants and children who are hard of hearing and the methods by which professionals can assess the effectiveness of these devices systematically. Assessment of amplification should be an on-going process that evolves as the child grows and his or her listening and communication needs develop. The overall goals of providing amplification for infants and children are highlighted, as well as strategies for hearing aid verification and outcomes validation.

RATIONALE FOR AMPLIFICATION FOR CHILDREN WHO ARE HARD OF HEARING

Without intervention, children with hearing loss either at birth or during childhood are likely to have delays in speech and language development, as well as diminished social opportunities and academic achievement. Until the advent of universal newborn hearing screening programs and early hearing detection and intervention programs, children who are hard of hearing were frequently not identified until after 18 to 24 months of age (Moeller, 2000). The developmental impact of delayed identification was severe and pervasive, as detailed in many early studies of children with hearing loss (Davis, 1977; Davis, Elfenbein, Schum, & Bentler, 1986). Hearing loss reduces access to acoustic cues and experience that are crucial for development. The negative developmental implications of hearing loss on listening and spoken language led to recommendations for early identification and intervention by the Joint Committee on Infant Hearing (JCIH; American Academy of Pediatrics, 2007). In addition to hearing screening by 1 month of age, diagnostic audiological assessment by 3 months of age, and enrollment in early intervention by 6 months of age, children identified with hearing loss also should receive appropriately fit amplification within 1 month of confirmation of hearing loss. Ideally, amplification can enhance acoustic access to communication and minimize the potential for delays. The extent to which amplification can be effective depends on two key factors: audibility and hearing aid use.

Speech Audibility

The term **audibility** is used to describe how much of the speech signal can be heard. Audibility can be expressed as either unaided—describing how much speech can be heard by the child based on his or her degree and configuration of hearing loss—or aided—based on the amount of speech that is audible with amplification. Speech audibility is often displayed graphically in an SPL-o-gram (Figure 10–1). The SPL-o-gram plots dB sound pressure level (SPL) as a function of frequency in hertz. Unlike the audiogram where the sound level increases from the top of the graph to the bottom, sound level is highest at the top of the SPL-o-gram. Hearing thresholds from the audiogram or other types of hearing assessment measured in dB HL are converted to an equivalent SPL. The speech spectrum is represented on the SPL-o-gram using the **long-term average speech spectrum** (LTASS). The LTASS represents the frequency range and level for a speech signal averaged over time and is plotted with the hearing thresholds in SPL to estimate audibility. The proportion of the LTASS that is above the hearing thresholds represents the audible portion of the speech spectrum. The LTASS is frequently referenced to an average conversational level for speech from 1 meter away, which is usually equivalent to an overall level of 60 or 65 dB SPL, but can also be used to represent speech at other levels (soft and loud).

Speech audibility can be quantified into a single numerical value using the **speech intelligibility index** [SII], (ANSI S3.5-1997). The SII is based on the idea that different frequency regions of the speech signal carry different amounts of

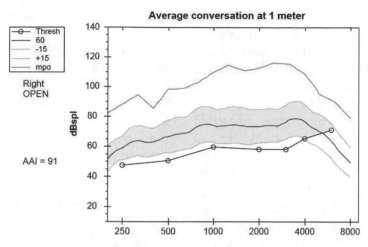

Figure 10–1. The SPL-o-gram is a graph that displays the hearing thresholds and output of the hearing aid as a function of frequency in dB sound pressure level (SPL). The circles connected by the solid line represent the hearing thresholds for the right ear. The dark black line represents the long-term average speech spectrum (LTASS) amplified by the hearing aid. The gray shaded area around the LTASS represents the peaks and valleys of the speech signal. The dark gray solid line represents the maximum output of the hearing aid.

importance for understanding speech. The SII is expressed as a proportion (between 0 and 1) or percentage (between 0 and 100), where higher values represent greater audibility of the speech signal. To calculate audibility using the SII, the speech spectrum is divided into discrete frequency bands. The proportion of the LTASS that is audible within each frequency band is multiplied by an importance factor for that band. Importance factors are derived from speech recognition experiments where frequency bands are removed using filters (Hirsch, Reynolds, & Joseph, 1954). The average amount of degradation in speech understanding that occurs when a frequency band is removed from the signal reflects that frequency region's importance. Importance factors have been derived for different types of

speech stimuli (syllables, words, and sentences) and talkers (male or female). The importance and audibility factors for all of the frequency bands are added to calculate the SII. Most of the importance functions that have been developed for the SII were derived from experiments with adults who have normal hearing. Whereas the SII has often been used to predict speech recognition in adults, predictions of speech recognition in children based on the SII tend to overestimate performance on average (McCreery & Stelmachowicz, 2011; Scollie, 2008).

Therefore, the primary purpose of the SII with children who are hard of hearing is to quantify the amount of speech information that is audible to the child with and without amplification. Unaided SII values can be used to quantify the impact of hearing loss on the audibility of speech without amplification. For estimates of unaided audibility, the unamplified LTASS is compared to hearing thresholds in SPL. Aided SII values are used to describe the amount of the LTASS that is audible with amplification based on the amplified speech signal, which is usually derived by measuring the output of the hearing aid in SPL with a stimulus that has the same spectral and temporal characteristics of the LTASS. The importance of documenting aided audibility using the SII has recently been highlighted by several studies of speech and language development in children who are hard of hearing. Development of vocabulary (Stiles, Bentler, & McGregor, 2012) and the structural aspects of language, including morphology and syntax (Koehlinger, Van Horne, & Moeller, 2013), have been shown to be higher in children with higher aided audibility than for peers who wear hearing aids that provide less aided audibility. Thus, the amount of the speech signal that is audible can directly impact the auditory access that the child has with his or her amplification and is a key component in the clinical assessment of amplification. Figure 10–2 displays examples of SPL-o-grams with different amounts of speech audibility.

Hearing Aid Use

For amplification to be effective, the devices must be used consistently. While this concept might seem overly simplistic, parents and caregivers can experience significant challenges in establishing and maintaining consistent hearing aid use in infants and young children. Older children and adolescents may experience decreased device use due to self-consciousness or bullying (Bauman

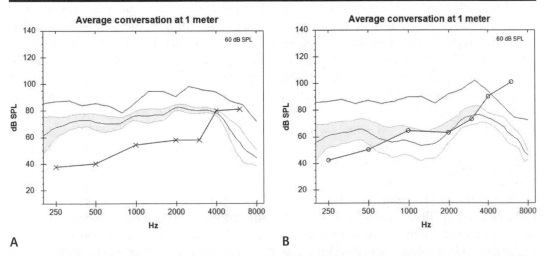

Figure 10–2. SPL-o-grams displaying a fitting that provides adequate audibility for speech (**A**) and a fitting that provides inadequate audibility for speech (**B**). In the left panel, most of the speech spectrum is above the hearing thresholds, except at frequencies above 4 kHz. Most of the speech spectrum in the right panel is below the listener's hearing thresholds, which indicates that these portions of the speech signal will not be audible to the listener at an average level.

& Pero, 2011; McKay, Gravel, & Tharpe, 2008). Despite the importance of consistent device use for supporting positive outcomes, surprisingly few studies have examined how much children are using their devices and what impact that might have on their development. An exploratory study by Moeller and colleagues (2009) sought to quantify the amount of hearing aid use among infants and young children who are hard of hearing and the factors that might support or limit consistent hearing aid use. For infants and toddlers, hearing aid use increased as a function of age, reflecting greater ease establishing a consistent wearing schedule as infants get older. Hearing aid use in infants and toddlers was also found to vary significantly across individuals and for listening situations such as the car and outdoors, potentially due to parental concerns for losing the devices in those situations.

In a later investigation by Walker et al. (2013), parent report about hearing aid use was compared to automated data-logging features on hearing aids, which report the average amount of time the hearing aid is on during the day. Parent report and data-logging were generally in strong agreement, with parents only over-estimating their child's hearing aid use by an average of 2 hours per day. Because data-logging systems vary across hearing aid manufacturers and have not been scientifically validated, the source of this discrepancy between data-logging and parent report cannot currently be resolved. Until evidence emerges to validate data-logging as a valid measure of average hearing aid use, both parent report and data-logging should be used by clinicians to monitor use.

The amount of hearing aid use that is sufficient to support positive outcomes in children who are hard of hearing has not been directly evaluated. Particularly in school-age children, hearing aid use is more consistent among children with greater degrees of hearing loss (McCreery, Walker, Spratford, Jacobs, & Hatala, 2013). Because children with greater degrees of hearing loss are more likely to experience suboptimal outcomes compared to children with milder hearing loss, establishing the amount of device use that is sufficient to support development while controlling for the amount of hearing loss is complicated. Bagatto et al. (2011) reported that a group of children who wore amplification but had risk factors including limited device use were often below normative values on several questionnaires of auditory development. Because of the potential impact of inconsistent device use on developmental outcomes and the fact that these devices can only benefit children when they are used, professionals should monitor the consistency of amplification use and help to develop strategies for overcoming challenges in use. Table 10–1 includes a list of strategies for supporting consistent hearing aid use.

GOALS OF AMPLIFICATION FOR CHILDREN

Because the primary goals of amplification in children are to restore audibility of the speech signal and promote consistent device use, the hearing aid assessment process for children should reflect these priorities. The following sections of the chapter describe the clinical process and theory of amplification assessment of children who are hard of hearing. The amplification assessment process starts

Table 10–1. Promoting Consistent Hearing Aid Use

1. **Quality time vs. quantity of time:** If parents are struggling to establish consistent hearing aid use for their child, encourage them to focus first on the listening situations where hearing aid use is less challenging at first. Highly communicative situations like reading or playing one-on-one can provide a foundation for increasing use in other situations.

2. **Recognize challenging situations:** Noisy listening environments, such as in the car or out in public, can be challenging to establish use because of difficulty listening and potential concerns for losing the devices. Counsel parents and caregivers to anticipate these challenges and provide additional support, such as FM systems or other hearing assistance technology, as needed.

3. **Provide retention devices:** Simple retention devices provided with the hearing aid care kit can reduce parent anxiety about losing the hearing aids and increase the likelihood that parents will be willing to have their children wear the hearing aids in a wide range of listening situations.

4. **Anticipate developmental changes:** Research suggests that children may experience a brief decline in the number of hours of hearing aid use per day between 6 and 12 months due to the development of fine motor skills, such as the pincer grasp, that allow children to take out their hearing aids (Walker et al., 2013). Encourage parents that these challenges are part of the normal developmental process and provide strategies to help parents avoid frustration during this phase.

with an accurate audiological evaluation of the child's hearing to establish the need for amplification. Following the diagnosis of hearing loss, pediatric validated **prescriptive methods** can be used to determine the amount of amplification needed. The device is then verified using objective, electroacoustic measures to ensure that the prescriptive recommendations are achieved. The parents, child, and caregivers are oriented to the daily use and function of the devices to help to establish consistent use. The outcomes with amplification are monitored to ensure that the child is meeting auditory, communication, and academic milestones. The amplification assessment process is ongoing and may change as the child grows and develops. The process is different for air conduction and bone conduction devices and the differences between the two modes of sound delivery are highlighted.

CANDIDACY FOR AMPLIFICATION

Hearing loss of nearly any type or degree can interrupt the process of listening and learning. Although children with greater degrees of hearing loss often have the most substantial delays (Ching, Johnson, et al., 2013), even children with milder degrees of hearing loss are more likely than peers with normal hearing to experience speech and language delays and academic challenges if amplification is not provided (Porter et al., 2013; Tharpe, 2008). Therefore, any child who is diagnosed with permanent hearing loss should be evaluated as a potential hearing aid candidate. Given the possibility of negative developmental consequences from hearing loss, hearing aids should be provided as soon as a diagnosis of hearing loss is confirmed. If the likelihood that a child will benefit for amplification is uncertain, clinicians should err on the side of providing amplification. Amplification can always been discontinued if determined to be ineffective; however, auditory experience that is missed related to hearing loss cannot be recovered once that time has passed. Some specific types of hearing loss, such as conductive hearing loss and auditory neuropathy spectrum disorder, or degrees of hearing loss, including unilateral and mild hearing losses, require special consideration when determining candidacy for amplification.

Type of Hearing Loss

Although sensorineural, mixed, conductive, and neural hearing losses can all negatively impact audibility, the type of hearing loss can influence the process of determining candidacy and providing amplification for children. Sensorineural hearing loss is the most frequent type of permanent hearing loss in children. Unlike adults who usually have high-frequency sensorineural hearing loss from noise-exposure or aging, children can have a wide range of audiometric configurations related to sensorineural hearing loss, consistent with the widely varying etiologies of hearing loss in children (Pittman & Stelmachowicz, 2003). Children with permanent conductive or mixed hearing losses should also be considered candidates for amplification, since these types of hearing loss also result in reduced access to auditory experience. Children with mixed and conductive hearing losses, however, may be more likely to experience fluctuations in hearing than children with sensorineural loss (Pittman & Stelmachowicz, 2003), so hearing should be monitored frequently. While all children diagnosed with hearing loss should be referred to an otolaryngologist for medical evaluation, the provision of amplification in children with conductive or mixed hearing losses should take into account the availability of other treatment options, including surgery or pharmacological intervention.

Children may be likely to experience temporary hearing loss related to chronic otitis media or other conditions. In most cases, children will receive prompt medical management of middle ear problems. In some cases, however, the child may not be eligible for surgical treatment of temporary conditions because of age, health status, or other factors. In cases where the duration of hearing loss is expected to exceed 3 months, amplification should be discussed as an option with the family, child, and medical care providers. Factors that may impact decisions about amplification for temporary hearing losses expected to exceed 3 months in duration include the degree and stability of hearing loss, related otologic complications such as ear drainage or external otitis media, and the child's age and developmental status. For temporary hearing losses, loaner hearing aids should be provided whenever possible. There is limited evidence in the literature to support or refute the efficacy of amplification in children with temporary hearing losses of extended duration, so professionals must take into account a wide range of individual factors when exploring candidacy for amplification.

Auditory Neuropathy Spectrum Disorder

Auditory neuropathy spectrum disorder (ANSD) is a type of hearing loss that occurs when there are problems with neural transmission of sound from the cochlear or auditory nerve. (See Rance, 2005 for a review.) Children are diagnosed with ANSD on the basis of having normal cochlear outer hair cell function, as measured by present otoacoustic emissions or cochlear microphonic responses on the auditory brainstem response, and abnormal auditory neural function, demonstrated with an absent wave V on the auditory brainstem response at the highest levels of stimulation. The etiologies of ANSD are highly varied in children (Rance, 2005). As a result, outcomes with hearing aids and cochlear implants are highly variable, with some children experiencing benefits similar to children with sensorineural hearing loss and some children with no demonstrable benefit from amplification both within and across studies (Roush, Frymark, Venediktov, & Wang, 2011). Because the amount of hearing aid benefit cannot be predicted on the basis on audiological characteristics such as degree of hearing loss, children diagnosed with ANSD should receive a trial with appropriately fit amplification. Unfortunately, because the auditory brainstem response that is the basis for early amplification is absent or significantly abnormal in children with ANSD, amplification cannot be provided until some behavioral measure of hearing can be estimated. Early behavioral measures of hearing are used as the basis for prescribing amplification and verifying that sufficient audibility for speech can be achieved. Children who do not progress in auditory and communication develop during the trial with amplification fit based on their behavioral audiogram should be referred promptly for cochlear implant candidacy.

Unilateral Hearing Loss

Some children have hearing loss that affects only one ear, known as unilateral hearing loss. Despite the fact that children with unilateral hearing loss have one ear with normal hearing, some may still experience greater developmental and academic deficits than peers with two normal-hearing ears. Approximately one third of children with unilateral hearing loss will be held back a grade (Lieu, 2004). Children with unilateral hearing loss may also experience difficulties listening in background noise and localizing the source of sounds in the environment (McKay et al., 2008). Developmental delays in speech and language skills are more common in unilateral hearing loss than in children with normal hearing, but less consistent than in children with bilateral hearing loss (Lieu, 2004). The factors that predict developmental and academic difficulties in children with unilateral hearing loss have not been reported in the literature; therefore, children with unilateral hearing loss should be evaluated as potential candidates for amplification in their impaired ear, unless there is clear evidence of limited benefit or obvious contraindications to using amplification.

Children with unilateral hearing loss can be divided into two groups with regard to candidacy for amplification. Children with mild to severe hearing loss are considered to have aidable hearing in their impaired ear and should be provided with a trial amplification in that ear. For children with profound unilateral hearing loss, the ability to provide audibility through amplification in the impaired ear is limited due to the reduced dynamic range between threshold and the level where sounds become uncomfortably loud. Even if some audibility can be provided with amplification, the sound quality relative to the ear with normal hearing may be poor. In cases of profound unilateral hearing loss, the **head shadow effect** may limit the audibility of sounds originating from the same side as the impaired ear (Shaw, 1974). The head shadow effect can result in 10 to 20 dB of attenuation for sounds that originate from the opposite side of the head (Figure 10–3). The head shadow effect occurs primarily for sounds greater than 2000 Hz, where the wavelengths of sounds are shorter than the distance between ears (the wavelength for sounds above 2000 Hz is greater than 6.78 inches). For individuals with significant unilateral hearing loss, effect devices that route sound to the normal hearing ear may be used to provide awareness of sounds that occur on the side of the impaired ear. The contralateral routing of sound (CROS) to the normal ear can occur through bone conduction or radio-frequency transmission. Bone conduction devices, such as bone conduction hearing aids or osseointegrated auditory devices, can be used to route sound to from the side with hearing loss to the ear with normal hearing by vibrating the bones of the skull. Finally, CROS hearing aids can also use radio-frequency transmission to send sound from a receiver on the impaired ear to a receiver on the ear with normal hearing. Research on these configurations with children is limited, although research with adults has suggested the CROS using radio-frequency transmission (Valente, Valente, & Mispagel, 2007) and bone conduction devices (Wazen et al., 2003) can result in improved outcomes with severe-to-profound unilateral hearing loss. If CROS devices with radio-frequency transmission are selected for children, occlusion of the normal-hearing ear by the receiver should be limited. With any CROS configuration, that the signals from each ear are still being received by

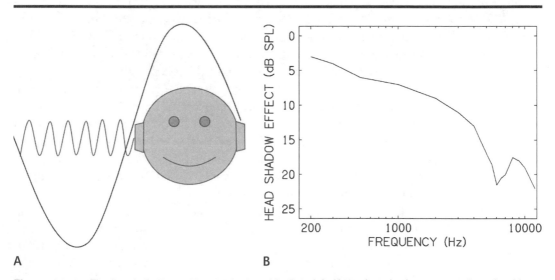

A   B

Figure 10–3. The head shadow effect is depicted in Panel A. Note that the longer wavelength of low-frequency sounds allows these sounds to be received at the opposite ear, whereas higher-frequency sounds with shorter wavelengths are obstructed by the head. Panel B displays the average magnitude of the head shadow effect as a function of frequency (from Shaw, 1974)

only one ear. Therefore, these configurations should not be expected to restore binaural hearing or experience the same perceptual benefits of having inputs from two ears.

SELECTION OF AMPLIFICATION FOR CHILDREN

Once children are determined to be candidates for amplification, the audiologist must make decisions about the type of amplification, style of device, earmold and what types of signal processing will be activated in the device. The selection process should focus on providing a device that is sufficiently flexible to change and adapt to meet the needs of the child as they grow and develop. The physical growth and development that children experience during early childhood and adolescence has an enormous impact on their ear canal size, particularly during the first year of life. The growth of the ear canal directly results in a decrease in the output of the hearing aid due to the acoustic effect of increased ear canal volume (Bagatto et al., 2005). The implication of normal growth means that the hearing aid output could decrease by as much as 20 dB over the first 3 years of life. The listening needs and environments of children over the next 5 years of their life should also be considered during the selection process. While the infant or toddler being fit with the hearing aid may not be using a phone or sitting in a classroom, the connectivity of the device to hearing assistance technology and telephones should be considered as those needs are likely to develop as the child enters preschool and school-age. Successful selection of amplification will ensure that chil-

dren can experience auditory access over a wide range of environments and listening situations as they grow and develop.

Routing of Signal

In most cases, air conduction hearing aids will be used to provide audibility for children who have mild to severe hearing loss. For children with severe or profound hearing loss or children who are not developing auditory and communication skills with appropriately fit amplification, cochlear implants are indicated and will be discussed in Chapter 11. In some cases, the external ear (pinna) or ear canal are not sufficiently developed to support a hearing aid. Conditions that can result in a small or malformed pinna or absent ear canal will prevent the use of air conduction hearing aids and require sound routing using bone conduction. Hearing devices are available that convert acoustic energy to mechanical vibrations to be transmitted to the cochlear via the skull through bone conduction. Bone conduction hearing aids can be coupled to the mastoid process behind the ear using a soft or rigid headband, similar to the coupling used for bone conduction testing during a standard audiological evaluation (Figure 10–4). Osseointegrated auditory devices (OAD) or bone-anchored hearing devices (BAHD) are similar to bone conduction hearing aids in the way they transmit acoustic energy through bone conduction; however, these devices are attached to the skull either via a magnet under the skin or surgical implant that is implanted into the temporal bone behind the ear and protrudes from the skull through the skin. Bone conduction routing of sound is only advisable in cases where the external ear and ear canal anat-

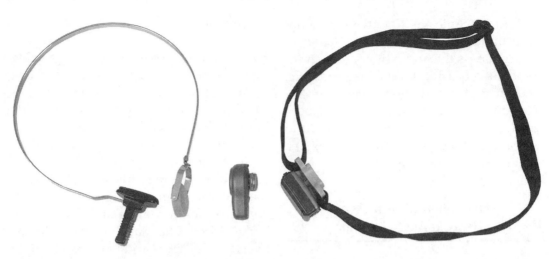

Figure 10–4. Coupling options for bone conduction devices. From left to right: (1) a hard bone conduction headband with an adapter for an osseointegrated auditory device processor; (2) an osseointegrated auditory device processor; (3) an osseointegrated auditory device processor coupled to a soft headband. Reprinted with permission, Ryan McCreery.

omy are not sufficient to permit air conduction routing of sound.

The Impact of Age-Related Differences in Ear Canal Acoustics on Candidacy

In order to evaluate whether or not a child is a candidate for air conduction amplification, the first step in the process is to convert the hearing thresholds from the audiogram from dB HL to dB sound pressure level (SPL) at the eardrum. Because the average threshold for normal hearing is not the same SPL at each frequency, dB HL was developed as a reference for audiometric assessment where the average threshold for normal hearing at every frequency is equal to 0 dB. Standard audiometric calibrations used to establish dB HL are referenced to a 2 cm³ coupler for insert earphones or a 6 cm³ earphone for headphone. These couplers are designed to approximate the residual

ear canal volume of those transducers coupled to an adult ear. Infants and children have smaller ear canals than adults, so the same transducer and sound level will produce a higher sound level in the child's ear canal than would be predicted from the adult calibration. The impact of these age-related differences in sound level on audiometric assessments is that children's thresholds referenced to dB HL may appear better (lower) than using a dB SPL-equivalent threshold that takes into account the child's individual ear canal acoustics. Converting dB HL thresholds to dB SPL at the eardrum allows for an assessment of the hearing loss and the impact on unaided audibility that takes into the account the child's ear canal acoustics. Acoustic differences between adult and child ears also will impact the output of the hearing aid in the child's ear canal, which will be discussed in a later section on hearing aid verification. Most clinical hearing aid verification systems will allow clinicians to enter the audiogram in HL and convert those values to SPL to assess the audibility of speech for the child's hearing levels. Free software, known as the Situational Hearing Aid Response Profile (SHARP), can also be used to convert audiometric thresholds to SPL and is discussed in greater detail in a later section of the chapter.

Fundamental Aspects of Hearing Aid Selection

Although there are many aspects of hearing aid selection, some fundamental principles will guide the selection process for most children who are hard of hearing. For example, hearing aids are recommended for both ears in children who have bilateral hearing loss to support the development of localization and other binaural skills that are supportive for listening in background noise.

Hearing Aid Style

For air conduction hearing aids, a wide range of hearing aid styles are available from behind-the-ear (BTE) to in-the-ear (ITE; Figure 10–5). BTE hearing aids have different receiver options including having the receiver-in-the-aid (RITA) or receiver-in-the-canal (RIC). In most cases, BTE hearing aids with RITA coupled to an earmold (Figure 10–6) will be the preferred device style for infants and children. The range of hearing losses over which BTE hearing aids can be fit is much larger than for ITE styles of hearing aids. A wide fitting range is important if the device will be flexible enough to provide more gain as the child gets older and their ear canal grows. The flexibility in fitting range provided by BTE hearing aids can also be beneficial in the event of progressive or fluctuating hearing loss, where the gain would need to be altered to accommodate changes in

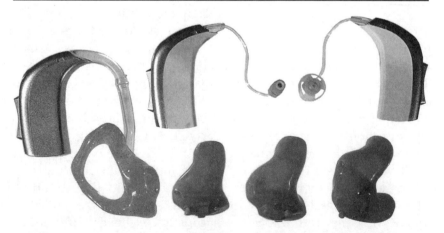

Figure 10–5. Hearing aid styles. *Top:* Behind-the-ear (BTE) hearing aid coupled to a custom earmold. BTE hearing aid with a receiver in the canal (RIC). BTE hearing aid with an RIC with a dome. *Bottom:* In-the-canal (ITC), half-shell in-the-ear (ITE), and full-shell ITE hearing aids. Reprinted with permission, Ryan McCreery.

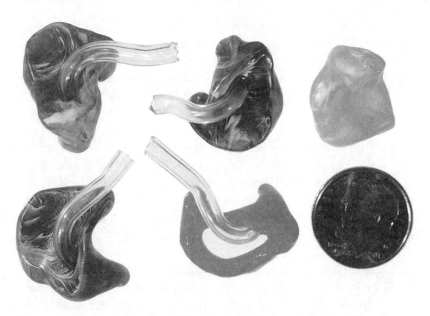

Figure 10–6. Earmolds. Five different earmolds from infants ranging in age from 2 to 6 months. Note the small size and lack of venting due to size constraints. Reprinted with permission, Ryan McCreery.

hearing. In general, BTE devices are also more durable and have greater battery life than other hearing aid styles, in addition to offering more options for connectivity. Because BTE hearing aids are coupled to an earmold, they can be easily adapted to ear canal growth over time by getting new earmolds, which is significantly less expensive than remaking the shell of an ITE hearing aid as the child's ear grows.

Children and their families should be given information about the advantages of BTE with RITA devices when making decisions about hearing aid style. Under specific circumstances, ITE or BTE with RIC hearing aid styles may be indicated for older school-age children and adolescents. While cosmetic appeal of hearing aids is a relatively minor consideration during infancy and early childhood, some older school-age children and adolescents will prefer smaller, more discrete devices.

Given that this period of development can be a challenging time to establish or maintain consistent hearing aid use, ITE or BTE with RIC might be considered options during this age as long as several conditions are met. First, the devices still must be able to provide adequate amplification for the child's degree and configuration or hearing loss. Second, the child must be at an age where ear canal growth has stabilized. The family must understand that a child fit with an ITE may be without his or her device if the hearing aid needs to be remade due to ear canal growth, which can take several weeks. Finally, the device should still provide options for connectivity with hearing assistance technology, phones, computers, gaming devices, or other systems and activities that the child enjoys. The cosmetic advantages of ITE and BTE with RIC hearing aids can quickly be offset by limited connectivity or problems using the devices with systems that are used to communicate with friends and family.

Hearing Aid Signal Processing

Another major aspect of the hearing aid selection process is to determine which hearing aid signal-processing features are appropriate for the child and will be activated in the fitting. In the past, decisions about whether or not to include hearing aid signal-processing features had to be made at the time the device was ordered, since many of these features were only available in specific models. With the advent of digital signal processing in hearing aids, even the most basic levels of hearing aid technology will include options for directional microphones, digital noise reduction, and frequency-lowering signal processing. As a result, the decision process has transitioned from which specific features will be ordered to which specific features will be activated in the fitting. Hearing aid signal processing features can be divided into two categories: inherent or activated. Inherent signal processing includes processing strategies and systems that are nearly always present and activated in the hearing aids. Although audiologists do not have to make deliberate decisions about whether or not to activate inherent processing, special consideration is still needed to determine the characteristics of these systems that will result in the greatest amount of audibility. Activated signal processing features are systems that the clinician can control whether or not the feature is active using programming software. Decisions about activated features are also made in an effort to enhance audibility, but the audiologist must also determine whether or not activated features are appropriate for a given child at the time of the fitting. Some decisions about activated features will depend on the age, degree of hearing loss, or other characteristics of the child. The two primary systems in the hearing aid that are inherent features are amplitude compression and feedback suppression. Both features typically are not deactivated in any modern hearing aid system. Clinicians, however, must make decisions about how to optimize these features to provide children with consistent audibility.

Amplitude Compression. Amplitude compression refers to automated systems that adjust the amount of amplification provided by the hearing aid based on the input level of sound received at the hearing aid microphone. Nearly two decades ago, many hearing aids provided linear gain as a function of input level. Linear gain is a system that provides 1 dB increase in the hearing aid output for a 1 dB increase in the input. At very high input levels (>85 dB SPL), some linear devices would substantially limit any increases in amplification to avoid loudness discomfort using output limiting. Linear amplification meant that adult hearing aid users were forced to adjust their volume controls to optimize audibility and listening comfort as the sound level in the environment varied (Leijon, 1990). In an effort to minimize the need to adjust the volume control when the sound level changed and optimize audibility over a wide range of input levels, wide dynamic range compression (WDRC) was developed (Kates, 2010). With WDRC, the hearing aid automatically and gradually reduces the amount of amplification that is provided as the input level increases for the range of input levels associated with communication (~45 dB SPL to 80 dB SPL). In effect, soft speech receives the most amplification, average speech sounds receive less, and loud speech sounds receive very little amplification. The perceptual effect of WDRC is that soft sounds are audible, but loud sounds are not uncomfortable, which means that the input to the hearing aid is audible and comfortable over a wide range of plausible input levels in different listening environments.

Infants and young children cannot reliably manipulate a volume control. Like adults, many older children and adolescents do not want to have to adjust the volume of the hearing aid because of changes in the sound level in the environment. Therefore, amplitude compression in the form of WDRC is a desirable feature for children to have in their hearing aids (see McCreery, Venediktov, Coleman, & Leech, 2012a for a review), as long as it is optimized to promote audibility across the range of speech inputs. Audiologists can verify that this goal is accomplished by measuring the audibility of speech at multiple input levels as part of the verification process. Amplitude compression can also help to promote consistent hearing aid use in children by balancing audibility with listening comfort across different listening situations where the level of noise in the environment might be uncomfortably loud with linear amplification.

Feedback Suppression. Acoustic feedback describes the whistling or buzzing sound that occurs when amplified sound from the hearing aid is picked up by the microphone and amplified again, creating a feedback loop. Although the feedback may not be audible to the hearing aid user, feedback can create annoyance and frustration for others, particularly for parents who may be trying to establish hearing aid use with their children. Before recent advancements in digital signal processing, acoustic feedback was a problem frequently reported by parents, particularly for children with severe or profound hearing loss who required significant amounts of amplification from their hearing aids to make speech audible. With these advances, most hearing aids now include **feedback suppression systems** that are automatically engaged as part of the fittings process. Some devices contain multiple types of feedback suppression, including passive systems that limit the amount of gain that can be provided in the hearing aid, to active systems that use phase cancellation or other approaches to limit feedback as it occurs. (See Dillon, 2012 for a review of feedback suppression approaches.)

Although very little research has been completed with feedback suppression and children who wear hearing aids, the benefits of this technology can be verified clinically and the potential disadvantages are relatively small. The advantages of feedback management can include reduced parent frustration while trying to establishing hearing aid use and improved audibility of high-frequency sounds, which may be limited when feedback was present. One potential negative consequence of feedback suppression is that the presence of feedback has been an indicator that earmolds need to be replaced. In fact, many feedback suppression systems are so affective that feedback may not occur even with a very poorly fitting earmold. While increasing the length of time that earmolds can be effective is positive overall, the acoustic consequences of a poorly fitting earmold can be substantial. Even if feedback suppression is effectively limiting the amount of feedback, a poorly fitting earmold will lead to decreased amplification due to sound leaking out of the ear canal and an increased residual volume. This limitation can be successfully avoided if clinicians monitor the fit of earmolds through both visual inspection and acoustic measurements during verification. Activating any feedback suppression systems in the hearing aid prior to the verification process will ensure that the effects of feedback suppression on speech audibility can be quantified.

Activated Hearing Aid Features

In addition to hearing aid features that are typically part of hearing aid signal processing, other hearing aid features must be activated in by the audiologist as part of the fitting, as well as being optimized to promote audibility. Three activated features have received significant attention in the literature: **directional microphones**, **digital noise reduction**, and **frequency lowering**. Some manufacturers have pediatric settings that will automatically determine which features are activated based on the age of the child entered into the programming software. Audiologists, however, should make individualized decisions about which features to activate for each child.

Directional Microphones. Listeners tend to face their conversational partner during verbal communication. Directional microphones take advantage of this fact by maintaining or enhancing amplification for sounds arriving from the front of the listener and reducing amplification for sounds arriving from behind the listener or from the sides. Directional processing is accomplished by using multiple microphones at different positions on the hearing aid or one microphone with mul-

tiple openings. The position of the sound relative to the listener is determined by comparing the time of arrival at different microphones. In adults, directional microphones have been shown to provide small, but consistent benefits for listening in background noise, particularly in situations where the listener is facing the talker of interest and the noise source is primarily behind or to the side of the listener (Amlani, 2001). For children, the benefits of directional microphones depend on the child's ability to orient towards the talker of interest. School-age children with hearing loss can accurately orient towards different speakers in classroom situations (Ricketts & Galster, 2008); however, evidence from infants and younger children with hearing loss is more limited. While infants and younger children do appear to locate the talker of interest in some listening situations, this age group is not in listening situations where the talker of interest is consistently located in front of them (Ching et al., 2009). For this reason, directional microphones may be appropriate for school-age children in specific listening situations where the talker of interest is likely to be in front or can be located by the child but not for infants and younger children who are exploring their world (McCreery, Venediktov, Coleman, & Leech, 2012b).

Digital Noise Reduction. Another signal processing strategy designed to limit the impact of noise on hearing aid users is digital noise reduction. Digital noise reduction describes a group of signal-processing strategies designed to detect the when noise is the predominant input to the hearing aid and reduce the amount of gain to improve listening comfort. Because most digital noise reduction systems reduce the amount of gain provided by the hearing aid, improvements in the signal-to-noise ratio that can occur with directional microphones are not possible with digital noise reduction. As a result, the primary improvements observed with adults are in improved listening comfort (Mueller, Weber, & Hornsby, 2006) or reduced listening effort in noise (Sarampalis, Kalluri, Edwards, & Hafter, 2009). Maintaining listening comfort in background noise can help to support hearing aid use in situations with background noise for children who wear hearing aids. Additionally, reduced listening effort has been documented in children with normal hearing using digital noise reduction (Gustafson, McCreery, Hoover, Kopun, & Stelmachowicz, 2014). Research describing digital noise reduction in children who wear hearing aids suggests that digital noise reduction does not have a negative impact on speech recognition (McCreery et al., 2012b; Stelmachowicz et al., 2010). Therefore, digital noise reduction may provide benefits to children as long as it does not reduce audibility for speech.

Frequency Lowering. Audibility of high-frequency speech sounds is important not only for understanding speech (Stelmachowicz, Pittman, Hoover, & Lewis, 2001), but also to support word learning (Pittman, 2008) in children who are hard of hearing. Limited audibility in the high frequencies for children has been implicated as a potential contributor to delays in both phonological (Moeller et al., 2007) and structural aspects (Koellinger et al., 2013) of speech and language development. These results suggest that even with appropriately fit amplification, the frequency range or bandwidth of hearing aids currently may not be suf-

ficient to maximize perception and developmental outcomes. As a result of this research, hearing aid manufacturers have attempted to extend the bandwidth of hearing aids, but have also introduced frequency-lowering signal processing as an alternative method of increasing access to high-frequency sounds. Frequency lowering refers to hearing aid signal-processing strategies that relocate high-frequency speech information to lower frequencies where hearing thresholds may be better or the hearing aid may provide more gain. Multiple frequency-lowering strategies are available in wearable hearing aids. (See Alexander, 2013 for a review of approaches to frequency lowering.)

Research on frequency lowering in children who wear hearing aids has grown rapidly in the past few years, but have shown mixed results for speech perception and communication development outcomes (McCreery et al., 2012c). Specifically, most studies suggest that frequency lowering outcomes are better than or equivalent to processing without frequency lowering. In determining individual candidacy for frequency lowering, audiologists must consider how much bandwidth is audible without frequency lowering and whether or not providing additional bandwidth is possible with frequency lowering. The audible bandwidth is an estimate of the highest frequency that is audible through the hearing aid. For conventional processing without frequency lowering, the audible bandwidth can be estimated by measuring the highest frequency whether the LTASS intersects the audiometric thresholds on the SPL-o-gram. With frequency lowering, the audible bandwidth can be estimated using software such as the SHARP (Brennan et al., 2013). Frequency lowering should only be implemented for children if the audible bandwidth can be increased compared to conventional processing. Because frequency lowering has the potential to distort the speech spectrum, audiologists should select frequency lowering settings that improve audibility with the least amount of spectral distortion.

VERIFICATION

Once the hearing aid and signal processing features have been selected, the audibility of speech can be verified for air conduction hearing aids using **probe-microphone measurements**. Probe-microphone systems measure or estimate the output of the hearing aid in the ear canal, taking into account the individual acoustic characteristics of the hearing aid fitting and ear. The results from probe-microphone verification can be plotted on the SPL-o-gram to evaluate audibility of the LTASS. Verification for advanced signal-processing features can also be completed as part of the verification process. The specific goals of hearing aid verification are to promote speech audibility and minimize the potential for loudness discomfort across a range of input levels. Because the child's ear canal will grow as part of normal development, verification should be completed every 3 months for children who are less than 3 years old and every 6 months for children between 3 and 5 years old. This schedule ensures that children are receiving measurements of the hearing aid in their ear frequently during the first few years of life when ear canal growth is particularly rapid and can be coordinated with on-going assessment of hearing thresholds and replacement of earmolds.

Probe-Microphone Verification

The cornerstone of verification for air conduction hearing aids is a measurement of a speech signal through the hearing aid at multiple input levels. A test signal is presented to the hearing aid via a calibrated loudspeaker. Probe microphone verification systems use two microphones to estimate the input to the hearing aid and the output of the hearing aid in the ear canal. The external microphone is placed on the ear and measures the unamplified signal that arrives at the ear. The internal or probe microphone is placed in the ear canal using a soft, thin tube that can be placed in the ear canal with the hearing aid and earmold (Figure 10–7). Measure-

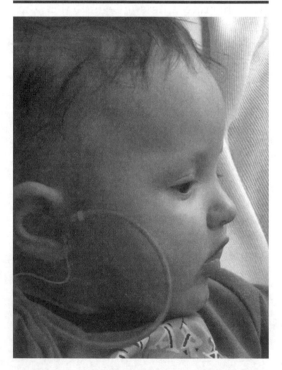

Figure 10–7. A probe microphone assembly used to measure the real ear or real-ear-to-coupler difference response from the ear canal. Reprinted with permission, Ryan McCreery.

ment of the hearing aid output in the child's ear canal with a probe-microphone system is known as in situ or real ear verification, because the hearing aid is measured on the ear. The SPL level of the LTASS with amplification from probe microphone measurements is plotted relative to the audiometric thresholds converted to SPL to estimate audibility. Unfortunately, many infants and young children cannot sit cooperatively for multiple probe microphone measurements in each ear or lack the head control that is required to sit in front of the loudspeaker. A reliable alternative to in situ measurements of hearing aid output are estimates based on the real-ear-to-coupler-difference (RECD); (Bagatto et al., 2005).

The RECD is a single measurement of a calibrated signal presented through the child's occluded earmold without the hearing aid to estimate the acoustic characteristics of the child's ear canal compared to a standard 2 cm^3 coupler (Figure 10–8). Subsequent hearing aid measurements in the 2 cm^3 coupler can be used to simulate the response of the hearing aid in the child's ear canal. The advantage of the RECD is that it requires minimal cooperation from the child and has been validated as an accurate predictor of in situ measurements across multiple studies (Bagatto, Scollie, Seewald, Moodie, & Hoover, 2002; Sinclair et al., 1996). In cases where the RECD cannot be measured, average RECD values are available in 1 month intervals for children under 5 years of age and in 1 year intervals between 5 to 12 years of age (Bagatto et al., 2005). Average RECD values should only be used if in situ

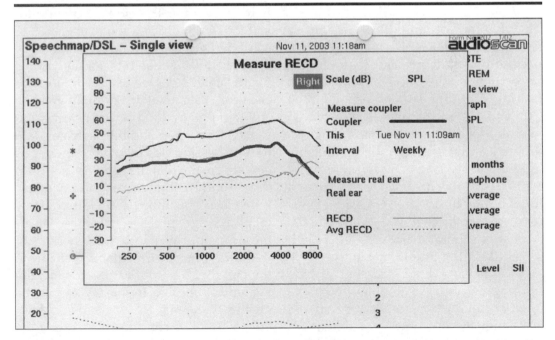

Figure 10–8. The real-ear-to-coupler-difference (RECD) measurement for hearing aid verification. The RECD (*gray line*) in dB as a function of frequency. The RECD is the difference between the broadband sound recorded in the child's ear canal (*thin black line*) compared to the same sound recorded in a 2 cm^3 coupler (*thick black line*). The average RECD for the child's age is displayed as the dashed line.

or measured RECD measurements are not possible, since the range around the average RECD can be ±10 dB, depending on the frequency and age of the child (Bagatto et al., 2002). Average RECD values were collected on children with normal middle ear conditions; therefore, average RECD values should be applied in cases of middle ear effusion or in children with tympanostomy tubes or tympanic membrane perforations, as those conditions will impact the acoustics of the RECD (Liu & Lin, 1999; Martin, Westwood, & Bamford, 1996). Using an average RECD with children who have abnormal middle ear conditions or obvious differences in ear canal size from age-matched children will lead to inaccurate predictions of hearing aid output.

Prescriptive Methods

The amount of amplification that is needed to make speech audible will depend on the degree and configuration of hearing loss. Prescriptive approaches to hearing aid fitting specify the amount of gain and output that should be achieved to make speech audible over a range on different input levels, while minimizing loudness discomfort. Two primary prescriptive approaches have been validated for children: the Desired Sensation Level (DSL v. 5; Scollie et al., 2005) and National Acoustics Laboratories (NAL-NL2; Keidser et al., 2011). Studies comparing DSL and NAL have suggested that a wide range of outcomes, including speech recognition, loudness perception and speech and language outcomes, are similar for children fit with either formula (Ching, Dillion, et al., 2013; Ching, Johnson, et al., 2013; Scollie et al., 2010). Therefore, either

fitting approach is reasonable to use with children. During the verification process, the gain and output of the hearing aid should be matched as closely as possible to prescriptive targets at each frequency. Both NAL and DSL include prescriptive targets for different speech input levels (soft, average and loud). Hearing aid fittings that are closely matched to prescriptive targets are much more likely to provide consistent audibility across a range of degrees of hearing loss than fittings where there are deviations from prescriptive targets greater than 5 dB (McCreery, Bentler, & Roush, 2013).

Verification Outcomes

Audiologists should document verification outcomes for each hearing aid fitting that they provide for children who are hard of hearing. The aided audibility for soft (50 or 55 dB SPL) and average (60 or 65 dB SPL) speech input levels should be reported and compared to normative data for the child's degree of hearing loss for each ear (Bagatto et al., 2011). In general, children with mild to severe hearing loss can achieve aided audibility greater than 65 with hearing aids fit to prescriptive targets. To ensure that the child has access to speech information across the frequency range, the maximum audible frequency for an average speech signal for each hearing aid should be reported as a measure of the audible bandwidth that is available to the child with amplification. Ideally, the maximum audible frequency should be greater than 6000 Hz or frequency lowering should be considered to extend the bandwidth to higher frequencies. Any deviations from prescriptive target greater than 5 dB should be noted and the reasons for these deviations (e.g., configuration of hearing loss, inadequate gain in the hearing aid) should be described.

Prior to the development of probe microphone measures for assessing the audibility of speech, audiologists were forced to rely on audiograms completed with the hearing aids in place to assess how the hearing aids functioned. Measuring the pure tone audiogram with hearing aids is no longer acceptable practice for a number of important reasons. First, measuring the behavioral response to pure tones does not provide information about whether or not speech is audible through the hearing aid. Additionally, the signal-processing systems in digital hearing aids do not process pure tones the same way that they process speech. In fact, many hearing aids will treat pure tone signals like feedback and alter the amount of amplification that is provided to those signals, which can lead to invalid results. Aided audiograms also do not test the maximum output of the hearing aid, nor do they allow for the assessment of advanced hearing aid features such as frequency lowering, digital noise reduction and directional microphones. For these reasons, aided audiograms are not recommended as part of the hearing aid verification process, as they do not provide a realistic measure of what the child is listening to with his or her hearing aids.

The Situational Hearing Aid Response Profile

Although the audibility of the average speech signal is often the primary focus of the hearing aid assessment process, children often are required to listen to speech under a wide range of listening conditions and from varying distances. The Situational Hearing Aid Response Profile (SHARP; Brennan et al., 2013) is a software program that allows simulation of alternative listening configurations that might be encountered by children. The SHARP program uses the verification data obtained for the standard average speech at 1 meter condition to make predictions for other potential listening situations where the input to the hearing aid may have a different spectrum than the LTASS (Figure 10–9A). For infants, both unaided and aided listening situations, such as being cradled and being held on the hip, can be used to demonstrate the effect of being closer to the talker. Classroom listening situations, such as being 4 meters from the teacher, can also be simulated to show how children who wear hearing aids can hear the teacher in a realistic classroom situation (Figure 10–9B). The head shadow effect can also be simulated acoustically to assess how sounds from the opposite side of the head are received at the ear with normal hearing in cases of unilateral hearing loss. The SHARP can be used for counseling parents or teachers about the effects of distance on audibility.

Verification of Bone Conduction Devices

Because the output of bone conduction devices is mechanical, verification of bone conduction devices currently cannot be measured using the same probe microphone approaches that are used for verification of air conduction amplification. Researchers, however, are currently developing objective measures to perform verification with bone conduction devices to ensure that speech audibility

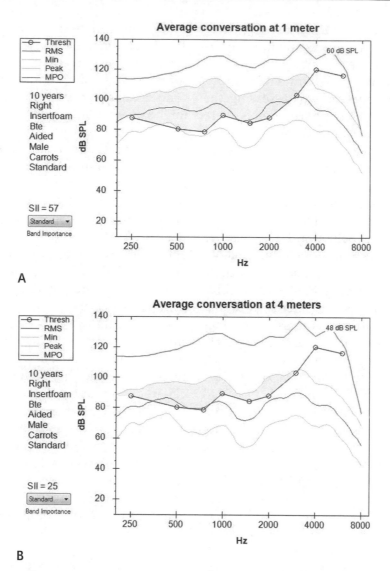

Figure 10–9. The effect of distance on audibility. Panel A displays the SPL-o-gram for an average speech signal at a distance of 1 meter. Panel B displays the same SPL-o-gram data for a speech signal at a distance of 4 meters. Note the reduction in audibility as distance increases. The Situational Hearing Aid Response Profile can be used to estimate the impact of distance on audibility across a wide range of realistic listening situations.

can be provided using these devices. An experiment using objective electromechanical assessment of bone conduction devices found improved speech percep-

tion and audibility compared to conventional ap-proaches (Hodgetts, Hagler, Hakansson, & Soli, 2011). While electromechanical interfaces for verifying bone conduction responses of hearing aids are not widely available at the present time, the use of objective verification measures for bone conduction devices should soon be feasible and would represent a significant improvement over methods that rely on subjective patient feedback.

HEARING AID ORIENTATION

One of the most integral parts of setting children and their parents or caregivers up for success with amplification is an on-going process of orientation to the use, maintenance, and function of amplification. Parents report that information about maintenance and promoting hearing aid use is their principle concern during the process of fitting amplification. Given that most children who are hard of hearing will be identified through universal newborn hearing screening and fit with amplification during infancy, parents or caregivers initially will be tasked with establishing routines for care and maintenance; however, the process of orientation should continue at each subsequent visit to identify challenges, provide support, and eventually transition the responsibility for maintenance to the child.

Care and maintenance of the hearing aid are extremely important as they can extend the life of the hearing aid and help to minimize the need for repairs. The parents should be provided with the tools that are necessary to ensure that the device is functioning on a daily basis, as well as basic materials to keep the hearing aids clean and free from moisture. Hearing aid care and maintenance kits are often complimentary or at minimal cost from hearing aid manufacturers (Figure 10–10). A care and maintenance kit

should include a hearing aid battery tester, a drying kit with desiccant for storage, a bulb for blowing out earmold tubing, a listening tube to perform listening checks, and a retention device. The function of the kit and a routine for care and maintenance should be introduced at the fitting and reviewed at subsequent appointments. Parents should be encouraged to check the hearing aid battery and listen to the hearing aid each day before the child wears the hearing aid to ensure that the device is functioning properly. The daily hearing aid listening check should include a visual inspection of the hearing aid and earmold. Visual inspection can often reveal problems with the hearing aid such as corrosion debris in the battery compartment or problems with the earmold such as wax or moisture occluding the sound bore or tubing. Parents can be instructed to use the listening tube to listen to the hearing aid while producing the sounds from the Ling Six-Sound Test (Agung, Purdy, & Kitamura, 2005). The Ling sounds includes the vowels /a/ (as in h<u>o</u>t), /i/ (as in b<u>ee</u>), /ʊ/ (as in b<u>oo</u>t) and consonants /m/ (as in <u>m</u>e), /s/ (as in <u>s</u>it) and /ʃ/ (as in <u>sh</u>ot). The purpose of the Ling Six-Sound Test is to produce speech sounds that represent the frequency range of speech in order to assess the sound quality of speech through the hearing aid. The use of signal-processing features such as frequency-lowering or directional microphones may affect the sound quality of the hearing aids or change the level of the sound through the hearing aid depending on where the sound source is during the listening check, so these processes should be discussed during orientation, if these features are present in the hearing aids. Parents will eventually learn to recognize how their child's hearing aid sounds and become adept at identifying problems

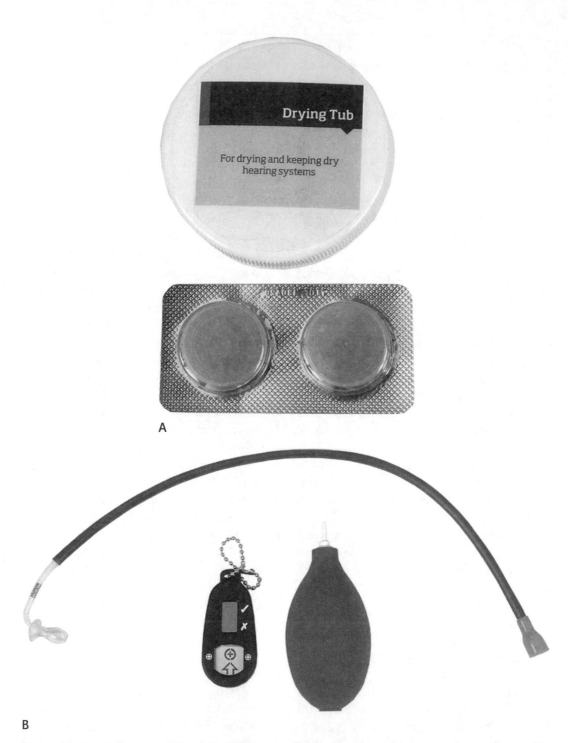

A

B

Figure 10–10. Components of a pediatric hearing aid care and maintenance kit. **A.** A desiccant drying tub where the hearing aids can be stored at night or when they are not in use. The desiccant tablets (*below*) absorb moisture from the hearing aids to prevent moisture-related malfunction. **B.** The other components of the hearing aid care and maintenance kit, including the listening tube (*above*), battery tester (*bottom left*), and earmold tubing blower (*bottom right*). Reprinted with permission, Ryan McCreery.

with sound quality. Providing ongoing support and orientation for parents and caregivers will ensure that they have the confidence to support their child's hearing aid use.

VALIDATION

The process of consistently verifying the hearing aids provides evidence that amplification provides consistent audibility as the child grows and develops, but the effects of amplification should be monitored periodically by the audiologist to ensure that the child is able to wear his or her devices consistently. In addition, auditory and communication development milestones should be evaluated periodically to ensure that the child's auditory skills are progressing as would be expected with amplification. Once a child reaches an age where speech recognition assessment is possible, aided speech recognition assessment should be completed to document that the audibility provided by the hearing aids has a positive impact on speech understanding.

Documenting Hearing Aid Use

Consistent hearing aid use is essential to achieve the positive benefits of amplification. Professionals who work with children who are hard of hearing and their families should assess hearing aid use at every point of contact with the family to help promote the importance of consistent use and identify potential barriers. An average estimate of daily hearing aid use can be obtained using the data-logging systems available through the program-ming software for most hearing aids. In addition, the child, parents, and caregivers should be asked to monitor and report the average amount of hearing aid use time per day. Specific questions about the situations where hearing aid use is consistent as well as those situations that are most challenging can lead to discussions about strategies for increasing use. The difficulty in establishing hearing aid use in infants and young children should be acknowledged and realistic expectations should be discussed. While families should be encouraged to establish and maintain consistent hearing aid use during waking hours, average hearing aid use per day increases as the child gets older, from 4 to 6 hours during infancy to 10 to 12 hours by age 3 to 4 years (Walker et al., 2013). Establishing consistent use may also be more challenging for children with milder degrees of hearing loss. Discussions about increasing hearing aid use should be supportive and should focus on solutions. In some cases, focusing on establishing hearing aid use in highly communicative times, such as one-on-one time reading or playing with family, can increase confidence that could generalize to other situations.

Aided Speech Recognition Assessment

Regular assessment of speech recognition can be an important tool for documenting auditory skill development and the benefits of amplification. Appropriate speech-recognition tasks should be developmentally appropriate in terms of the child's language and cognitive abilities and use materials that have been validated with children. Speech-recognition assessment with amplification can be completed through a sound field speaker in the audiometric test booth at levels that simulate conversational levels. Choosing levels for speech-recognition assessment that correspond with the input levels used for verification (soft speech: 50 or 55 dB SPL; average speech: 60 or 65 dB SPL) can allow clinicians to more directly assess the relationship between audibility and speech recognition.

In children who are hard of hearing without additional developmental concerns, speech- recognition testing can start as early as 2 years of age using point-to-body-part tasks or point-to-picture tests, such as the Early Speech Perception Test (ESP; Geers & Moog, 1990). The Phrases-in-Noise Test (Schafer et al., 2012) is another option for speech-recognition assessment for young children, as it uses a play task that requires the child to act out basic phrases in quiet or with background noise using a doll. A wide range of clinical assessment tools that assess speech perception have been developed. Speech-recognition materials are available that have a varying range of linguistic complexity from phonemes and syllables to sentences, depending on the linguistic skills of the child.

Assessment of general aided speech recognition is important; however, speech-recognition testing may also be used to answer specific clinical questions about the child's auditory skills or hearing aid signal-processing features. For example, an assessment with speech in front of the child and noise from the sides or behind the child with and without directional microphones activated can be used to demonstrate the benefits of this technology. Assessment tools such as the UWO Plurals Test (Glista & Scollie, 2009) can be used to target perception of high-fre-quency phonemes such as /s/ and /z/ to measure the impact of the bandwidth of a child's hearing aids or the impact of frequency-lowering technology. Varying the linguistic content of the stimulus (words vs. sentences) can help to determine how children may use their language skills to support speech recognition. Speech-recognition testing can provide valuable information for monitoring outcomes with amplification.

Outcomes Assessment Questionnaires

Assessment of language and communication skills in children who are hard of hearing can be primarily accomplished by the child's speech language pathologist. Outcomes assessment questionnaires, however, can provide supplemental information about the development of auditory abilities that may not be directly assessed through standardized assessments of speech and language. These tools also provide important information about how children use their auditory skills in their everyday lives and listening environments. Auditory outcomes questionnaires typically can be completed by the parents, teachers, and/or the child. Many questionnaires are available that fall into at least two categories: auditory development questionnaires and listening behavior questionnaires (Table 10–2).

Auditory development questionnaires are typically used with infants and young children who wear hearing aids in order to monitor the progression of early auditory skills. Examples of early auditory development questionnaires include the Infant-Toddler Meaningful Auditory Integration Scale or Meaningful Auditory Integration Scale (IT-MAIS/MAIS;

Table 10–2. Outcomes Questionnaires for Children Who Wear Hearing Aids

Scale	Age Range*	Features	More information
Infant-Toddler Meaningful Auditory Integration Scale (IT-MAIS)	0–2 years	Short interview for parents about auditory development for infants.	http://tinyurl.com/bsdqszj
Early Listening Function (ELF)	0–2 years	Questions about auditory awareness and behavior in infants and toddlers.	http://tinyurl.com/chgbaa3
Children's Home Inventory for Listening Difficulties (CHILD)	3–12 years	Everyday listening situations are rated on a 1–8 scale.	http://tinyurl.com/bqch4ct
LittlEARS, EARS TeenEARS	0–2 years 2–12 years 13+ years	Questionnaires about auditory development that span age range of childhood and adolescence.	http://tinyurl.com/broq4ro
Screening Instrument for Targeting Educational Risk (SIFTER)	3–18 years	Assesses classroom listening and behavioral skills. Preschool, elementary, and secondary versions available.	http://tinyurl.com/mrh8aow
Parents'/ Teachers' Evaluation of Aural/Oral Performance in Children (PEACH/TEACH)	2–18 years	Questions about listening in different realistic listening environments, including quiet and noise subscales.	http://tinyurl.com/cz32qjv
Speech, Spatial, and Qualities of Hearing (SSQ)	6–18 years	Originally developed for adults; Adapted for parents, teachers or school-age children to ask questions about a range of listening skills and environments.	http://tinyurl.com/mlpkh4v

Note. *Suggested age range assuming typical development.

Zimmerman-Phillips, Osberger, & Robbins, 2001) or the LittlEars auditory development questionnaire (Tsiakpini et al., 2004). Auditory development questionnaires ask parents to rate or describe their child's auditory abilities such as responding to his or her name, auditory awareness of sounds in the environment, or other early auditory skills that should be evident in children who are hard of hearing once they receive amplification. In addition to tracking the child's auditory skill development during the first two years of life, these scales also can provide parents with a framework for what types of behaviors their child may be exhibiting as they develop. One of the most significant limitations of these questionnaires is that children who have additional developmental delays may not exhibit significant progress in terms of auditory skill development even if amplification is providing some benefits. Clinicians should use their clinical judgment about the use and timing of early auditory development questionnaires in children who are hard of hearing with additional disabilities.

Listening behavior questionnaires are used to assess how children who are hard of hearing use their listening skills to function in realistic situations. Teachers, parents, and the child may complete these scales to assess listening in background noise, ease of listening, and to identify listening situations where listening may be particularly difficult. Listening behavior questionnaires often ask about listening in public places or classroom environments and are most appropriate for school-age children. Examples of listening behavior questionnaires include the Parents (or Teacher) Evaluation of Aural/Oral Performance in Children (PEACH or TEACH; Ching & Hill, 2007) and adaptations of the Speech, Spatial, and Qualities questionnaire (SSQ; Gatehouse & Noble, 2004) for children, parents, and teachers (Galvin, Mok, & Dowell, 2007). Questionnaires that assess the child's listening skills from multiple perspectives can be informative, not only for looking at performance in different listening situations (home vs. at school), but also for assessing the child's perceptions of his or her own auditory abilities. Children, however, must be old enough to understand basic acoustical terminology like noise and reverberation to answer questions about these concepts, which may not be possible until the child is 6 or 7 years old. See Chapter 4 for a comprehensive list of questionnaires used.

SUMMARY

Clinical assessment of hearing aids for children is a continuous process that involves selection and activation of appropriate hearing aid features, verification of audibility, providing orientation to parents and children, and monitoring auditory developmental outcomes. Professionals who serve children who are hard of hearing face the challenging task of working with parents and caregivers, many of whom have no experience with hearing loss or hearing aids, and providing informational and support counseling to ensure that the child receives consistent access to their auditory environment to develop speech, language and cognitive skills that will provide a foundation for academic and social success later in childhood. By maintaining consistent hearing aid use and audibility for speech during the child's development, audiologists can have a significant positive impact on the development of children with hearing loss and who use hearing aids.

REFERENCES

Agung, K. B., Purdy, S. C., & Kitamura, C. (2005). The Ling sound test revisited. *Australian and New Zealand Journal of Audiology, 27*(1), 33.

Alexander, J. M. (2013). Individual variability in recognition of frequency-lowered speech. *Seminars in Hearing, 34*, 86–109.

American Academy of Pediatrics. (2007). Joint Committee on Infant Hearing. Year 2007 position statement: Principles and guidelines for early hearing detection and intervention programs. *Pediatrics, 120*(4), 898–921.

American National Standards Institute. (1997). *American National Standard: Methods for calculation of the speech intelligibility index.* Melville, NY: Acoustical Society of America.

Amlani, A. M. (2001). Efficacy of directional microphone hearing aids: A meta-analytic perspective. *Journal of the American Academy of Audiology, 12*(4), 202.

Bagatto, M., Moodie, S., Scollie, S., Seewald, R., Moodie, S., Pumford, J., & Liu, K. R. (2005). Clinical protocols for hearing instrument fitting in the Desired Sensation Level method. *Trends in Amplification, 9*(4), 199–226.

Bagatto, M. P., Moodie, S. T., Malandrino, A. C., Richert, F. M., Clench, D. A., & Scollie, S. D. (2011). The University of Western Ontario pediatric audiological monitoring protocol (UWO PedAMP). *Trends in Amplification, 15*(1), 57–76.

Bagatto, M. P., Scollie, S. D., Seewald, R. C., Moodie, K. S., & Hoover, B. M. (2002). Real-ear-to-coupler difference predictions as a function of age for two coupling procedures. *Journal of the American Academy of Audiology, 13*(8), 407–415.

Bauman, S., & Pero, H. (2011). Bullying and cyberbullying among deaf students and their hearing peers: An exploratory study. *Journal of Deaf Studies and Deaf Education, 16*(2), 236–253.

Brennan, M. A., McCreery, R. W., & Lewis, D. E. (2013). *An update to the Situational Hearing Aid Response Profile (SHARP).* Poster presentation at the American Auditory Scoeity Meeting, Phoenix, AZ.

Calderon, R., & Low, S. (1998). Early social-emotional, language, and academic development in children with hearing loss: Families with and without fathers. *American Annals of the Deaf, 143*(3), 225–234.

Ching, T. Y., Dillon, H., Hou, S., Zhang, V., Day, J., Crowe, K., . . . Thomson, J. (2013). A randomized controlled comparison of NAL and DSL prescriptions for young children: Hearing aid characteristics and performance outcomes at three years of age. *International Journal of Audiology, 52*(Suppl. 2), S17–S28.

Ching, T. Y., & Hill, M. (2007). The parents' evaluation of aural/oral performance of children (PEACH) scale: Normative data. *Journal of the American Academy of Audiology, 18*(3), 220–235.

Ching, T. Y., Johnson, E. E., Hou, S., Dillon, H., Zhang, V., Burns, L., . . . Flynn, C. (2013). A comparison of NAL and DSL prescriptive methods for paediatric hearing aid fitting: Predicted speech intelligibility and loudness. *International Journal of Audiology, 52*(S2), S29–S38.

Ching, T. Y., O'Brien, A., Dillon, H., Chalupper, J., Hartley, L., Hartley, D., . . . Hain, J. (2009). Directional effects on infants and young children in real life: Implications for amplification. *Journal of Speech, Language, and Hearing Research, 52*(5), 1241–1254.

Davis, J. (2001). *Our forgotten children: Hard-of-hearing pupils in the school* (3rd ed.). Bethesda, MD: SHHH Publications.

Davis, J. M., Elfenbein, J. L., Schum, R. L., & Bentler, R. A. (1986). Effects of mild and moderate hearing impairments on language, educational, and psychosocial behavior of children. *Journal of Speech and Hearing Disorders, 51*(1), 53–62.

Dillon, H. (2012). *Hearing aids.* New York, NY: Thieme.

Galvin, K. L., Mok, M., & Dowell, R. C. (2007). Perceptual benefit and functional outcomes for children using sequential bilateral cochlear implants. *Ear and Hearing, 28*(4), 470–482.

Gatehouse, S., & Noble, W. (2004). The speech, spatial and qualities of hearing scale (SSQ). *International Journal of Audiology, 43*(2), 85–99.

Geers, A. E., & Moog, J. (1990). *Early Speech Perception Test Battery.* St. Louis, MO: Central Institute for the Deaf.

Glista, D., & Scollie, S. (2009). Modified verification approaches for frequency lowering devices. *Audiology Online,* 1–11. Retrieved from http://www.audiologyonline.com/articles/modified-verification-approaches-for-frequency-871

Gustafson, S., McCreery, R. W., Hoover, B., Kopun, J. & Stelmachowicz, P. G. (2014) Listening effort and perceived clarity for normal hearing children with the use of digital noise reduction. *Ear and Hearing.* Advance online publication.

Hirsh, I. J., Reynolds, E. G., & Joseph, M. (1954). Intelligibility of different speech materials. *The Journal of the Acoustical Society of America, 26,* 530.

Hodgetts, W. E., Hagler, P., Hakansson, B. E., & Soli, S. D. (2011). Technology-limited and patient-derived versus audibility-derived fittings in bone-anchored hearing aid users: A validation study. *Ear and Hearing, 32*(1), 31–39.

Kates, J. M. (2010). Understanding compression: Modeling the effects of dynamic-range compression in hearing aids. *International Journal of Audiology, 49*(6), 395–409.

Keidser, G., Dillon, H. R., Flax, M., Ching, T., & Brewer, S. (2011). The NAL-NL2 prescription procedure. *Audiology Research, 1*(1), e24.

Koehlinger, K. M., Van Horne, A. J. O., & Moeller, M. P. (2013). Grammatical outcomes of 3- and 6-year-old children who are hard of hearing.

Journal of Speech, Language, and Hearing Research, 56(5), 1701.

Leijon, A. (1990). Preferred hearing aid gain in everyday use after prescriptive fitting. *Ear and Hearing, 15*, 299–305.

Lieu, J. E. C. (2004). Speech-language and educational consequences of unilateral hearing loss in children. *Archives of Otolaryngology–Head & Neck Surgery, 130*(5), 524.

Liu, T. C., & Lin, K. N. (1999). Real-ear to coupler difference in patients with eardrum perforation. *ORL; Journal for Oto-Rhino-Laryngology and Its Related Specialties, 61*(6), 345–349.

Martin, H. C., Westwood, G. F. S., & Bamford, J. M. (1996). Real ear to coupler differences in children having otitis media with effusion. *British Journal of Audiology, 30*(2), 71–78.

McCreery, R. W., & Stelmachowicz, P. G. (2011). Audibility-based predictions of speech recognition for children and adults with normal hearing. *The Journal of the Acoustical Society of America, 130*(6), 4070.

McCreery, R. W., Venediktov, R. A., Coleman, J. J., & Leech, H. M. (2012a). An evidence-based systematic review of amplitude compression in hearing aids for school-age children with hearing loss. *American Journal of Audiology, 21*(2), 269.

McCreery, R. W., Venediktov, R. A., Coleman, J. J., & Leech, H. M. (2012b). An evidence-based systematic review of directional microphones and digital noise reduction hearing aids in school-age children with hearing loss. *American Journal of Audiology, 21*(2), 295.

McCreery, R. W., Venediktov, R. A., Coleman, J. J., & Leech, H. M. (2012c). An evidence-based systematic review of frequency lowering in hearing aids for school-age children with hearing loss. *American Journal of Audiology, 21*(2), 313.

McCreery, R. W., Walker, E. A, Spratford, M., Jacobs, S., & Hatala, E. (2013) *Speech recognition for children who are hard of hearing*. Poster presented at the American Auditory Society Meeting, Scottsdale, AZ.

McKay, S., Gravel, J. S., & Tharpe, A. M. (2008). Amplification considerations for children with minimal or mild bilateral hearing loss and unilateral hearing loss. *Trends in Amplification, 12*(1), 43–54.

Moeller, M. P. (2000). Early intervention and language development in children who are deaf and hard of hearing. *Pediatrics, 106*(3), e43.

Moeller, M. P., Hoover, B., Peterson, B., & Stelmachowicz, P. (2009). Consistency of hearing aid use in infants with early-identified hearing loss. *American Journal of Audiology, 18*(1), 14.

Moeller, M. P., Hoover, B., Putman, C., Arbataitis, K., Bohnenkamp, G., Peterson, B., . . . Stelmachowicz, P. (2007). Vocalizations of infants with hearing loss compared with infants with normal hearing: Part I–Phonetic development. *Ear and Hearing, 28*(5), 605–627.

Mueller, H. G., Weber, J., & Hornsby, B. W. (2006). The effects of digital noise reduction on the acceptance of background noise. *Trends in Amplification, 10*(2), 83–93.

Pittman, A. L. (2008). Short-term word-learning rate in children with normal hearing and children with hearing loss in limited and extended high-frequency bandwidths. *Journal of Speech, Language and Hearing Research, 51*(3), 785.

Pittman, A. L., & Stelmachowicz, P. G. (2003). Hearing loss in children and adults: Audiometric configuration, asymmetry, and progression. *Ear and Hearing, 24*(3), 198.

Porter, H., Sladen, D. P., Ampah, S. B., Rothpletz, A., & Bess, F. H. (2013). Developmental outcomes in early school-age children with minimal hearing loss. *American Journal of Audiology, 22*(2), 263–270.

Rance, G., & Aud, D. (2005). Auditory neuropathy/dys-synchrony and its perceptual consequences. *Trends in Amplification, 9*(1), 1–43.

Ricketts, T. A., & Galster, J. (2008). Head angle and elevation in classroom environments: Implications for amplification. *Journal of Speech, Language, and Hearing Research, 51*(2), 516.

Roush, P. A., Frymark, T., Venediktov, R., & Wang, B. (2011). Audiological management of auditory neuropathy spectrum disorder in children: A systematic review of the literature. *American Journal of Audiology, 20*(2), 159–70.

Sarampalis, A., Kalluri, S., Edwards, B., & Hafter, E. (2009). Objective measures of listening effort: Effects of background noise and noise reduction. *Journal of Speech, Language, and Hearing Research, 52*(5), 1230.

Schafer, E. C., Beeler, S., Ramos, H., Morais, M., Monzingo, J., & Algier, K. (2012). Developmental effects and spatial hearing in young children with normal hearing sensitivity. *Ear and Hearing, 33*(6), e32–e43.

Scollie, S., Seewald, R., Cornelisse, L., Moodie, S., Bagatto, M., Laurnagaray, D., . . . Pumford, J. (2005). The desired sensation level multistage input/output algorithm. *Trends in Amplification, 9*(4), 159–197.

Scollie, S. D. (2008). Children's speech recognition scores: The Speech Intelligibility Index and proficiency factors for age and hearing level. *Ear and Hearing, 29*(4), 543–556.

Scollie, S. D., Ching, T. Y., Seewald, R. C., Dillon, H., Britton, L., Steinberg, J., & King, K. (2010). Children's speech perception and loudness ratings when fitted with hearing aids using the DSL v. 4.1 and the NAL-NL1 prescriptions. *International Journal of Audiology, 49*(S1), S26–S34.

Shaw, E. A. G. (1974). Transformation of sound pressure level from the free field to the eardrum in the horizontal plane. *The Journal of the Acoustical Society of America, 56*, 1848.

Sjoblad, S., Harrison, M., Roush, J., & McWilliam, R. A. (2001). Parents' reactions and recommendations after diagnosis and hearing aid fitting. *American Journal of Audiology, 10*(1), 24.

Stelmachowicz, P., Lewis, D., Hoover, B., Nishi, K., McCreery, R., & Woods, W. (2010). Effects of digital noise reduction on speech perception for children with hearing loss. *Ear and Hearing, 31*(3), 345.

Stelmachowicz, P. G., Pittman, A. L., Hoover, B. M., & Lewis, D. E. (2001). Effect of stimulus bandwidth on the perception of /s/ in normal-and hearing-impaired children and adults. *The Journal of the Acoustical Society of America, 110*, 2183.

Stiles, D. J., Bentler, R. A., & McGregor, K. K. (2012). The speech intelligibility index and the pure-tone average as predictors of lexical ability in children fit with hearing aids. *Journal of Speech, Language and Hearing Research, 55*(3), 764.

Tharpe, A. M. (2008). Unilateral and mild bilateral hearing loss in children: Past and current perspectives. *Trends in Amplification, 12*(1), 7–15.

Tomblin, J. B., Oleson, J., Ambrose, S. E., Walker, E. A. & Moeller, M. P. (2014) The influence of hearing aids on speech and language development in children with hearing loss. *JAMA Otolaryngology–Head & Neck Surgery, 140*(5), 403–409.

Tsiakpini, L., Weichbold, V., Kuehn-Inacker, H., Coninx, F., D'Haese, P., & Almadin, S. (2004). *LittlEARS auditory questionnaire.* Innsbruck, Austria: MED-EL.

Valente, M., Valente, M., & Mispagel, K. (2007) *Fitting options for adult patients with single sided deafness.* Retrieved from http://www.audiologyonline.com/articles/fitting-options-for-adult-patients-980

Wake, M., Hughes, E. K., Collins, C. M., & Poulakis, Z. (2004). Parent-reported health-related quality of life in children with congenital hearing loss: a population study. *Ambulatory Pediatrics, 4*(5), 411–417.

Walker, E. A., Spratford, M., Moeller, M. P., Oleson, J., Ou, H., Roush, P. & Jacobs, S. (2013). Predictors of hearing aid use time in children with mild-to-severe hearing loss. *Language, Speech, and Hearing Services in Schools, 44*, 73–88.

Wazen, J. J., Spitzer, J. B., Ghossaini, S. N., Fayad, J. N., Niparko, J. K., Cox, K., . . . Soli, S. D. (2003). Transcranial contralateral cochlear stimulation in unilateral deafness. *Otolaryngology–Head & Neck Surgery, 129*(3), 248–254.

Zimmerman-Phillips, S., Osberger, M. J., & Robbins, A. M. (2001). *Infant-Toddler Meaningful Auditory Integration Scale.* Sylmar, CA: Advanced Bionics.

CHAPTER 11

Cochlear Implant Assessment

Tamala S. Bradham and K. Todd Houston

KEY POINTS

■ As the Food and Drug Administration (FDA) guidelines continue to change, more parents are choosing cochlear implantation for their children diagnosed with severe and profound bilateral hearing loss.
■ Cochlear implants provide access to audition, and children often achieve listening and spoken language outcomes that are comparable with their hearing peers—when appropriate follow-up and intervention services are in place.
■ Cochlear implantation requires careful candidacy assessment to determine if this procedure is appropriate for the child with hearing loss.
■ Ongoing assessment of the pediatric cochlear implant recipient is crucial to measure progress and to determine if the technology is functioning appropriately and is programmed correctly.
■ Red flags, indicators that a different course of intervention may be required, occur when the child's developmental or communicative progresses is limited or delayed after cochlear implantation.

INTRODUCTION

Families who have chosen a listening and spoken language outcome for their children with hearing loss have a variety of options to help their children access speech and environmental sounds. With significant advancements in hearing aid technologies and real ear fitting techniques, children can hear unlike ever before (see Chapter 10). There are times, however, that even with an appropriately fit hearing aid technology, children cannot access critical speech information that can help them with the development of spoken language. At this critical juncture, a cochlear implant may be recommended.

Why would a cochlear implant be of interest? Cochlear implants have been shown to improve outcomes in speech, language, and literacy (Geers, Nicholas, & Moog, 2007; Nicholas & Geers, 2007). Children with 2 years experience with a cochlear implant were mainstreamed at *twice* the rate of children of the same age and with the same hearing loss who do not have cochlear implant (Francis, Koch, Wyatt, & Niparko, 1999). Furthermore, children with cochlear implants generate a cost savings from kindergarten to 12th grade that is estimated to be between $30,000 and $200,000 (Francis et al., 1999).

One of the Public Health Application and Outreach goals from Healthy People 2020, Objective ENT-VSL-3 is to increase the number people who are deaf or very hard-of-hearing who use cochlear implants (U.S. Department of Health and Human Services, 2011). Despite the substantial benefit this treatment can provide recipients, cochlear implantation is an underused service (Shapiro & Bradham, 2012). The National Institute on Deafness and Other Communication Disorders' (NIDCD) Healthy Hearing Progress Report noted that in 2004, only 2 of every 1,000 adults who are deaf or very hard of hearing received a cochlear implant (National Institute of Health [NIH], 2010). For children ages 1 through 6, Bradham and Jones (2008) reported that only 55% of the children who were appropriate for cochlear implantation were recipients of this technology.

To address this national healthcare issue, there has been significant emphasis on educating practitioners on candidacy criteria for cochlear implants, programming of the device, outcomes, and red flags (Cosetti & Waltzman, 2012; Ganek, Robbins, & Niparko, 2012; Shapiro & Bradham, 2012). The purpose of this chapter is to review factors in determining cochlear implant candidacy, verification and validation of cochlear implant programming and monitoring, and counseling expectations.

Vignette #1

The audiologist, Dr. Button, received a report from the speech-language pathologist, Ms. Gab, that Abel has not been hearing [s] or [sh] for about a month now. Ms. Gab also noted in the most recent speech-language evaluation that Abel was having difficulties with morphologic markers such as [-s] as in cat versus cats. Abel is about to enter kindergarten in about six months.

After checking Abel's hearing aid settings using simulated real ear measures, Dr. Button realizes a change in access to sounds. The hearing aid settings were no longer reaching prescriptive targets. Abel has minimal access to sounds in the mid frequencies and relatively no access to high frequency sounds. Abel has one of the most powerful digital hearing aids on the market. Now, Dr. Button has to tell the parents:

"Mr. and Mrs. Trend, based on today's measures with Abel's hearing aids and the speech-language report, Abel can hear low frequency sounds like [m] and [o] but cannot adequately hear [s] or [sh] in quiet listening environments. In noisy places, based on these findings, Abel is probably having difficulties hearing and communicating with you at home. You might recall that when we first started with hearing aids, we mentioned a technology called a cochlear implant. Do you have time to hear more about this as an option to explore?"

COCHLEAR IMPLANT

A cochlear implant is a biomedical device that can help provide sounds to a person with significant hearing loss. The cochlear implant consists of two parts: an external portion that sits behind the ear and an internal portion that is surgically placed under the skin and in the cochlea, the hearing organ (Figure 11–1). The external device contains the microphone, speech processor, transmitter, and battery. The internal device houses the receiver/stimulator and electrode array. Unlike a hearing aid, which amplifies sounds to be detected by impaired cochleas, the cochlear implant bypasses areas within the inner ear that do not stimulate the hearing organ for sound recognition and directly stimulates the viable auditory nerve (U.S. Department of Health & Human Services, 2013). The cochlear implant converts acoustical signals into highly processed electrical patterns. These patterns are then relayed to the electrodes that are inserted into the cochlea.

It is important to note that neither a hearing aid nor a cochlear implant restores a child's hearing to normal. This technology, however, allows children to hear sounds not previously heard without it.

Cochlear implants are regulated as Class III devices by the Food and Drug Administration (FDA). Once the cochlear implant is approved by the FDA, it means that it has gone through several processes, specifically the product development protocol (PDP) and the premarket approval (PMA) process, that is required to confirm that the device is safe and effective (FDA, 2014). Based on the application submitted by the cochlear implant manufacturer, the FDA will approve those

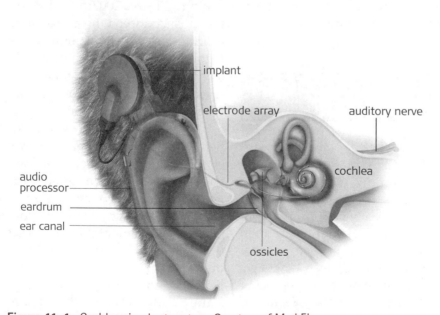

Figure 11–1. Cochlear implant system. Courtesy of Med El.

manufacturer-defined parameters. The cochlear implant manufacturer can only promote the approved parameters. The cochlear implant center, though, can recommend a cochlear implant to a patient outside these predefined parameters. As stated by the FDA (2011):

> Good medical practice and the best interests of the patient require that physicians use legally available drugs, biologics and devices according to their best knowledge and judgment. If physicians use a product for an indication not in the approved labeling, they have the responsibility to be well informed about the product, to base its use on firm scientific rationale and on sound medical evidence, and to maintain records of the product's use and effects. (para. 1)

While advertisements cannot take place to encourage off-label use, off-label usage is allowed if determined by the cochlear implant team that it would be beneficial to the child. Ultimately, the family makes the final decision to proceed with the cochlear implant and the interventional program to follow.

GOALS OF COCHLEAR IMPLANTATION FOR CHILDREN

The primary goal for cochlear implantation in children with hearing loss is to obtain communicative competence (Ganek et al., 2012). For those children who receive limited or no benefit from amplification, cochlear implantation is often a viable option with associated positive outcomes in listening, spoken language, literacy, and social/emotional well-being (Fryauf-Bertschy, Tyler, Kelsay, Gantz, &

Woodworth, 1997; Geers, 2008; Geers & Moog, 1994; Geers, Tobey, & Moog, 2008). Improved hearing sensitivity, as provided by cochlear implant(s), however, does not guarantee the ability to discriminate between sounds or to perceive speech for spoken communication, so children who receive cochlear implant(s) require intensive auditory, speech, and language training (Wilkins & Ertmer, 2002). Thus, there is increasing demand for speech and language services for children who are cochlear implant recipients, especially from well-trained early interventionists and speech-language pathologists (SLPs).

For infants, toddlers, and young children with cochlear implants who are learning to listen and develop spoken language through **auditory-verbal therapy**, a developmental approach is often employed. In this scenario, once the child has been fit with amplification or cochlear implants and has gained access to audition, typical neurodevelopment can be facilitated, often leading to the acquisition of age-appropriate auditory, speech, and language milestones (Cole & Flexer, 2007; Estabrooks, 2006). For most children who are identified with hearing loss as infants, immediate use of amplification will allow the development of early auditory milestones until they reach the appropriate age, size, or weight for cochlear implantation.

Some children, however, are identified with hearing loss later, received inadequate audiological management, and/or were provided inappropriate early intervention services, resulting in delayed acquisition of listening and spoken language developmental targets. These children may still be candidates for cochlear implantation. Their performance age in listening and spoken language may be significantly delayed when compared to their chronological age. For these children, an auditory-verbal approach may still be viable. Weekly auditory-verbal sessions can then be scheduled with the parents or caregivers to model strategies that can be used to close the language gap. Through direct coaching, parents and caregivers can learn techniques and appropriate language modeling that facilitate auditory learning and spoken language, especially during daily routines encountered by the child with hearing loss.

For children with cochlear implants who are acquiring spoken language through audition, it is vital that the early interventionists and/or speech-language pathologists have the knowledge and skills to accurately assess the child's present level of functioning to determine whether the child's communication development is simply delayed or if the child's speech and language have become disordered. Through precise assessment of speech, language, and functional listening skills, early interventionists and/or speech-language pathologists can identify both short- and long-term goals that can be targeted through intervention and/or weekly auditory-verbal sessions. Depending on the case, assessments repeated at 6-month or yearly intervals can be used to measure the child's progress. These assessments will yield standard scores to determine if the child is reaching age-appropriate communication milestones, especially when compared to same-age hearing peers. For those children with delayed language, periodic assessments can be used to determine if the child is beginning to close the gap between his or her language performance and his or her chronological age. And finally, comprehensive assessments can be used to determine a child's eligibility to qualify for intervention or specialized services. In other cases, assessments may be used to document that a child has made sufficient progress and no longer needs the same level of service delivery.

Because of early identification of hearing loss, early intervention, and the use of advanced hearing technology, no degree of hearing loss should preclude auditory brain development (Cole & Flexer, 2007). That is, because children with hearing loss now have the opportunity to develop spoken language through audition and remain in synchrony with typical developmental processes, these children—even those with severe and profound sensorineural hearing losses—acquire spoken language in same manner as their hearing peers. For this reason, most experienced early interventionists and SLPs serving these children will use speech and language assessments that are standardized on typical hearing children, with only a few exceptions. If the child with hearing loss is acquiring spoken language, the early interventionist and SLP should use assessments that compare the child's performance to what is considered to be typical development.

While a cochlear implant is a viable option for many children, it may not be appropriate for all children with significant hearing loss. The usage of a cochlear implant does not guarantee that a child will develop listening and spoken language. By using evidence-based practices, families can be counseled about known factors that contribute to communication competence. There are, however, factors that are unique to the child that may be unknown at the time of cochlear implantation. For these reasons, it has become a standard of care for a child to undergo an interdisciplinary approach in determining cochlear implant candidacy.

Vignette #2

Mr. and Mrs. Trend listened to Dr. Button describe a cochlear implant and potential outcomes. They wanted Abel to listen, talk, read, and access a mainstream classroom. Because of the EVA diagnosis, they understood it was possible that Abel's hearing loss would progress, but they thought they had more time. According to Dr. Button, his practice does not provide services for a cochlear implant, so he has to refer them to another place. He said Abel would have to be seen by another audiologist, otolaryngologist, radiologist, speech-language pathologist, and a psychologist. He said there may be other providers who will need to see Abel to determine if he is a candidate. What did they mean by a "candidate," and why so many people?

COCHLEAR IMPLANT CANDIDACY PROCESS: IT IS MORE THAN A HEARING A TEST!

One of the most important elements of cochlear implant success within the pediatric population is patient and family selection (Daya et al., 1999). A hearing test alone will not determine if a patient is a candidate or not. As mentioned above, the FDA provides the parameters in which the devices have been approved for usage and can be used as guidelines for selecting a cochlear implant candidate (Table 11–1). As part of the evaluation, the following questions have to be answered:

- Are there other noninvasive technologies available that can make sounds accessible to develop listening, spoken language, literacy, and social skills?
- Are there qualified intervention providers and family support services to help maximize the child's ability to learn how to listen and communicate?
- Are there any safety issues that should be considered to minimize

any potential risk for this surgery, programming, and/or intervention?

As the child and the family progress through the cochlear implant candidacy testing, in addition to the above questions, the interdisciplinary team members are trying to determine:

- Does the child meet the criteria for a cochlear implant based on the FDA labeling?
- If not, based on the research and clinical observations, could the child receive more benefits if he or she received the cochlear implant? What are those benefits?
- Does the family have realistic expectations?

To answer these questions, the cochlear implant team will not only look at the audiologic and medical results but will be evaluating the "whole" child and family unit (Winter & Phillips, 2009). The first part of the evaluation is to obtain a comprehensive history. The medical examination conducted by a neuro-otologist/pediatric otolarynologist/otologist will examine the viability of the auditory nerve and

Table 11–1. General FDA Cochlear Implant Guidelines

Company	Device Name	Pediatric Approval Guidelines
Advanced Bionics	HiRes90K/Naida CI Q70/Neptune	12 months–17 years
		Profound, bilateral sensorineural hearing loss; Used appropriately fit hearing aids and receives little or no benefits
		<4 years: failure to reach appropriate developmental milestones as measured by IT-MAIS or MAIS and/or <20% word recognition testing
		>4 years: <12% on word recognition testing and <30% on sentence recognition testing
Cochlear	Nucleus CI24RE Cochlear Implant/ Nucleus 5	2–17 years
		Severe to profound sensorineural hearing loss; Limited benefits from binaural hearing aid trial with word recognition scores ≤30%
		12–24 months
		Profound sensorineural hearing loss; Limited benefits from binaural hearing aid trial
Med El	Maestro Cochlear Implant Systems— Med El Concert/ Rondo/Opus 2	12 months to 17 years
		Bilateral, profound sensorineural hearing loss; Little or no benefits from appropriately fit binaural hearing aids
		Lack of progress in developing auditory skills
		Scoring <20% on speech recognition tests

surgical candidacy. The audiologic assessment should include both physiologic and behavioral assessments to determine ear-specific degree and type of hearing loss. Furthermore, the audiologic assessment should include baseline auditory functional assessments. These functional assessments can include questionnaires like the Infant Toddler-Meaningful Auditory Integration Scales (IT-MAIS; Zimmerman-Phillips, Robbins, & Osberger, 2000) and/or LittlEARS (Coninx et al., 2009) questionnaires as well as aided testing in the sound booth and real ear measures. A speech-language pathologist will assess auditory skills, speech production, and receptive and expressive language skills. The psychologist on the team, at the minimum, will attain a nonverbal intelligence (i.e., IQ) score with appropriate testing. These team members will also discuss realistic expectations regarding what a cochlear implant can and cannot do. Some teams also have a social worker who can evaluate the needs of the family, identify stressors, and counsel them on parenting skills. Another essential component of the cochlear implant candidacy testing includes evaluation of the educational setting. With the family's consent, the early intervention program, child care program, and/or school of choice should be consulted to determine the educational needs of the child (Table 11–2). Additional assessments may be required to determine candidacy for the cochlear

Table 11–2. Educator's Questionnaire

Educator's Questionnaire
Child's name: _____ Date: _____
Educator's name: _____ School name: _____
School placement: _____ Grade: _____
Do you have any experience with CI?   Yes   No _____
Do you have any experience with hearing loss?   Yes   No _____
What is the child's usual mode of communication? Sign   Aural/Oral   Other _____
Days absent? _____   Reason (if known) _____
Mood toward school _____
Peer relations?   Good   Fair   Poor/Few friends _____
Work/Study habits?   Good   Fair   Poor _____
Do think that the child is motivated to perform well?   Yes   No _____
Does the child complete homework, papers come back signed, etc.?   Yes   No _____
Does the child wear his or her hearing aids to school?   Yes   No _____
Do you think that the child benefits from wearing his or her hearing aids?   Yes   No _____
Does the child wear an FM system at school?   Yes   No _____
Do the parents attend the IEP meeting?   Yes   No _____
How much contact do you have with the parents? _____
Describe the types and availability of support services at school. _____ _____
Describe your feelings and expectations for cochlear implant. _____ _____
What can we do here to help you? _____ _____
Candidate for CI?   Yes   No _____

implant, depending on the needs of the child or family. Table 11–3 provides a brief description of the evaluations a child and a family may undergo to determine candidacy. During the candidacy evalu- ation, the family will learn about what a cochlear implant can do and what it does not do. The family, and the child if he or she is old enough, may be asked to complete an expectation questionnaire to

Table 11–3. Descriptions of Cochlear Implant Candidacy Evaluations

Audiological Evaluation:	A comprehensive hearing assessment completed with and without the child's hearing aids. This may require more than one visit. It is essential that the child brings his or her hearing aids and ear molds to the evaluation. If the child does not have a hearing aid, then the cochlear implant center should have stock/loaner hearing aids available to complete the aided testing.
Sedated Auditory Brainstem Response and Otoacoustic Emissions Tests:	Per the JCIH statement, the child should have at least one objective measure of hearing sensitivity. Some children require sedation to obtain these test results. If an ABR has not been completed, then one may be recommended by the cochlear implant team.
CT Scan/MRI:	A specialized x-ray to evaluate the anatomy of the inner ear. Some children are sedated for this procedure. It is important to determine the status of the internal auditory meatus.
Medical Examination:	The otologist/otolaryngologist will take a medical history, review the CT scan, and determine if there are any medical contraindications that would prohibit surgery.
Speech-Language Evaluation:	Formal and informal assessment of the child's communication abilities with his or her hearing aids. Communication goals are usually discussed at this appointment.
Developmental/ Cognitive/Psychological Evaluation:	For children, formal and informal assessment of the child's developmental milestones and capacity to learn.
Social Work Evaluation:	To evaluate parent stressors and family support, the social worker will work with the family to navigate services needed to maximize the child's outcomes. Family expectations also will be discussed.
Educational Assessment:	The child's school will be contacted regarding educational placement, support, and the need, if any, for inservice on cochlear implants.
Other Assessments:	A genetic evaluation and ophthalmology examination may also be recommended. Since 40% of children with hearing loss may have additional special needs, genetic testing may assist the family in making a decision about how to proceed.

assist the professionals in counseling (Figure 11–2). Once the evaluations are completed, then the cochlear implant team members review the findings and make a recommendation to the family.

Many factors can help guide the cochlear implant team in making an appropriate prognosis. Using a candidacy checklist can help identify these factors that may influence the outcomes (Table 11–4). The Graded Profile Analysis (GPA; Daya et al., 1999), the Children's Implant Profile (CHIP; Hellman et al., 1991), the Cochlear Implant Candidacy—Children (CICC; Bradham, Lambert, Turick, & Swink, 2003), or the Modified ChIP (Barnes, Lundy, Schuh, Foley, & Maddern, 2000) are such tools that guide the team in their discussions about whether or not to recommend a cochlear implant to a family for consideration. It is important to note that it is not about the number received on these measures, but the identification of potential issues that could negatively impact meeting the family's goals and expectations. Furthermore, in the era of having to justify

Revised Pediatric Cochlear Implant Expectations Questionnaire

When using a Cochlear™ Nucleus ® Implant, my child:

☐ May no longer need speech therapy

☐ May have to see someone's face to understand words

☐ May not be able to appreciate music

☐ May continue to have difficulty understanding speech in the presence of background noise

☐ May not demonstrate an improvement in speech production/articulation

☐ May be able to notice many everyday sounds

☐ May need to have the sound processor programmed on an ongoing, regular basis

☐ May be able to tell the difference between some, but not all, voices

☐ May not be able to use their device while swimming or bathing

☐ May need to continue to wear a hearing aid on the opposite ear

☐ May be able to attend a mainstream educational setting immediately

☐ May immediately show an improvement in speech

☐ May be able to hear their own voice

☐ May be able to locate the direction of sounds

☐ May need some time to adjust to new aspects of hearing

Hear now. And always   Cochlear·

Figure 11–2. Expectation questionnaires. Courtesy of Cochlear.

payment for services, these measures can serve as an objective tool in making the case for payment.

Once the team has decided, they will make a candidacy recommendation to the family. The recommendations fall into

Table 11–4. Cochlear Implant Candidacy Checklist for Children

Circle the number that corresponds to the level of concerns where 1 is no concern, 2 slight concerns, 3 mild concerns, 4 moderate concerns, and 5 significant concerns.						
Team impression of the factors important to implant use and success						**Comments**
Demographics:						
Chronological Age	1	2	3	4	5	
Duration of Deafness	1	2	3	4	5	
Medical/Radiological	1	2	3	4	5	
Multiple Handicap	1	2	3	4	5	
Psychological/Expectations:						
Cognition Learning Style	1	2	3	4	5	
Family Structure & Support	1	2	3	4	5	
Expectations (Patient)	1	2	3	4	5	
Expectations (Family Members)	1	2	3	4	5	
Audiometric:						
Hearing Loss Stability	1	2	3	4	5	
Hearing Aid Usage	1	2	3	4	5	
Speech & Language:						
Speech & Language Abilities	1	2	3	4	5	
Communication Strategies	1	2	3	4	5	
Availability of Support Services	1	2	3	4	5	
Other:	1	2	3	4	5	

Recommendations:

_____ Yes: Implant: _____   Ear: Right   Left   Color: _____

_____ No: _____

_____ Hold Status: _____

_____

Note. The lower the CICC score, meaning no to slight concerns, the greater the amount of improvement, whereas the higher the CICC score, meaning greater concerns, the lower the amount of improvement. Children scoring above 40% on the CICC showed the slowest amount of improvement.

three categories: proceed with the cochlear implant, do not proceed (and why), or wait (and why). It is also not uncommon for families to get a second opinion. Every effort should be made to assist the family when they are seeking additional advice from other healthcare providers.

If the child is considered to be a cochlear implant candidate, a determination will be made regarding which device to use. This varies by cochlear implant center. In some cases, the surgeon will make a recommendation of a particular device based on the medical and radiologic examination. Some centers only offer the option of the cochlear implant system available from one manufacturer, whereas other centers offer makes and models by all companies. It is incumbent on the cochlear implant team to ensure that the family has access to unbiased information about each of the cochlear implants systems available and approved by the FDA. It is also very helpful for a family to talk with other families who have children with a cochlear implant. While this portion of the cochlear implant candidacy process can be time intensive and not reimbursable by insurance companies, it is an essential part of the process.

Another consideration prior to surgery is to determine if the child should be a **bimodal listener** (i.e., with a hearing aid in one ear and a cochlear implant in the other ear) or **bilateral listener** (i.e., should receive cochlear implants in both ears). If it is decided to proceed with two cochlear implants, the family and the surgeon will need to discuss sequential versus simultaneous cochlear implantation. Factors that will determine how to proceed include the age of the child, degree of residual hearing in the nonimplant ear, family choice, and financial coverage/reimbursement rates.

Finally, some cochlear implant centers complete a cochlear implant candidacy agreement with the family that outlines the family's responsibilities and the cochlear implant team's responsibilities. Having clear expectations from all parties in the beginning can minimize potential miscommunication later. See Table 11–5 for a sample candidacy agreement.

Cochlear implant surgery is done under general anesthesia as an outpatient procedure. For young children, a pediatric anesthesiologists should be a member of the surgical team. The surgery is approximately 1 to 2 hours. The risks of cochlear implant surgery include those of general anesthesia as well as risks unique to ear operations, including infection, bleeding, facial nerve injury, cerebral spinal fluid leakage (CSF leak), dizziness after surgery, rupture of the tympanic membrane, and failure to secure the cochlear implant. While these all can occur, they are very rare, occurring in less than 1 out of 100 people (Loundon, Blanchard, Roger, Denoyelle, & Garabedian, 2010). One common report following surgery, however, is the change in taste of foods that can last up to 6 months following surgery.

The internal part of the cochlear implant is designed to last a lifetime; however, the external devices require periodic upgrades due to changes in technology, and cochlear implant recipients often are responsible for upgrade costs. Approximately 2 to 4 weeks following surgery, the patient returns for fitting and activation of the cochlear implant system(s). This is the first time the patient hears with the cochlear implant.

PROGRAMMING AND VERIFICATION

Programming the cochlear implant system requires special training and is com-

Table 11–5. Sample Cochlear Implant Candidacy Agreement

I/we _____ am/are the parent(s) of _____,

who will be receiving a cochlear implant through _____.

Expectations of Parents:

1. Recognition of importance of audition and its implications for the development of hearing and speech.

2. Commitment to providing a learning environment which enhances the use of audition and spoken communication.

3. Assume responsibility for the child's cochlear implant system.

   a. Attend scheduled programming and speech-language-auditory therapy sessions.

   b. Maintain the equipment including daily monitoring for proper functioning, timely repairs, and regular contact with an audiologist.

   c. Provide the school with back-up supplies to make sure that your child has access to sounds during the day (i.e., batteries, cable).

4. Work with all professionals to optimize coordination and consistency of program.

5. Maintain records, such as a journal, regarding child's auditory learning to assist with monitoring child's progress and to determine appropriate goals.

6. Participate in family support programs and speech-language therapy sessions.

7. Discuss with the CI Team any concerns about the child's auditory needs.

Expectations of CI Team:

1. Provide information regarding importance of audition and its implications for the development of hearing and speech.

2. Provide opportunities and support for parents to learn about cochlear implants, auditory development, and auditory learning principles including appropriate activities to support auditory learning.

3. Provide a positive, supportive, and nonjudgmental atmosphere for communication which encourages parents to participate as team members to promote their child's development.

4. Provide assessments to monitor child's progress and determine appropriate goals.

5. Program the cochlear implant system to maximize audibility and comfort.

6. Provide a loaner sound processor or supplies, when available, while the personal system is being repaired.

Expectations of Child:

1. Child wears cochlear implant(s) during all waking hours.

2. Child goes to school wearing the cochlear implant system. A note should be provided if the cochlear implant system is/are not working.

3. Report to the parents, teachers, audiologist, and/or speech-language pathologist when the device is not functional, when age appropriate.

4. Make communicative attempts.

pleted by an audiologist. The audiologist must be able to program 8 to 22 electrodes that will simulate the approximate 3,000 inner hair cells and 30,000 auditory neurons (Rubinstein, 2004; Zeng, 2004) for speech detection and understanding to occur. How does one tell if the child has an appropriate program? How does the audiologist tell when it is time to reprogram?

As mentioned in Chapter 4, due to changes in health care, there has to be a documented need why the audiologist reprogrammed the sound processor. Previously, it was standard for a child to have set appointment times at least the first 6 months, if not the first year, post surgery for programming sessions with the audiologist (Bradham, Snell, & Haynes, 2009). Today, however, with improved coding strategies, streamlined programming techniques, limited programming audiologists with increased demands, and poor reimbursement (Wolfe & Schafer, 2010), the audiologist should design the follow-up program session around the needs of the patient. Since a toddler or young child may not be able to share what he or she can and cannot hear, it is important to aggressively monitor them to ensure that he or she is receiving sounds and making progress with listening and spoken language. The speech-language pathologists and teachers of the deaf and hard of hearing play a critical role in monitoring the progress of the toddler or young child and should alert the family and the audiologist if they observe any concerns.

To determine if a child has an appropriate program and if the child's sound processor should be reprogrammed, the audiologists should administer a functional assessment and sound field and speech perception measures to verify the audibility of a cochlear implant system and to ensure an optimized program. With age-appropriate testing procedures as described in Chapter 4, appropriate sound field thresholds should show a flat configuration in the range of 25 to 35 dB HL. Working to achieve thresholds softer than this range by adjusting the program

or sensitivity settings may create a more desirable audiogram, but may not result in optimal speech understanding in day-to-day life. Better examples for verifying audibility and program optimization include speech perception testing in quiet and noise, or, for a small child, a Ling Six-Sound detection audiogram (Shapiro & Bradham, 2012). This testing documents that audibility provided by the cochlear implant is having a positive impact on speech comprehension. Telemetry testing should be completed during each visit to verify proper function of all channels and electrodes. Also, any signs of discomfort during programming and usage should be addressed immediately and documented. Any electrode(s) that are causing distress and/or facial stimulation should be disabled or clipped.

In order to diagnose any possible problems with the program, the audiologist must be aware of the typical progress a child can achieve with a cochlear implant. In addition, the family should be counseled on appropriate expectations. The preoperative counseling is essential to help guide the family's expectations and performance over time with a cochlear implant. Another simple, but very effective tool, is having the family complete a guided journal and track first words, first phrases, alerting to new sounds, and other developmental and communicative milestones. If the family sees changes in what the child once heard and is no longer hearing, then they should contact the audiologist for an evaluation.

VALIDATION

Unfortunately, there are no real ear measures or prescriptive targets as described in Chapter 10 to help verify appropriate settings of the cochlear implant system. Thus, the process of validating the programs is more challenging. Parental involvement is essential for validating cochlear implant benefits. Performing daily listening checks, Ling Six-Sound tests, and monitoring the child's behavior are key in early detection of possible problems. The speech-language pathologist and teachers of the deaf or hard of hearing should monitor auditory and communication development milestones to ensure that the child's auditory skills are progressing as would be expected with cochlear implant(s). Both normed-referenced and criterion-referenced testing should be completed to monitor closing the gap between the chronological age and the language age. Language sampling is also critical in evaluating subtle changes in spoken communication. At any point, if any changes are observed, the child should be seen by the programming audiologist for evaluation and reprogramming if needed.

Red Flags

While vast improvements have been made in the early identification of hearing loss in young children, coupled with the use of advanced hearing technology such as cochlear implants, some children fail to reach their developmental, communicative, and academic potential even when comprehensive, timely, and well-coordinated family-centered early intervention services have been provided. Practitioners—especially early interventionists, speech-language pathologists, and pediatric audiologists—should be aware of the red flags that may signal either minor or more serious factors that could be impacting the child's progress.

Often, these red flags require an immediate response so that the child does not experience any further delays in acquisition of spoken language (Bell & Houston, in press).

According to Robbins (2005, p. 2), *"it is important to note that what we term a red flag is not a diagnosis of a problem or a statement of permanent disability, but a notice to pay attention to the skill."* For any practitioner serving young children with hearing loss who are cochlear implant recipients, extensive knowledge of typical development is required, especially if the parents' desired communication outcomes are for their child to be on par with their hearing peers who use spoken language. The practitioner should not compare the developmental progress of the child with hearing loss to other children with a similar diagnosis. Rather, the child with cochlear implants should be compared to typical developing peers and the corresponding developmental milestones in listening, speech, language, cognition, and conversational competence.

Progress toward achieving a range of developmental and communicative milestones can be facilitated through the early diagnosis, audiological management, and early intervention that provided to young children with hearing loss and their families. More importantly, progress, or in some cases the lack thereof, can be assessed using a range of formal and informal diagnostic measures. If a child has failed to master a developmental milestone, then questions should be asked as to why, answers sought, and corrective steps in the intervention plan initiated. Too often, however, practitioners take "a wait and see" approach in hopes of spontaneous learning of new skills. Similarly, some practitioners may assume that addressing these deficits is someone else's responsibility. This is a sign of a professional's lack of training, apathy, or possibly a combination of the two. As most seasoned early interventionists and speech-language pathologists working with this population of children acknowledge, these milestones rarely are acquired without direct intervention with the child that also involves parents and caregivers. A proactive approach to understanding why a child is failing to meet his or her developmental milestones will only lead to more direct intervention tailored to the child's specific situation and learning needs.

When concerns are raised about a child's progress, practitioners can sort and prioritize which developmental areas or skills should be targeted based on two primary factors: (1) the length of the delay, and (2) the number of skills delayed (Robbins, 2005). Because parents, caregivers, and practitioners are keenly aware of the targeted developmental milestones in the child's intervention plan, failing to acquire one or more skills should raise concern. Robbins (2005, p. 2) states, *"The greater the number of skills that are delayed at an interval, the more substantial the concern."* A common term, **red flag**, is often used to signal a concern, a problem, or an undesirable characteristic that demands attention and should be addressed or corrected. An issue garnering one red flag may be relatively minor and easily remediated, while two red flags elicit a stronger cause for alarm and require more focused attention and intervention (Tables 11–6, 11–7, and 11–8).

For example, a child with hearing loss who has a 3-month delay in a speech, language, and listening may be viewed as one red flag. While any delay is viewed as significant, this case would be a mild concern.

Table 11–6. Tracking Auditory Progress in Cochlear Implant Kids, Group 1

Group 1: Children Implanted at Age Four Years or Earlier					
Skill	1 mo	3 mos	6 mos	9 mos	12 mos
1. Full time use of CI*	▓				
2. Changes in spontaneous vocalizations with CI use		▓			
3. Spontaneously alerts to name 25% of the time		▓			
4. Spontaneously alerts to name 50% of the time			▓		
5. Spontaneously alerts to few environmental sounds			▓		
6. Performance in audio booth consistent with what is reported at home				▓	
7. Evidence of deriving meaning from many speech and environmental sounds					▓
8. Major improvement in language					▓

*Cochlear implant

Note. Children are credited only for skills in listening-alone condition. Spontaneous means without prompting or modeling and when not in a listening set. The shaded area is the time postimplant activation that the child should be demonstrating the skill (Robbins, 2005). Used with permission by Advanced Bionics.

Table 11–7. Tracking Auditory Progress in Cochlear Implant Kids, Group 2

Group 2: Children Implanted at Age Five Years or Older (Some residual hearing, consistent hearing aid use prior to CI*, primarily oral)					
Skill	1 mo	3 mos	6 mos	9 mos	12 mos
1. Full time use of CI	■				
2. Understands some words or phrases closed set		■			
3. Understands many words or phrases closed set			■		
4. Spontaneously alerts to name 50% of the time			■		
5. Understands familiar phrases in everyday situations when listening auditory alone				■	
6. Spontaneous recognition of own name versus names of others				■	
7. Knows meaning of some environmental or speech signals when heard auditory only sounds					■
8. Major improvement in language					■

*Cochlear implant

Note. Children are credited only for skills in listening-alone condition. Spontaneous means without prompting or modeling and when not in a listening set. The shaded area is the time postimplant activation that the child should be demonstrating the skill (Robbins, 2005). Used with permission by Advanced Bionics.

Table 11–8. Tracking Auditory Progress in Cochlear Implant Kids, Group 3

Group 3: Children Implanted at Age Five Years or Older (Limited or no residual hearing, limited or no hearing aid use, heavily rely on visual cues or signs)					
Skill	1 mo	3 mos	6 mos	9 mos	12 mos
1. Full time use of CI*	■				
2. Begins to discriminate patterns of speech (syllable numbers, stress length, etc.)		■			
3. Understands some words in closed set			■		
4. Begins to spontaneously respond to name			■		
5. Reports when device is not working (i.e., dead battery)				■	
6. Understands many words or phrases in closed set					■
7. Understands a few things open-set					■
8. Major improvement in language					■

*Cochlear implant

Note. Children are credited only for skills in listening-alone condition. Spontaneous means without prompting or modeling and when not in a listening set. The shaded area is the time postimplant activation that the child should be demonstrating the skill (Robbins, 2005). Used with permission by Advanced Bionics.

Often, in one red flag situations that involves slight delays in skill acquisition, clinicians can model, coach, and provide intervention strategies to the child's parents or caregivers. Likewise, the practitioner can determine if all prerequisite skills were achieved. Perhaps earlier developing skills should be readdressed to establish greater meaning and more consistent use in the child. When done in a timely fashion, mastering all of the prerequisite skills can lead to the natural development of later skills, the closing of developmental delays, and requiring relatively minimal direct intervention or facilitation.

Clinicians also should assess the child's listening environment to determine if the child is given opportunities to use the skill that is considered to be a red flag. For example, the child may have decreased or delayed expressive vocabulary compared to same-age peers. The clinician's next step should be to assess if the child is encouraged to use expressive language at home or if the parent or a sibling speaks for him, inhibiting language output. A plan of action, consistent data kept on progress, and a reassessment every 3 months should be used by a qualified clinician (Robbins, 2005).

A six-month delay of skills warrants two red flags and may point to a general lack of progress in the child (Robbins, 2005). Weekly progress monitoring is critical when targeting listening and spoken language in children with cochlear implants. The clinician must develop a comprehensive but convenient process for collecting performance data during regular intervention sessions and comparing that performance to typical developmental norms. Several developmental scales and other standardized measures are available to track progress (see Houston & Caraway, 2010 for a suggested list of evaluation measures; Appendix A). The clinician should take immediate steps to understand the contributing factors that may be impacting the child's ability to acquire the designated developmental and communicative milestones. When the clinician is assessing a general lack of progress, significant concerns would necessitate immediate action, such as the maintenance and functioning of the cochlear implant(s), reduced parent engagement with intervention, the training of the interventionist, and/or the overall intervention plan. And, as Caraway and Elder (2008) report, children enrolled in a listening and spoken language program often make more than a year of progress in their language development during a 12-month period of intervention. Increasingly, this rate of progress (or higher) is achievable when proper hearing technology (i.e., cochlear implants) is used throughout all waking hours, the parents are actively engaged in language facilitation during daily routines, and the well-trained clinician offers focused guidance and modeling of developmentally appropriate communication targets.

SUMMARY

Cochlear implants continue to create new opportunities for children with significant hearing loss to access audition and achieve spoken language outcomes that rival their hearing peers. The criteria and guidelines for pediatric cochlear implantation continue to evolve and are being expanded. Looking forward, more children with severe and profound hearing loss will receive cochlear implants, and if worldwide trends in age of implantation are indicators, they will obtain these devices at younger and younger ages, often as infants.

Professionals, especially early interventionists, speech-language pathologists, pediatric audiologists, cochlear implant teams, and physicians, share a responsibility to ensure that children with cochlear implants and their families have access to timely, coordinated, and evidence-based intervention and habilitation from well-trained providers. To adequately serve these children, diligent monitoring of their developmental, communicative, and academic progress is required, which entails regular use of standardized assessments as well as ongoing tracking of skill acquisition. Failure to reach specific milestones often necessitates a change in the intervention plan, modification of the cochlear implant mapping/programming, securing services from other well-trained service providers or clinicians, or a combination of these and other variables.

Children who use cochlear implants are achieving outcomes that continue to impress those who serve them and their families. The technology is truly revolutionary and has allowed more children with significant hearing loss a means by which to learn spoken language and vastly improve the quality of their lives. Cochlear implant technology will continue to evolve, new communication assessments will be developed, candidacy criteria will continue to change and expand, and intervention and habilitation strategies will be shaped by research. For professionals, this is an exciting time to be in the field. And, for children with severe and profound hearing loss, the future is full of unlimited possibilities.

REFERENCES

Barnes, J., Lundy, L., Schuh, M., Foley, J., & Maddern, B. (2000, February). *Modified children's implant profile (ChIP 2000): Nine factors import to implant use and success for children up to 12 years of age.* Paper presented at the 6th International Cochlear Implants Conference, Miami, FL.

Bell, A., & Houston, K. T. (in press). Red flags: Barriers to listening and spoken language in children with hearing loss. *Perspectives on hearing and hearing disorders in childhood.* American Speech-Language-Hearing Association.

Bradham, T. S., & Jones, J. (2008). Cochlear implant candidacy in the United States: Prevalence in children 12 months to six years of age. *International Journal of Pediatric of Otorhinolaryngology, 72*(7), 10232–11028.

Bradham, T. S., Lambert, P. R., Turick, A., & Swink, N. (April, 2003). *New tool in determining cochlear implant candidacy: Preliminary data using the children implant candidacy criteria (CICC).* Cochlear Implants in Children 9th Symposium, 38, Washington, DC.

Bradham, T. S., Snell, G., & Haynes, D. (2009). Current practices in pediatric cochlear implantation. Perspectives on hearing and hearing disorders in childhood. *American Speech-Language-Hearing Association, 19*(1), 32–42.

Caraway, T. H., & Elder, T. H. (2009). Doing what it takes: Advancing outcomes for children with hearing loss. Perspectives on hearing and hearing disorders in childhood. *American Speech-Language-Hearing Association, 18*(2), 69–73.

Cole, E., & Flexer, C. (2007). *Children with hearing loss: Developing listening and talking–birth to six.* San Diego, CA: Plural.

Coninx, F., Weichbold, V., Tsiakpini, L., Autrique, E., Bescond, G., Tamas, L., . . . Brachmaier, J. (2009). Validation of the LittlEARS® Auditory Questionnaire in children with normal hearing. *International Journal of Pediatric Otorhinolaryngology, 73*(12), 1761–1768.

Cosetti, M. K., & Waltzman, S. B. (2012). Outcomes and cochlear implantation: Variables affecting formants in adults and children. In J. T. Roland & D. S. Haynes (Eds.), *Cochlear implants: Adult and pediatric.* Philadelphia, PA: W. B. Saunders.

Daya, H., Figueirido, J. C., Gordon, K. A., Twitchell, K., Gysin, C., & Papsin, B. C. (1999). The role of a graded profile analysis in determining candidacy and outcome for cochlear implantation in children. *International Journal of Pediatric Otorhinolaryngology, 49*(2), 135–142.

Estabrooks, W. (Ed.). (2006). *Auditory-verbal therapy and practice*. Washington, DC: Alexander Graham Bell Association for the Deaf and Hard of Hearing.

Food and Drug Administration (FDA). (2011). *Regulatory information: "Off-label" and investigational use of marketed drugs, biologics, and medical devices* [Information sheet]. Retrieved from http://www.fda.gov/regulatoryinformation/guidances/ucm126486.htm

Food and Drug Administration (FDA). (2014). *Medical devices: PMA approvals*. Retrieved from http://www.fda.gov/MedicalDevices/ProductsandMedicalProcedures/DeviceApprovalsandClearances/PMAApprovals/default.htm

Francis, H. W., Koch, M. E., Wyatt, J. R., & Niparko, J. K. (1999). Trends in educational placement and cost-benefit considerations in children with cochlear implants. *Archives of Otolaryngology-Head & Neck Surgery, 125*(5), 499–505. doi:10.1001/archotol.125.5.499

Fryauf-Bertschy, H., Typer, R. S., Kelsay, D. M. R., Gantz, B. J., & Woodworth, G. G. (1997). Cochlear implant use by prelingually deafened children: The influences of age at implant and length of device use. *Journal of Speech, Language, and Hearing Research, 40*(1), 183–199. doi:10.1044/jslhr.4001.183

Ganek, H., Robbins, A. M., & Niparko, J. K. (2012). Language outcomes after cochlear implantation. In J. T. Roland & D. S. Haynes (Eds.), *Cochlear implants: Adult and pediatric.* Philadelphia, PA: W. B. Saunders.

Geers, A. E. (2008). *Long-term outcomes of cochlear implantation in early childhood: A mid-term report.* Paper presented at the 10th International Conference on Cochlear Implants and Other Implantable Auditory Technology, San Diego, CA.

Geers, A. E., & Moog, J. S. (1994). Spoken language results: Vocabulary, syntax, and communication. *Volta Review, 96*(5), 131–148.

Geers, A. E., Nicholas, J. G., & Moog, J. S. (2007). Estimating the influence of cochlear implantation on langue development in children. *Audi-*

ological Medicine, 5(4), 262–273. doi:10.1080/16513860701659404

Geers, A. E., Tobey, E., & Moog, J. S. (2008). Long-term outcomes of cochlear implantation in the preschool years: From elementary grades to high school. *International Journal of Audiology, 47*(S2), S21–S30. doi:10.1080/14992020802339167

Hellman, S. A., Chute, P. M., Kretschmer, R. E., Nevins, M. E., Parisier, S. C., & Thurston, L. C. (1991). The development of a Children's Implant Profile. *American Annals of the Deaf, 136,* 77–81.

Houston, K. T., & Caraway, T. (2010). For children with hearing loss: The times, they are a-changin'. *Perspectives on hearing and hearing disorders in childhood, 20*(2), 48–55.

Loundon, N., Blanchard, M., Roger, G., Denoyelle, F., & Garabedian, E. N. (2010). Medical and surgical complications in pediatric cochlear implantation. *Archives of Otolaryngology-Head and Neck Surgery, 136*(1), 12–15. doi:10.1001/archoto.2009.187

National Institute for Health (NIH). (2010). *Healthy people 2010 hearing health progress review.* Washington, DC: National Institute on Deafness and other Communication Disorders.

Nicholas, J. G., & Geers, A. E. (2007). Will they catch up? The role of age at cochlear implantation in the spoken language development of children with severe to profound hearing loss. *Journal of Speech, Language, and Hearing Research, 50*(4), 1048–1062.

Robbins, A. M. (2005). Clinical red flags for slow progress in children with cochlear implants. *Loud & Clear, 1,* 1–8. Retrieved from http://www.bionicear.com

Rubinstein, J. T. (2004). How cochlear implants encode speech. *Current Opinion in Otolaryngology & Head and Neck Surgery, 12*(5), 444–448.

Shapiro, W. H., & Bradham, T. S. (2012). Cochlear implant programming. In J. T. Roland & D. S. Haynes (Eds.), *Cochlear implants: Adult and pediatric.* Philadelphia, PA: W. B. Saunders.

Wilkins, M., & Ertmer, D. (2002). Introducing young children who are deaf or hard of hearing to spoken language: Child's voice, an oral school. *Language Speech Hearing Services in Schools, 33*(3), 196–204.

Winter, M. E., & Phillips, B. N. (2009). Clinical management of cochlear implants in children: An overview. In L. S. Eisenberg (Ed.), *Clinical management of children with cochlear implants.* San Diego, CA: Plural.

Wolfe, J., & Schafer, E. C. (2010). *Programming cochlear implants.* San Diego, CA: Plural.

United States Department of Health & Human Services. (2011). *Healthy people 2020: Hearing and other sensory or communication disorders.* Washington, DC: Author.

United States Department of Health & Human Services, National Institute on Deafness and Other Communication Disorders. (2013).

Cochlear implants. Retrieved from https://www.nidcd.nih.gov/health/hearing/pages/coch.aspx

Zeng, F. G. (2004). Trends in cochlear implants. *Trends in Hearing, 8*(1), 1–34. doi:10.1177/108471380400800102

Zimmerman-Phillips, S., Robbins, A. M., & Osberger, M. J. (2000). Assessing cochlear implant benefit in very young children. *Annals of Otology, Rhinology, & Laryngology Supplement, 185,* 42–43.

PART III

Beyond the Assessments: Components to Consider

CHAPTER 12

Supporting Families Through the Assessment Process and Beyond

*Joni Alberg, Janet DesGeorges, Patti Martin,
and Tamala S. Bradham*

KEY POINTS

- The primary reason to engage in family centered-care is to maximize outcomes and to help the child reach his or her fullest potential. This requires not only appropriate services by qualified professionals but partnerships with significant family involvement.
- Family-centered care recognizes the critical roles families play to ensure the health and wellbeing of each family member. In the field of pediatric hearing loss, researchers have found that family-centered care strongly influences family and child outcomes for children with hearing loss.
- Family members play many roles in raising children that include care giving, nurturing, and protecting the child. During the assessment process additional significant roles are required of parents such as

"informant," "observer," "decision maker," "role model," "teacher," and "advocate." The most important role they play, however, is parent.
- Engaging the family in the assessment process and creating a partnership is key in developing a family-centered model of care.
- Partnering with the family for creation of the roadmap that the family will travel is essential. There is no "right" way, and there are no "short cuts" as every journey is unique. While there may be detours and new ways of getting to the final destination, it is important to have the right team, optimal access to sound, and family support and involvement for a successful journey.

INTRODUCTION

When an infant is born, new parents look for ten fingers and ten toes. They look lovingly upon this new life in the midst of extreme exhaustion. Regardless of where an infant is born, at some point, the medical community will evaluate him or her. Lots of screenings and exams will be completed on this new life—and more will be conducted later as the baby grows. During this assessment process, some parents or caregivers will learn that their child has a special need. There is no set response as to how a parent will react to learning their child has a special need. When a parent learns his or her child has a hearing loss, the lives of the family members are forever changed. This invisible condition may be questioned by some or may provide a confirmation of suspicion by others. As a professional, it is essential to remember the diagnosis is but one part of the child and family.

The successful acquisition of listening and spoken language is dependent on the family, as a whole, working together towards this common goal in partnership with a team of professionals. It is essential for parents to understand what information the assessment(s) provides and how the assessment results will be used to guide the services and educational planning for the acquisition of listening and spoken language.

This chapter discusses the importance of including the family in all aspects of the assessment. Specifically, this chapter discusses the valuable information parents provide to guide the assessment administration and interpretation, how to explain assessment results to parents for optimal understanding, helping parents understand how assessment results will be used to promote listening and spoken language acquisition, and how assessments will be used to create a guide or "road map" for the child's future.

THE FAMILY

Parents and caregivers are integral to the assessment process and should be included throughout, rather than relegated to a waiting area. A professional should always remember that the parents know their child best and are truly the experts when it comes to reporting their child's strengths and areas of concern. Parents and caregivers wear many different hats; they are *police officers* trying to teach their child right from wrong. Other times, they function as *peacekeepers*, helping siblings to get along. Additionally, in many homes, one or both parents may work outside the home, serve as the *caregiver* for elderly or sick parents, and/or parent several children (Alberg & Bradham, 2013).

During and after the assessment process, the parents or caregivers will be looking to the professional for guidance and direction. Although the focus of the assessment is on the child, it will be the parents who will be responsible for implementing the recommendations and strategies for developing listening and spoken language. Professionals are there to not only assess and report, but also to coach and mentor parents and caregivers as they take on many additional roles such as:

- Informant. The parents and caregivers have unique knowledge about their child, and they can provide detailed information both during the diagnostic process and at specific intervals throughout the intervention stages.
- Observer. During assessment, parents and caregivers will be able to report if the behavior(s) experienced during the assessment

are typical and consistent with what the child does on a daily basis. As services are implemented, parental observations regarding incorporation of new skills into daily living help determine the success of the intervention strategies as well as determine the need for modifications or changes.

- Decision maker. It is incumbent upon professionals to ensure that parents, as decision makers, understand the assessment results and how this information can be used to set goals and future expectations. In addition, it behooves professionals to assure parents that decision making is not a one-time process, but rather ongoing and fluid depending on the child's progress.
- Role model and teacher. Most parents recognize that they are role models for their child, but most do not label themselves as the "first teacher" without encouragement from professionals. Because parents are with their child more than any service provider, helping parents incorporate instruction into daily activities by demonstrating and teaching both language and social skills necessary for their child to achieve their goals is paramount.
- Student. When their child is diagnosed with hearing loss, parents suddenly find themselves in the role of student. There is a new vocabulary to learn, "lingo" to understand, and an array of professionals to meet that they did not anticipate needing to know. Professionals must always remember that for most families the information being presented will need to be clearly explained and, perhaps, presented in more than one way.
- Advocate. One of the most important goals of the assessment and intervention process is to assist parents to become the advocates for their child and family. Well-informed and involved families make the most effective advocates for services and supports to help achieve the goals set for their children.

For many families, this is the first time they have ever met someone with a hearing loss. Ninety-two percent of children with permanent hearing loss are born to two hearing parents (Mitchell & Kramer, 2004). They do not have a guidebook, and they may not have any emotional support to help them deal with the myriad of feelings and emotions they will probably experience during the assessment process.

Despite the many hats worn by parents of children with hearing loss, the primary role is to be their parent. This may seem obvious, but it may not always feel that way to the parent. In addition to the overwhelming amount of information provided to them about what their child can and cannot hear, other evaluations needed, appointments they must make and keep, as well as what must be done if the child is to learn to listen and speak, families will probably be dealing with their own uncertainties and grief, not to mention those of their spouse or partner, extended family, friends, and neighbors. The most important question for professionals to ask every time they see a family member will be "How are *you* doing?"

So much of the attention professionals provide is on the child and his or her needs. Families may be struggling with feelings they may not be comfortable sharing unless asked. They may feel guilt, fear, sadness, anger, or denial. In addition, they may be dealing with many other issues peripheral to their child's hearing loss, such as loss of a job, eviction from their home, rejection by loved ones, trying to make financial ends meet (Crais, 2009). It is important to know potential obstacles that can impede family-centered care (Crais, 1994).

Professionals will be teaching families about hearing loss, language development, audiologic management, and providing them with strategies they will be required to implement for their child. Knowing how adults learn, including one's own learning style as the professional, is an important tool to have. One of the biggest challenges faced by professionals is making sure information presented to parents and caregivers is in *their* preferred mode of learning even though it may be different from how they themselves best learn.

Much has been written about adult learning styles and the literature contains a variety of labels to classify learners. Here are some common descriptions of adult learning styles (Caraway, 2010; Thurbur, 2003):

- Dynamic learners want to "jump in" and start doing things. They do not want to spend time reading and learning the reasons for doing; they just want to get started. These learners may also be called accommodating, because they adapt to, or accommodate, immediate circumstances. They want to see immediate results.

- Analytic learners prefer to read background information and develop an intellectual understanding of what they will be doing and why. Knowledge is organized so they can focus on specific problems and converge on the correct solution.

- Common sense learners prefer to understand basic facts about what they are expected to do and then take action. They will want to know the theory behind the action they are being asked to take.

- Imaginative learners prefer to talk about possibilities and will want to engage in brainstorming solutions to the issue at hand.

Knowing preferred learning styles will be important, because individuals have a tendency to present information in their own preferred style. This works well if the family member with whom the professional is working has the same learning style as the professional, but the situation can be a disaster if the learning styles are different. Analytic learners have a tendency to give families a great deal of materials to read and study before they are ready to discuss strategies and demonstrate specific activities for the families to use with their child. If the family member is a dynamic learner and wants to "jump right in" immediately, he or she will be frustrated that the professional won't show the family member what to do and will probably not read all the materials given to him or her. This may result in a "disconnect" between the professional and the family member from the start, a disconnect that can be difficult to repair (Table 12–1).

Supporting families involves meeting parents and caregivers where they are

Table 12–1. Reflecting on Working With Families

- What are your feelings about working with families?

- What do you enjoy about it and what is hard?

- What do you consider your strengths in working with families?

- Do you have questions, worries, or concerns about building partnerships with families?

in their child's hearing loss journey and equipping them with skills, disciplines, and knowledge so that they can reach their desired outcome for their child (Caraway, 2010).

FAMILY-CENTERED CARE

While the focus of the assessments is on the child, the impact of how the assessment is performed and findings presented will affect the entire family. Thus, partnering with the family throughout the assessment process and during the planning of the follow-up care is recommended. While recognizing that this is a shift away from traditional patient-based services, family-centered care recognizes the critical role families play to ensure the health and wellbeing of each family member (Crais, 1994; Institute for Patient and Family Care, 2010). The services, therapies, and interventions prescribed should be based on the concerns and priorities of the family, not just the diagnosis alone (*Medical Dictionary for Health Professionals and Nursing*, 2012; Table 12–2).

Family-centered care, which has gained acceptance as the standard for providing medical services to children with special healthcare needs and their

Table 12–2. Core Principles of Family Centered Care

Family-centered care is based on a set of core principles including:

- Understanding and respect for personal preferences and values, knowledge, and beliefs; family situations and lifestyles; and cultural traditions.

- Presenting accurate, complete information in an unbiased and timely manner so families can effectively participate in decision making.

- Involving families as a member of the "care/intervention" team in development, implementation and evaluation of the care/intervention plans.

- Empowering families by providing necessary tools and support.

- Ensuring coordinated and efficient transitions between and among providers.

Source: Institute for Patient and Family Care, 2010; Memorial Healthcare System, 2014.

families, grew out of the consumer and family support movements of the mid 20th century (Kuo et al., 2000). In the past, families played a more passive role as observers rather than as participants. In medicine, there are several studies that report positive effects when family-centered care is incorporated in the patient's medical home. Damboise and colleagues (2003) showed that family-centered care positively affected anxiety levels and cardiovascular health, which lead to fewer medical interventions. In the field of childhood deafness, researchers have found that family-centered care strongly influences family and child outcomes for children with hearing loss (Calderon, 2000; Calderon, Bargones, & Sidman, 1998; Moeller, 2000). Family-centered care has been shown to relate positively to better communication exchanges between parents and children (Calderon et al., 1998), more advanced language outcomes in kindergarten-aged children (Moeller, 2000) and later educational development (Calderon, 2000; Calderon & Naidu, 2000; Yoshinaga-Itano, Coulter, & Thomson, 2000). But even today, some research suggests that there is still a disconnect between actual family participation and the desired participation in which families want to participate more in the care of the child but often are not afforded this opportunity (Crais, Roy, & Free, 2006; Romaniuk, O'Mare, & Akhtar-Danesh, 2014). The core of family-centered practice today is professionals and families working hand-in-hand to provide services to achieve optimal outcomes for the child.

Family-centered care is endorsed by the American Academy of Pediatrics (AAP) as a critical component of the medical home (AAP, 2002); the Maternal and Child Health Bureau of the U.S. Department of Health and Human Services endorses family-centered care as a core objective for the care of children with special healthcare needs (Goode & Jones, 2006); and the Joint Committee on Infant Hearing (JCIH) lists family-centered care as a core principle of early hearing detection and intervention programs (JCIH, 2007). It is essential, therefore, that all assessments be approached as one component of the overall family-centered care provided to families.

ENGAGING THE FAMILY IN THE ASSESSMENT PROCESS

Raising a successful child with hearing loss is a complex, individualized journey for each family. Parents rely on both subjective and objective information to make decisions and provide for their child's success. This requires a parent's ability to collate facts, feelings, and data across a variety of domains in a child's development to set goals towards positive achievement. Professionals can support this process by ensuring a family understands and participates in assessing their child's development through all stages of growth.

When provided with family-centered care, parents can participate meaningfully as engaged partners in the assessment process. Each family will demonstrate involvement in different ways. It is important for professionals not to judge families for a perceived "lack of involvement" but to work on strategies for bringing families along the continuum of involvement. Additional factors may contribute to a parents' ability to be involved and may need to be addressed including, but not limited to:

- Emotional resources and acceptance level of the hearing loss;
- Confidence level in decision making and parenting one's own child;
- Understanding and perception of the impact of hearing loss;
- Confidence and trust in the professional with whom the family is working; and
- Individual family capacity due to life stressors (e.g., time constraints, money, family, work, school).

Identifying the obstacles for both the parent and professional are essential to meeting the needs and expectations of the child receiving care (Table 12–3).

To engage the parents and caregivers, it is important to deliver key messages at the right time. Four tools found to be effective for engaging families are AIDET (the

Table 12–3. Obstacles to Family-Centered Care

Obstacles for Families

- Family stresses about money, time, sleep, housing, transportation, balancing work and family, parenting decisions, medical expenses, food.

- Feelings
  - Protective Feelings
    - How can I keep my child safe?
    - Is this provider too young? Too old? Experienced?
    - Can this provider help me with my child if she is not a parent herself?
  - Guilt
    - I'm not a good parent if I don't do all of the care for my child.
  - Gate-keeping
    - If someone else has to tell me how to help my child, does that mean I'm not doing a good enough job?
  - Resentment and jealousy
    - He does what the provider asks but not for me.
  - Frustration
    - I'm always in such a hurry. There is just not enough time to do everything that the providers tell me to do.
  - Other feelings may include
    - intimidation; feeling stupid in front of the therapist; out of respect, parents may not feel able to express their own ideas, beliefs, experiences.

Obstacles for the Provider

- Expected to be culturally and linguistically competent.

- Lack of experience and/or training with building family-centered care.

- Adult learning styles.

- Productivity and documentation.

- Feeling unappreciated for their expertise and the hard work they do.

- Not being a parent themselves/Being a parent themselves.

- Lack of respect from the family because the provider is younger than the parents.

- Managing graduate students in their sessions.

five fundamentals of patient communication: **A**cknowledge, **I**ntroduce, **D**uration, **E**xplanation, **T**hank you), GIVER (**G**reet, **I**ntroduce, **V**erify, **E**ngage, **R**eview), teach-back, and motivational interviewing (Always Use Teach-back!, 2014; Bradham, 2014; Miller & Rollnick, 1991; Studer, 2003).

AIDET, GIVER, and Case History

When professionals are meeting a new parent or caregiver, the use of AIDET can be a great tool to guide professionals on how to format their time with the family (Studer, 2003; Table 12–4).

Table 12–4. AIDET (Studer, 2003)

Acknowledge "You are important." Make eye contact, shakes hand, acknowledges everyone in the room, get down to the child's level, ask or make a relationship-building question/statement (e.g., "Ms. Smith, your daughter has beautiful eyes." Or, "your shirt says 'University of South Carolina,' my brother went to school there.").

Introduce "You are in good hands." Give your name, specialty, years of experience, and may mention a referring physician to position colleagues well. Example: "I'm Dr. Jane Doe, your audiologist. I want you to know that I've worked with more than 500 families who have children with hearing loss during the past 20 years I've been in practice in this specialty area. I also see that Dr. Smith referred you to me. We've worked together for many years. You're fortunate to have such an excellent doctor."

Duration "I anticipate your concerns." Tell the patient what to expect (e.g., how long will the test take, what will happen, can they bring a special toy, when will they know the test results, does insurance cover this, etc.).

Explanation "I want you to be informed and comfortable." Carefully listen to your patient's story and use language the patient can understand when describing the assessment tools used, what you expect from the child during the assessment, and what was learned from the assessment.

Thank You "I appreciate the opportunity to care for you." Thank the patient for choosing your clinic, for waiting and for coming in today. In closing, ask, "What other questions do you have?"

Another tool to assist professionals in introducing themselves and engaging the parents and caregivers is called GIVER.

- Greet: "Greet the patient!" Make him or her feel comfortable. Smile, shake hands, and make eye contact! Essentially, use your manners!
- Introduce: "Tell the family who you are!" Let them know your specialty and "manage up" the referring provider. At the minimum, give them your business card. Even better, give them a biosketch card with your picture!
- Verify: "Do you have the right patient?" The Joint Commission requires that the professionals use two identifiers to make sure they have the right patient.
- Engage: "Let's talk and listen to one another!" Family engagement is central to improving healthcare outcomes. Listen to what the family is saying, pause briefly, and then

respond to the family. Sometimes it is helpful to summarize what was said to show that you are an active listener and that you care. This is also an excellent time to obtain the case history.
- Review: "Review what will happen during the visit." Based on your case history and what the patient has shared with you, tell them your plan for that visit and what to expect from you and your practice. (Bradham, 2014)

While not all of the family's stress will dissipate, these tools do provide some direction that will help the family navigate often uncharted waters. When you start to use GIVER or AIDET, start with one letter and over time, gradually add the other letters to your practice.

Whether AIDET or GIVER is used, a case history should be completed to guide the assessment process. Furthermore, the case history is a good way to engage the family to share their story. For example, during an audiological evaluation, the family could be asked what they think their child hears or does not hear, and/or to describe specific instances where they have witnessed their child "hearing" or "not hearing." If a speech-language evaluation is being conducted, it is effective to ask the parents how they communicate with their child and how they know if he or she understands what they are communicating. Families will be able to provide rich, real-world information about their child that the evaluator must consider when conducting assessments. This information will be especially important if the assessment results reveal something contradictory to what the family members have reported and may require the evaluator to dig deeper.

Teach-Back

Because parents are the primary language role models and teachers of listening and spoken language for their child, it is essential for professionals to make sure parents understand what they are hoping to teach them. The "teach-back method" is an effective way of assessing whether a parent understands the information presented (Table 12–5). Instead of asking, "Do you have any questions?" the professional should ask open-ended "what" and "how" questions such as:

- "I want to be sure I explained everything clearly. Can you please explain the information back to me so I can be sure that I did?"
- "What will you tell your wife (husband/partner/child/etc.) about what you learned today?"

Table 12–5. Teach-Back Tips

1. Be aware of your body language and make appropriate eye contact.
2. Monitor your voice and tone; be caring without being condescending.
3. Do not use jargon.
4. Avoid yes and no questions; use open ended questions.
5. Use printed or video materials to support learning.
6. Document the use of and patient responses in your report.

Source: Adapted from Schillinger et al., 2003.

- "We've gone over a lot of information today. In your own words, please review for me what we talked about. How will you apply these strategies at home?"
- "Tell me more about how you will share these results with the child's mother and next steps (NC Program on Health Literacy)."

Use of the teach-back method may be a new skill to incorporate into the assessment battery. Incorporating this practice with every family will allow it to become a habit over time. As you are preparing to use this method, it is important to mentally rehearse, "What is the most important item that I want to be sure this family understands?" and "How would I ask them to teach-back?" (Always Use Teach-back!, 2014). Parents may need help to learn how to "teach-back." Professionals can demonstrate how they themselves might share information with others, modeling this for the parents and then asking them to do the same. The teach-back method should be used every time new information is presented or when the professional suspects information presented previously has been forgotten. Using this method, the professional becomes the learner rather than a teacher and he or she will find out whether his or her communications have been effective (Schillinger Bindman, Wang, Stewart, & Piette, 2004).

Professionals may ask themselves, "How can I do this? I don't have enough time now to spend with each of my clients/patients? How can I possibly find time to ensure parent understanding?" For professionals who find the directive of "slowing down" in opposition to the reality of a 15 to 17-minute office visit, it's worth considering the potential practice benefits of patient-centered care, including:

- Improved outcomes (Berkman, Dewalt, Pignone, Sheriden, & Lohr, 2004; Kinmonth, Woodcock, Griffin, Spiegal, & Campbell, 1998; Schillinger et al., 2004; Stewart, 1995);
- Greater likelihood that patients/clients will follow a treatment/intervention plan; and
- Better communication between staff and patients/clients.

Professionals who have good collaborative partnerships with families use their skills to recognize which of these areas may need to be addressed (Table 12–6). In addition, highly effective professionals understand that families often receive support beyond the professional spectrum and link the family to other resources.

Motivational Interviewing

Two questions professionals ask are, "How can I best help my patient and their family that I serve?" and "When a fam-

Table 12–6. Characteristics of a Collaborative Partnership

- All acknowledge that each possesses unique skills and knowledge that benefit the partnership.
- All demonstrate trust and respect for one another.
- Professionals recognize the decision-making power of parents in the partnership.

Source: Dinnebeil, Hale, and Rule, 1996.

ily is struggling with follow-through on recommendations, how can I best engage them and help them in this journey?" Along with teach-back, **motivational interviewing** (MI) is another technique that can be used to help engage the family in the assessment and therapeutic process. MI is a patient-centered counseling style that uses specific techniques to elicit intrinsic motivation for behavioral change (Miller & Rollnick, 1991). Contrary to confrontational styles in which the professional advises a patient about changes that need to be made to address the health concern, MI provides a structure to create a collaborative atmosphere where the patient's internal motivations are discovered and discussed instead of the patient being on the defense. The professional respects the families' goals and values, and these are fully considered when assessing a child (Rollnick & Miller, 1995). MI is founded on the principles of partnership, acceptance, compassion, and evocation (Stowe, Stringer, & Wells, 2013). When using MI, the professional applies a range of well-timed techniques (i.e., open-ended questions, affirmations, reflective listening, and summary statements) to evoke and reinforce motivation. One MI technique called the ruler technique uses a scale from 0 to 10 to explore a patient's perceptions about their confidence, and can be used to monitor degree of motivation and understanding (Miller & Roll-nick, 2002). To illustrate this technique, the professional could ask: "How confident are you that you could explain the test results today _____? On a scale from 0 to 10, where 0 is not at all confident and 10 is extremely confident, where would you say you are?" (Miller & Rollnick, 2002, p. 113). To motivate the family member and to promote understanding, the use of a follow-up, open-ended question can be helpful: "Why are you at a _____ and not a 0?" or "What can we do to move you from (current number) to (future number)?" (Miller & Rollnick, 2002, p. 114). This inquiry allows the family member to reflect on the information presented and ask for further clarification and support.

It is important to recognize that when giving advice and directions, the information provided may be premature because the family is not ready to receive it. Stowe and Wells (2013) provide an excellent illustration of this point:

> The city has experienced a mild tremor. As you walk through your home, you see many of your personal treasures knocked over by the tremor. Your natural tendency is to "right them," to set them back in place. But what if you walked through the home of someone else. You might want to "help" by "righting things," but how would you know where they should go? (p. 33)

EXPLAINING ASSESSMENT RESULTS TO THE PARENTS AND CAREGIVERS

The hearing loss journey brings a vast amount of new information for parents to learn. Assessment results, especially those measuring language, intellectual potential, and academic achievement, can be very confusing to parents. Parents or caregivers may focus only on one result or score. There will be criterion-referenced and norm-referenced tests; there may be medical diagnoses; they will hear about "standard," "age-equivalent," "grade-equivalent," and "percentile" scores; they will learn about receptive and expressive language and how "language" is not the same as "speech." In short, they may become overwhelmed with all the test results they are given for their child.

It is up to the professional to carefully and clearly explain the terms used to "describe" to the family how their child performed at this particular point in time. It must be explained that norm-referenced tests will measure how their child compares to the many, many children who were given the test during its development and from which the test's "norms" were developed. It should be explained if the test developers included children with hearing loss in the "norm" group. This information could be helpful to the interpretation of a child's test results.

When a norm-referenced test is administered, the results of each subtest and/or the test as a whole will be reported in **standard scores**. These are the scores that should be shared with parents as they most accurately reflect how an individual child performs compared to the population of children on whom the test was "normed." The child's standard scores can be easily depicted on a bell curve and clearly show how a child compares to his or her typically hearing peers of the same age.

Using a **bell curve**, professionals can plot standard scores from the test and the family can quickly see if their child's results are within the "normal" range, that is, between 85 and 115 (Figure 12–1).

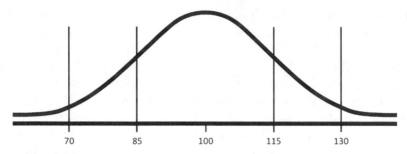

| 70 | 85 | 100 | 115 | 130 |

Figure 12–1. Bell curve of standard scores used to explain assessment to parents and caregivers.

If one or more scores lie below 85, the specific skill addressed by this test will likely become a focus of treatment/therapy and the professional must determine the strategy that will be recommended to teach the skill. Additionally, any scores falling above 115 may be strengths that can be used to address the skill(s) needing attention.

It is important to use caution in discussing age/grade-equivalent and percentile scores with parents when providing the results of norm-referenced testing. These scores can be misleading due to their variability. (See Chapter 2.) It is, however, important for families to understand that these scores may be used by the educational system to justify why a child does or does not qualify for special services. Families who are well informed about assessment results by the professionals conducting the assessments will be able to advocate appropriately for their child.

Some of the tests professionals will administer will be criterion-referenced. These tests measure specific skills and whether or not a child has acquired them. They are useful to determine what a child does and does not know, and whether or not a child has gaps in the development of specific skills. A child's scores on a criterion-referenced test are not compared to other children of the same age but only measure an individual child's knowledge and skill acquisition.

Families need to know why assessments are being done (purpose) and how the information will guide development of a therapy or intervention plan. Bradham and Alberg (2013) offer the following tips to ensure a successful partnership between parents and the professionals who administer and/or present data to them.

- Talk about it. Professionals should make sure that the lines of communication are open when discussing the focus of a particular assessment, such as the limitations (i.e., what it may or may not be able to show); to explain how the assessment may guide the family in understanding and setting a plan as a result of test scores; and to make sure the goals of the family have been addressed and are being respected. As information is delivered, it may be important to monitor tone of voice, body language, and rate of speech. Parents can be asked, "What are *your* expectations?" and then discuss with the professional how their expectations "fit" with the clinician's expectations.

■ Avoid and/or explain acronyms and other testing jargon. The professional should use "teach-back" when explaining test scores to confirm understanding. It is important to avoid delivering test scores only through complicated matrices and percentiles, abbreviations, and acronyms. Delivery of the test results in a way parents can understand is the goal.

■ Don't make assumptions or generalizations. Every family is unique with very specific needs; all options should be presented in an unbiased manner. Families should not be "labeled" nor should other professionals.

■ Create true partnerships. The elements of true partnership include respect, trust, encouragement, honesty, patience, non-judgmental attitude, and unbiased support in family decision making. Also, helping families learn the appropriate words to use to "report back" findings to other family members and loved ones may augment parent–professional partnerships.

■ Respect objective and subjective "data" families use and need. Families use both intuition/gut feeling and hard data to make decisions regarding their child. Professionals must understand that sometimes families may not be able to prove on paper what they know their child needs. Professionals must respect the parent's intuition and follow the parent's decisions.

Parents' efforts and strengths should be acknowledged, showing the parents they are being listened to by the professionals. It is important, though, that the professional continue to provide unbiased information so the parents can make informed decisions.

■ Consistency of information. Keep in mind families likely will see a variety of specialists and each will provide an opinion about what the parents should do. At times, these opinions may be in opposition to one another. "This strategy is better because . . . " or "You should try this." These various opinions can be confusing and overwhelming for the family. Professionals working with the family must help parents sift through all the information they have collected and guide them as they, the parents, decide what choices and options will work best for them and their child. (Bradham & Alberg, 2013)

FAMILY SUPPORT

A family's "team" of support often includes many different professionals with different areas of expertise and training to support the family, including providing assessments in their particular area of proficiency. In addition, families may receive support from other parents, adults with hearing loss, and others (Figure 12–2).

Families need to have a baseline of emotional availability in order to effectively participate in objective testing of their child. Assessment, at its core, shows where an individual child is at a given

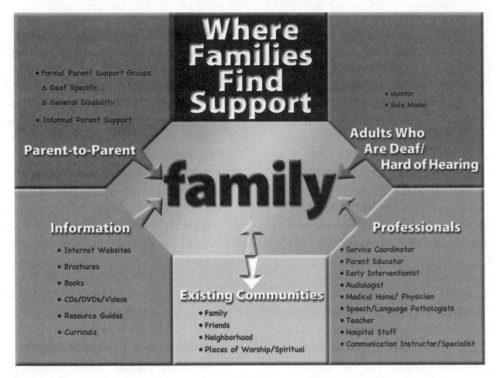

Figure 12–2. A family's team of support, which includes many different professionals with different areas of expertise and training. *Source:* Alberg, Hutsell, Martin, and Seaver, 2008. Used with permission.

time. If a child lags behind where he or she should be, the parents must have the emotional fortitude to deal with this reality, yet have the confidence and seek support to set goals for their child and reach for them. A parent's ability to set high expectations and reach for them is also inherently connected to the factors previously stated.

CREATING A ROADMAP FOR THE FUTURE

Assessments provide a critical reference point for evaluating change and impact over time. They establish a basis for com-

paring the child's level of skill before and after an intervention, therapy, and/ or choice. Using assessment data, parents and professionals can make decisions about the next steps and make adjustments to the strategies being used with a particular child. Assessments are a crucial element in any planning, monitoring and evaluation framework. They are powerful tools for families when they understand how assessment data are used to create a roadmap to ensure successful outcomes for their child. This roadmap can provide hope and satisfaction for families by giving them signposts to show they are on the right path and to help them veer back on to the right path when things are not going well.

Parent Perspective

"I have three children; my middle child and youngest child are hearing impaired. Both children had their first assessments at three months of age and have been regularly assessed since. The assessments are a valuable tool. They help me to have an objective view of how my children are doing and how I am doing. The assessments show in what areas my children are doing well, and in what areas my children need work. When the assessments come back, my children's service providers and I are able to update our goals and decide if we need to change our plan of action. The assessments are a good motivation for me. If the results aren't as good as I would like, I'm motivated to work harder because I know my children are capable of doing better, but they need my help. If the results are as good as I expected, I'm motivated because it's so rewarding to see how good intervention pays off. If a fundamental part of language acquisition is missed early on, it will have life long consequences. The assessments help to make sure our team isn't missing anything."

—Jeannene Evenstad (*The Hands & Voices Colorado Hearing Resource Guide,* 2011). Used with permission.

From the time a child with hearing loss is identified through the diagnostic process in a hospital or audiology office and later through early intervention and the school years, assessment and testing will be a part of a family's life. Whether or not the process of data gathering will help a family to be meaningfully involved in success for their child is partly dependent on a professional's ability to include the family in understanding and using the information generated from the testing.

Welcome to Holland

A family's ability to move forward emotionally in having a child with hearing loss is reflected in this often cited essay—**Welcome to Holland** By Emily Perl Kingsley:

I am often asked to describe the experience of raising a child with a disability—to try to help people who have not shared that unique experience to understand it, to imagine how it would feel. It's like this . . .

When you're going to have a baby, it's like planning a fabulous vacation trip—to Italy. You buy a bunch of guide books and make your wonderful plans. The Coliseum. The Michelangelo David. The gondolas in Venice. You may learn some handy phrases in Italian. It's all very exciting.

After months of eager anticipation, the day finally arrives. You pack your bags and off you go. Several hours later, the plane lands. The stewardess comes in and says, "Welcome to Holland." "Holland?!?" you say. "What do you mean Holland?? I signed up for Italy! I'm supposed to be in Italy. All my life I've dreamed of going to Italy."

But there's been a change in the flight plan. They've landed in Holland and there you must stay. The important thing is that they haven't taken you to a horrible, disgusting, filthy place, full of pestilence, famine and disease. It's just a different place. So you must go out and buy new guide books. And you must learn a whole new language. And you will meet a whole new group of people you would never have met. It's just a different place. It's slower-paced than Italy, less flashy than Italy. But after you've been there for a while and you catch your breath, you look around . . . and you begin to notice that Holland has windmills . . . and Holland has tulips. Holland even has Rembrandts.

But everyone you know is busy coming and going from Italy . . . and they're all bragging about what a wonderful time they had there. And for the rest of your life, you will say "Yes, that's where I was supposed to go. That's what I had planned." And the pain of that will never, ever, ever, ever go away . . . because the loss of that dream is a very very significant loss. But . . . if you spend your life mourning the fact that you didn't get to Italy, you may never be free to enjoy the very special, the very lovely things . . . about Holland.

WELCOME TO HOLLAND by Emily Perl Kingsley. © 1987 by Emily Perl Kingsley. All rights reserved. Reprinted with permission of the author.

CONCLUSION

Assessment testing can support professionals in their own work by ensuring that their limited energy and time are used to the fullest for creating the most impact for success. There is no *one* road traveled in this journey as there are many ways for a family to reach their final destination. For the family who has chosen listening and spoken language, having qualified professionals who incorporate family-centered practices, suitable family support, and appropriate access to sounds are key components to support a family on their journey. The power of good data can inform, support, encourage, prod, and challenge families in a positive way to create progress for the child with hearing loss—a goal that both parents and professionals can share together.

REFERENCES

Alberg, J., & Bradham, T. (2013, November 1). Overheard: Getting parents on your side. *The ASHA Leader*. Retrieved from http://www.asha.org/Publications/leader/2013/131101/Overheard--Getting-Parents-on-Your-Side.htm

Alberg, J., Hutsell, G., Martin, P., & Seaver, L. (2008). *Investing in family support: Taking it to the next level*. Presentation at the Early Hearing Detection and Intervention Conference, New Orleans, LA.

Always Use Teach-back! (2014). *Coaching*. Retrieved from http://www.teachbacktraining.org/assets/files/PDFS/Teach%20Back%20-%20Coaching.pdf

American Academy of Pediatrics. (2002). The medical home 2002. *Pediatrics, 110,* 184–186.

Berkman, N. D, Dewalt, D., Pignone, M. P., Sheridan, S. L., Lohr, K. N., Lux, L., Sutton, S. F., . . . Bonito, A. J. (2004). *Literacy and health outcomes. Evidence Report/Technology Assessment No. 87* (Prepared by RTI International–University of North Carolina Evidence-based Practice Center under Contract No. 290-02-0016). AHRQ Publication No.04-E007-2. Rockville, MD: Agency for Healthcare Research and Quality. Retrieved from http://archive.ahrq.gov/downloads/pub/evidence/pdf/literacy/literacy.pdf

Bradham, T., & Alberg, J. (2013, May 21). *The top 10 take-aways for CSD work with families.* Retrieved from http://blog.asha.org/author/tamalabradham/

Bradham, T. S. (2014). *How do you greet your patient? Are you a GIVER?* Retrieved from http://lean care.wordpress.com/2014/08/18/how-do-you-greet-your-patient-are-you-a-giver-by-tamala-s-bradham-ph-d/

Calderon, R. (2000). Parental involvement in deaf children's education programs as a predictor of child's language, early reading, and social-emotional development. *Journal of Deaf Studies and Deaf Education, 5*(2), 140–155.

Calderon, R., Bargones, J., & Sidman, S. (1998). Characteristics of hearing families and their young deaf and hard of hearing children. Early intervention follow-up. *American Annals of the Deaf, 143*(4), 347–362.

Calderon, R., & Naidu, S. (2000). Further support for the benefits of early identification and intervention for children with hearing loss. *The Volta Review, 100*(5), 3–84.

Caraway, T. (2010). *Adults are not just big babies.* Presentation at Investing in Family Support Conference, Scottsdale, AZ.

Crais, E. (1994). Moving from "parent involvement" to family-centered services. *Hearsay, 9*(2), 12–15.

Crais, E. (2009). *The role of parents in assessing young children with disabilities: How family-centered are we?* [PowerPoint presentation]. Retrieved from http://www.ohioslha.org/pdf/Convention/2009%20Handouts/Elizabeth%20Crais-Roles%20of%20Parents%20Child%20L

Crais, E. R., Roy, V. P., & Free, K. (2006). Parents' and professionals' perceptions of the implementation of family-centered practices in child assessments. *American Journal of Speech-Language Pathology, 15*(4), 365–377.

Damboise, C., & Cardin, S. (2003). Family-centered critical care: How one unit implemented a plan. *American Journal of Nursing, 103*(6), 56AA–56EE.

Dinnebeil, L. A., Hale, L. M., & Rule, S. (1996). A qualitative analysis of parents" and service coordinators" descriptions of variables that influence collaborative relationships. *Topics in Early Childhood Special Education, 16*(3), 322–347.

Evenstad, J. (2011). *Colorado resource guide for families of children who are deaf/hard of hearing in Colorado* (p. 20). Boulder, CO: Colorado Families for Hands & Voices. Retrieved from http://www.cohandsandvoices.org/docs/CoResourceGuide2011.pdf

Goode, T., & Jones, W. (2006). *A guide for advancing family-centered and culturally and linguistically competent care.* Washington, DC: National Center for Cultural Competence, Georgetown University Center for Child and Human Development. Retrieved from http://mchb.hrsa.gov/grants/fcclcguide2007.pdf

Institute for Patient- and Family-Centered Care. (2010). *Frequently asked questions.* Retrieved from http://www.ipfcc.org/faq.html

Joint Commission on Infant Hearing. (2007). *2007 Joint Committee on Infant Hearing position statement executive summary.* Retrieved from http://www.jcih.org/ExecSummFINAL.pdf

Kingsley, E. P. (1987). "Welcome to Holland." Retrieved from http://www.our-kids.org/Archives/Holland.html

Kinmonth, A. L., Woodcock, A., Griffin, S., Spiegal, N., & Campbell, M. J. (1998). Randomized controlled trial of patient centered care of diabetes in general practice: Impact on current well-being and future disease risk. *British Medical Journal, 317*(7167), 1202–1208.

Kuo, D. Z., Houtrow, A. J., Arango, P., Kuhlthau, K. A., Simmons, J. M., & Neff, J. M., (2012). Family-centered care: Current applications and future directions in pediatric health care. *Maternal and Child Health Journal, 16*(2), 297–305.

Medical dictionary for the health professions and nursing. (2014). Retrieved from http://medical-dictionary.thefreedictionary.com/family-centered+care

Memorial Healthcare System. (2014). *Patient-family-centered care.* Retrieved from http://www.mhs.net/patients/patient-care/

Miller, W. R., & Rollnick, S. (1991). *Motivational interviewing: Preparing people to change addictive behavior.* New York, NY: Guilford Press.

Miller, W. R., & Rollnick, S. (2002). *Motivational interviewing: Preparing people for change* (2nd ed.). New York, NY: Guilford Press.

Mitchell, R. E., & Karchmer, M. A. (2004). Chasing the mythical ten percent: Parental hearing status of deaf and hard of hearing students in the United States. *Sign Language Studies, 4*(2), 138–163.

Moeller, M. P. (2000). Early intervention and language development in children with hearing loss. *Pediatrics, 106*(3), E43–E51. doi:10.1542/peds.106.3.e43

North Carolina Program on Health Literacy. (n.d.). *The teach-back method.* Retrieved from http://www.nchealthliteracy.org/toolkit/tool5.pdf

Rollnick, S., & Miller, W. R. (1995). What is motivational interviewing? *Behavioral and Cognitive Psychotherapy, 23,* 325–334.

Romaniuk, D., O'Mare, L., & Akhtar-Danesh, N. (2014). Are parents doing what they want to do? Congruency between parents' actual and desired participation in the care of their hospitalized child. *Issues in Comprehensive Pediatric Nursing, 37*(2), 103–121. doi:10.3109/0146086 2.2014.880532

Schillinger, D., Bindman, A., Wang, F., Stewart, A., & Piette, J. (2004). Functional health literacy and the quality of physician-patient communication among diabetes patients. *Patient Education and Counseling, 52*(3), 315–323.

Schillinger, D., Piette, J., Grumbach, K., Wang, F., Wilson, C., Daher, C., Leong-Grotz, K., . . . Bindman, A. (2003). Closing the loop: Physician communication with diabetic patients who have low health literacy. *Archives of Internal Medicine, 163*(1), 83–90.

Stewart, M. A. (1995). Effective physician-patient communication and health outcomes: A review. *Canadian Medical Association Journal, 152*(9), 1423–1433.

Stowe, D. L., Stringer, P., & Wells, S. P. (2013). Facilitating change through motivational interviewing. *Volta Voices, 20*(5), 32–35.

Studer, Q. (2004). *Hardwiring excellence* (pp. 94, 142–153. Gulf Breeze, FL: Fire Starter.

Thurber, J. (2003). Adult learning styles. *National Property Management Association, 15*(1), 17–18.

Yoshinaga-Itano, C., Coulter, D., & Thomson, V. (2000). The Colorado newborn hearing screening project: Effects on speech and language development for children with hearing loss. *Journal of Perinatology, 20*(8 Pt. 2), S132–137.

CHAPTER 13

Assessment Considerations for Children With Hearing Loss Who Are Culturally and Linguistically Diverse

Michael Douglas

KEY POINTS

■ Professionals in the fields of speech-language pathology and audiology delivering services to children with hearing loss who live in other-language-speaking homes need to consider a host of issues while completing appropriate speech and language assessments.

■ When professionals are preparing for assessment with children with hearing loss and come from other-language-speaking homes, information about the child's history, language environments, and proficiency with language(s) will guide the selection of assessments and the extent each language should be investigated.

■ Use of trained interpreters, if necessary, is an acceptable and lawful way to complete speech and language assessment in this population.

■ When conducting assessments on children who have hearing loss and live in other-language-speaking homes, clinicians need to include a combination of measures that accurately reflect each child's communicative abilities.

■ When interpreting assessments, clinicians must consider results from all methods of assessments in the context of developing listening and spoken language goals for children with hearing loss.

■ During the development of the recommendations, the information from the assessments must address issues related to bilingual development in children with hearing loss, and indicators to monitor during treatment.

■ Professionals who understand the expected course of both monolingual and bilingual language acquisition will be better prepared to analyze pertinent data crucial for facilitating each child's success.

INTRODUCTION

Although the United States' majority language is English, it is not a monolingual country. More than 60 million people age 5 years and older speak a language other than English, with 21% of them not speaking English "well" or "not at all"(Ryan, 2013). The U.S. Census Bureau (2013) reports 39 languages into four major groups: Spanish, other Indo-European languages, Asian and Pacific Island languages, and all other languages. Of the 60 million who were reported to speak another language other than English, Ryan (2013) reported Spanish to lead the others at 62%, followed by other Indo-European languages at 18%. These are shadowed by Asian and Pacific Island languages at 15% and 5% by other languages (e.g., Native American, Arabic, African languages). The U.S. Census Bureau also projected the Hispanic population to increase to 39% by the year 2060 compared to 22% in 2008 (U.S. Census Bureau, 2008). With a higher prevalence of hearing loss in the pediatric U.S. Hispanic-American population compared to most children, bilingualism will continue to be a growing necessity for many families, including those who have children with hearing loss (Keamy, Eavey, & Mehra, 2009).

There is mounting evidence in the literature to suggest that encouraging minority language development neither impairs the language of a child with hearing loss nor prevents him or her from learning the majority language in the presence of adequate speech perception and an effective immersion process (Bunta & Douglas, 2013; McConkey-Robbins, 2007; McConkey-Robbins, Green, & Waltzman, 2004; Teschendorf, Janeschik, Bagus,

Lang, & Arweiler-Harbeck, 2011; Thomas, El-Kashlan, & Zwolan, 2008). **Minority language** is defined here as any other language spoken in a country that is not that country's majority language (e.g., Mandarin in the United States) where a **majority language** is considered to be the language spoken by the majority population in any one country (e.g., English in the USA).

Bilingual achievement (i.e., the ability to understand and use a majority and minority language) for children with hearing loss, however, is neither uniform nor easy (Bunta & Douglas, 2013). It is further complicated by a host of factors related to hearing loss, including a myriad of social and linguistic influences related to multilingual learning that need to be carefully considered (Bunta & Douglas, 2013; Douglas, 2011; Goldstein, 2012). Specifically, professionals need to thoughtfully consider influences of chronological age and duration of deafness, the health of the child, the presence or absence of normal inner ear anatomy, use and benefit of hearing technology (e.g., digital hearing aids, cochlear implants, and FM systems), the child's behavior and desire to communicate, family support, educational placement, and the impact of additional disabilities (Chute & Nevins, 2002; Easterbrooks, O'Rourke, & Todd, 2000; McClatchie & Therres, 2003; Niparko, 2000). Additional social and linguistic factors include socioeconomic status, type and amount of linguistic input in other languages, the child's innate ability to acquire language, immigration status, years away from home country, parental education, beliefs and attitudes, and differing aspects of culture (Goldstein, 2012; Iglesias & Rojas, 2012).

When professionals are providing multilingual assessment to children with hearing loss, standard protocols used in the assessment of children from other-language-speaking families will likely have to be modified and/or extended to reflect the added factors professionals must contemplate when hearing loss is present. Integrating these considerations starts with a comprehensive examination process that includes appropriate speech and language assessment (Kohnert & Derr, 2012).

Appropriate assessment should be designed according to its purpose, which may include one or more of the following:

■ determining whether a speech and/or language impairment versus a speech and/or language difference is present;

■ establishing baseline measurements;

■ determining progress;

■ gathering data that will help the clinician determine a prognosis (in other words, is the impairment likely to decrease with intervention and if so, to what degree?);

■ identifying the best intervention model that will most appropriately & reasonably meet the child's needs; and/or

■ designing an appropriate treatment plan.

The purpose of this chapter is to offer additional considerations that need to be kept in mind when conducting assessments with children who have hearing loss and are **culturally and linguistically diverse** (CLD). Children with hearing loss who are CLD are those who are either (1) exposed to another language, (2) conversant in another language beside English, or (3) bilingual. They may (a) be exposed to and learn more than one lan-guage before the age of 3 or (b) have already learned a language before the age of 3 and are starting to learn another language. Some may come from a bilingual home where the family speaks both English and another language, while others come from a monolingual home where the family only speaks a language other than English (Douglas, 2011). Effectively assessing this population is a multifaceted, dynamic task that requires an ongoing commitment to learning (Austin et al., 2005). It relies on programming flexibility and support from all personnel, including administrators, as well as support among departments in agencies that treat children with hearing loss (Rhoades, Perusse, Douglas, & Zarate, 2008). This chapter is in no way meant to be a comprehensive guide; rather it covers an initial set of useful points for clinicians to consider when (a) preparing for assessment, (b) determining the language of assessment, (c) administering the assessment, and (d) interpreting the results of the assessment.

PREPARING FOR ASSESSMENT

This section discusses certain activities that need to be completed to help clinicians prepare for an appropriate speech and language assessment on children with hearing loss who are culturally and linguistically diverse (CLD). These include:

■ selecting the method of evaluation,
■ gathering a case history, and
■ completing a caregiver interview.

Each of these is discussed briefly in the following sections.

Selecting the Method of Evaluation

The American Speech-Language-Hearing Association (ASHA, 2004) has identified three ways a child who is CLD may be evaluated. Ideally, a bilingual speech-language pathologist trained in CLD issues and fluent in the individual's native language and as well as in English completes the assessment. If this option is not feasible, ASHA recommends the consideration of two other options. The first allows a trained monolingual speech-language pathologist to conduct the assessment with assistance from a trained bilingual ancillary examiner. The **ancillary examiner** is one who has received in-depth training in the measure(s) to be used and who administers testing in the native language in the presence of the speech-language pathologist. The speech-language pathologist is responsible for scoring and analyzing all testing data. The other method allows a trained monolingual speech-language pathologist to conduct the assessment, assisted by a trained interpreter. Information regarding the use of interpreters for speech-language pathologist can be found in the resources section under Langdon (2002).

Case History and Caregiver Interview

In order to capture supporting factors and attend to areas of concern for children with hearing loss who are CLD, a thorough case history (i.e., medical, neurological, developmental, and social) should be completed. A case history usually begins with a questionnaire designed to quickly and efficiently capture referring concerns, supporting factors, and pertinent background information regarding a potential child with hearing loss who is CLD (See Appendix 13–A). Typically, the form is completed by the family member prior to the appointment, either online, or in the waiting room. Once the clinician has an initial case history, he or she will need to:

- interview the caregiver,
- understand the clients' linguistic profile, and
- calculate certain age indices.

Interviewing the Caregiver

Prior to meeting with the family, clinicians should take some time to get to know the culture of the family, being aware that the family's regard for the examiner's personal qualities will vary based on their cultural background. For example, some Spanish-speaking families are likely to place value on certain persona, such as approachability and genuine concern the professional shows in the family whereas Asian and Middle Eastern cultures appreciate a more professional demeanor. Responding appropriately to these differences can potentially reduce a family's sensitivity to certain questions (Roseberry-McKibbin, 2002). The "Self-Assessment for Cultural Competence" on the ASHA website (2014) can be referred to for reflection of the examiner's current level of cultural competence and to improve service delivery with CLD populations.

During the meeting, a semistructured interview should be conducted in the language with which the family is most comfortable. This type of conversational interview allows the family to share information that is most important to them and can tell the examiner information about the family's goals, the child's culture, and language practices. In the case of school-age children, information about their communication abilities in other environments and changes in language use across time will need to be gathered from parents and teachers through parent/teacher questionnaires or semi-structured interviews (Anderson, 2012; Gutierrez-Clellen & Kreiter, 2003; Hammer et al., 2012; Restrepo & Gutierrez-Clellen, 2012). The invitation of a friend to serve as an interpreter is inappropriate and should be avoided to prevent discomfort in sharing personal information with a family's peer (Hammer et al., 2012). Providing interpreters and access to health care, however, is consistent with U.S. civil rights nondiscrimination policies and more specifically Title VI of the Civil Rights Act of 1964 (Department of Justice, 1964, 2014).

Understanding the Child's Linguistic Profile

The distinction between simultaneous and sequential bilingual acquisition should be considered when taking a case history (Rhoades, 2006). The distinction between the two is important as each type of bilingualism may present with small differences in developmental patterns (Guiberson, Barrett, Jancosek, & Yoshinaga Itano, 2006). This can be done based on the age the child began exposure to each language. **Simultaneous language learners** will have been exposed to or have learned more than one language before the age of 3 years. **Sequential language learners** have learned one language before the age of 3 years and will begin, or have begun, exposure and learning of the second language after the age of 3 years (Goldstein, 2012; Roseberry-McKibbin, 2002). This

information will also guide the selection of assessments for the examination.

In order to make the most appropriate recommendations, the clinician will also need to discern whether the child being evaluated comes from a monolingual, other-language family, or a bilingual, English-speaking family. These distinctions are important, because each home environment may facilitate differing developmental patterns and guide the selection of tests as well. This information can be gathered through a home language survey (Appendix 13–A).

A home language survey is a questionnaire, given prior to an assessment, that gathers information on the language or languages used in the home. The survey may include questions about the family's country of origin and length of time the family and child have been in or plan to stay in the United States. A schedule of when and how the child learned the languages and that delineates the extent and nature of exposure to each language may be included. Additionally, queries on the academic and/or educational placement as well as the family's perception of the individual's current communication abilities will be important components of the home language survey. The home language survey will help the clinician prepare to meet with the family, gather appropriate assessments, and determine language(s) to examine that will yield the most meaningful results (Austin et al., 2005; Guitierrez-Clellen & Kreiter, 2003).

The home language survey will further help the clinician determine which language(s) to evaluate. It is best to select the language(s) based on which information will yield the most diagnostically meaningful results as well as results that adequately address the referring concerns of the family.

Calculating Certain Age Indices

Indices such as **hearing age (HA)** and **intervention age (IA)** can be better measurements to determine either baseline, present level of performance, or an adequate amount of development rather than using chronological age alone (Buhler, DeThomasis, Chute, & Decora, 2007; Chin & Lento-Kaiser, 2002; Dorman, 2007). These indices are important parts of the case history and should be determined during this phase of data collection. Hearing Age (HA) refers to the time difference between the date of the examination and the date that the child received a hearing aid or his or her cochlear implant was activated (Kühn-Inacker, Weichbold, Tsiakpini, Coninx, & D'Haese, 2003). Intervention Age (IA) is the time difference between the date of the examination and the date that the child received consistently appropriate, auditory-based intervention. Knowing how long a child has had his or her hearing devices and/or has been in intervention will help the clinician develop an initial gauge of the child's linguistic level for the appropriate selection of certain tests. For example, if the child with severe-profound hearing loss who presented with a hearing age of 24 months using a cochlear implant and an intervention age of 18 months, the clinician may want to prepare by considering assessments that capture the presentence and/or simple sentence skills of the child.

This section has presented some initial activities that prepare speech-language clinicians for an appropriate assessment with children who have hearing loss and are CLD. When speech-language pathologists engage in these activities, they are likely to increase the accuracy of their test selection and identify the language(s) that need to be assessed.

DETERMINING LANGUAGES OF ASSESSMENT

Regardless of the presence or absence of hearing loss, determining the language(s) of assessment for children with hearing loss who are CLD is the primary responsibility of the clinician completing the assessment. Additional issues that need to be considered when reviewing information obtained during the case history and caregiver interview include:

- federal mandates on speech/language assessment procedures and
- certain linguistic proficiencies.

Considering the Law

When conducting assessment with school-aged children who have hearing loss and are CLD, examiners need to consider federal law. Federal laws mandate that in public schools, assessment of speech and language disorders of **Limited English Proficient** (LEP) speakers should be provided and administered in the child's native language or other mode of communication in the form most likely to yield accurate information on what the child knows and can do academically, developmentally, and functionally, unless it is clearly not feasible to do so (IDEA, 2004). Therefore, clinicians must evaluate the child in all languages the child is exposed to or reportedly speaks, and the evaluation should occur across a variety of situations, if possible.

Considering Language Proficiency

When selecting assessments for school-aged children, clinicians also must take into account certain language proficiency levels in each language, such as Basic Interpersonal Communication Skills (BICS) and Cognitive Academic Language Proficiency (CALP; Baker, 2006). BICS refers to the ability to understand and use basic words and phrases with context-embedded language in everyday conversational speech. This requires 1 to 2 years of exposure to develop. CALP refers to the ability to understand and use language in academic settings for the development of reading and writing. This can take from 5 to 7 years to develop when there is support for the language and up to 10 years without such support (Roseberry-McKibbin & Brice, 2005).

BICS and CALP are important to consider when preventing the mistake of continuing the assessment solely in English or with an assessment that requires CALP skills. For example, a school-aged child with hearing loss who emigrated 1 year ago should be tested differently than a similar child who had been immersed in an English learning program for 5 years. For bilingual school-aged children, formal and/or informal data must be gathered to provide preliminary information about an individual's BICS and CALP levels in both languages (Douglas, 2011). This knowledge will further assist in determining the extent to which skills in each language must be measured. To fully capture the strengths and needs of bilingual, school-aged children, assessment might be completed over a period of 2 to 3 visits.

Conversely, for infants and those in earlier stages of language development, BICS and CALPS may not play a significant role in determining the language of assessment. In these cases, clinicians can consider the language of assessment administration to be the preferred language of the family while addressing the other language to the extent that seems appropriate.

Overall, determining the languages of assessment is the primary responsibility of the examining clinician. Simply stated, if there is another language indicated during the home language interview, that other language must be assessed in the evaluation to whatever extent appropriate. Considering the child's exposure and proficiency in each language will help the examiner predict whether the child is performing at the preverbal, presentence, simple sentence, or complex sentence level, thereby aiding in the selection of appropriate tests. There are several formal and informal methods of appropriate assessment discussed in the subsequent sections of this chapter.

ADMINISTERING ASSESSMENT

For any assessment to be meaningful and useful, it must be thorough, incorporating as much relevant information as possible. It should include a combination of assessment tools that truly evaluate the intended skills and accurately reflect the child's communicative abilities. Most important, the assessment should be tailored to each individual child (Shipley & McAfee, 2009). In this section, initial guidelines regarding the following assessment activities are discussed:

- audiological assessment,
- formal and informal language assessment,
- assessment of low-incidence languages,
- assessment for bilingual children who show no language dominance, and
- articulation assessment.

Audiological Assessment

Ideally, a full audiological evaluation should preface all speech and language assessment so the clinician can consider unaided and aided ear-specific detection thresholds during analysis of assessment results. When appropriate, speech perception testing should be gathered in all languages to which the child is exposed. A listening device check also should be completed by an appropriately trained professional to confirm that the child's hearing technology is in good working order.

Formal and Informal Assessment

A variety of formal and informal assessment procedures should be utilized relative to the child's hearing and intervention experience in order to thoroughly describe the individual's speech and language skills while detailing what language was tested under what conditions (Goldstein, 2012; Pena & Kester, 2012).

Standardized testing may be conducted in the native language if appropriate measures are available. However, the standardization sample may not be representative of the individual tested because of the child's hearing loss and influences from his or her community (Anderson, 2012). Instead, parent questionnaires or the child's strengths and weaknesses demonstrated on test tasks can be analyzed as raw scores or criterion-referenced assessments (Bunta & Douglas, 2013; Pena & Kester, 2012). It will be the examining professional's responsibility to obtain and select the most appropriate assessment, which more often than not may be a nonstandardized, non-norm-referenced test.

Examiners should also be aware that a bilingual child's choices for language

use in a particular setting are determined by his or her perceptions of the situation and the topic in addition to the language of the conversational partner (Goldstein, 2012). Therefore, a variety of conversational partners should be used to determine how a child's performance varies across functional language environments (Douglas, 2011).

Informal testing such as speech and language sampling, dynamic assessment, structured observation, and narrative assessment can be conducted (Guiterrez-Clellen, 2012).

- Authentic language samples need to include a variety of situations and linguistic tasks (narratives, conversations, etc.) that are consistent with the child's experiences. When gathering language samples, the following measures can be documented in each language:

1. Mean length of utterance (MLU)—is a quantitative measure for morpho-syntactic complexity. It indicates how many **words** and grammatical elements (e.g., plurals, past tense markers, etc.) a child uses per utterance. To calculate MLU, count the total number of words and morphemes in a child's spontaneous utterance, and then divide it by the total number of utterances.
2. Type-Token Ratio (TTR)—a ratio of the number of different words compared to the total number of words used.
3. Mean sentence length (MSL)—the average number of words per sentence.

For example: The girl watched the girl run. The girl run again. The girl smiles. This example has a MLU of 5 (13 words + 2 morphemes = 15/3 utterances), a TTR of 6:13 and an MSL of 4.3.

- Dynamic assessment embeds treatment into testing, allowing the assessor to determine the client response to the intervention. It consists of an informal pretest, intervention, and then a post-test.

- Structured observation is the act of noting certain behaviors in a contrived setting and recording them for assessment purposes. The assessors actively witness the behaviors without manipulating or prompting the examinee.

- Narrative assessment can be done by asking the child to retell a story from a wordless picture book. The clinician aims to determine the child's comprehension while collecting the child's language samples in both languages.

When combined, dynamic assessment and language samples will help to determine successful learning contexts and aid in the collection of different linguistic structures (Anderson, 2004; Patterson & Pearson, 2004). The results of these measures, especially when they are done in a context where the child interacts most frequently, can and should be considered more accurate indicators of a child's linguistic function than standardized measures (Austin et al., 2005; Douglas, 2011).

Articulation Assessment

Assessment of articulation skills may be conducted formally or informally solely in the individual's first language when the exposure to the other language(s) is determined to be negligible (Austin et al., 2005). For bilingual children, formal assessments of articulation skills compared to monolingual children are not appropriate. Informal articulation/phonological assessment in both languages will provide more information on how their combined phonological systems impact production compared to their bilingual counterparts and may be more sensitive to the identification of speech disorders (Goldstein, 2004). Stimulability probing (teaching efforts made during assessment to improve correct speech production) will help the clinician determine the most appropriate intervention targets and understand the child's cueing needs. Stimulability probes are teaching efforts made during assessment to improve correct speech production. When gathering articulation samples, the following measures can be documented in each language:

- Phonological mean length of utterance (pMLU): measures mean whole word phonological complexity.
- Proportion of whole-word proximity (PWP): measures how closely the child's production matches the adult target (Ingram, 2002).

To calculate pMLU, choose 25 random words uttered. Assign one point for each consonant and vowel in the word. Each correctly produced consonant is assigned an additional point. To calculate PWP, calculate the pMLU for each word in the list. The PWP is the ratio between the pMLU for the target words in the sample and the child's PMLU for the same sample. For example, pMLU for "spoon" is 7, a child's response of /pun/ is 5. The PWP is .71

For bilingual children, determination of articulation errors cannot be based only on the phonology of the majority language. When the sounds of the home language are "filtered" through the sounds of the majority language, the result is considered an accent or a dialectical variation. These differences cannot be considered articulation errors (Austin et al., 2005; Douglas, 2011).

Assessing Low-Incidence Languages

In cases where low-incidence languages are assessed, the results of informal assessments will provide a more accurate indicator of the child's linguistic abilities. Clinicians can use the information gained during the case history and caregiver interview to determine the best method of informal assessment (e.g., semistructured interview combined with structured observation and/or probes, etc.) that will yield the most meaningful results. Examiners should keep in mind that a host of social factors such as years away from home country, socioeconomic status, immigration status, parents' education status and acculturation status will have a significant impact on the language-learning experiences of the examinee. Such factors may also contribute to a varying ability among children to perform on certain tests and can be revealed for each child during the case history and/or family interview.

In addition, due to lack of available instruments in low-incidence languages, examiners may have the option of translating items from English measures to assess targeted skills such as sentence rep-

etition tasks. Although these translations may provide insights into a child's abilities, they should be completed with caution as there will be items that cannot be directly translated. Furthermore, the need to translate items automatically renders the child different from the test sample. It will never be appropriate to report any scores in these situations (Austin et al., 2005; Roseberry-McKibbin, 2002).

Assessing Bilingual Children Who Show No Language Dominance

When professionals are assessing *bilingual* children with hearing loss, each language should be assessed to whatever extent appropriate while considering the limitations of standard scores (Goldstein, 2004). Standard scores reflect the performance of children who receive consistent exposure and use of the language being tested. Therefore, such scores from tests designed for monolingual-speaking children will not be as useful as a raw score analysis because monolingual children may be expected to use different language forms than bilingual children (Bedore, Cooperson, & Boerger, 2012; Pena & Kester, 2012).

Additionally, standard assessments of how many words every 2- or 5-year-old should know in one language are not appropriate for children who have their vocabulary knowledge distributed across two languages (Patterson & Pearson, 2012). Some bilingual children may even lose native language skills due to lack of use. In these cases, informal assessment procedures combined with raw score analysis of formal assessments and/or pre/post-test comparison would provide more meaningful results than standard scores because the child would not be representative of the test sample (Anderson, 2004; Bunta & Douglas, 2013). A host of social factors such as those mentioned at the beginning of this chapter will also have a significant impact on the language-learning experiences of the examinee and contribute to a varying ability between children to perform on certain tests which can be determined during the case history and/or caregiver interview.

Assessment Methods Sensitive to Language Impairment

If the goal of assessment is to determine the presence of language impairment, the use of a combination of assessment procedures can be used to determine the nature and severity of any language disability (Restrepo & Gutierrez, 2012). The following assessments are sensitive to such impairment and include:

- nonword repetition performance,
- sentence repetition tasks,
- spontaneous language samples,
- structured probes, and
- dynamic assessment (Gutierrez-Clellen, 2012; Kohnert, 2012; Restrepo & Gutierrez-Clellen, 2012).

Nonword repetition tasks help to distinguish children as language impaired versus children who are developing language typically with a high degree of accuracy (Dollagahn & Campbell, 1996). In other words, it is difficult for children with language impairment to imitate nonwords. Likewise, sentence repetition tasks help to predict linguistic competence and are sensitive to language impairment (Semel, Wiig, & Secord, 2013). Bilingual children with language disorders have deficits with narratives and comprehension and limited syntax complexity in both languages; therefore, the use of spontaneous language sample analysis is an excellent method of evaluating language production (Gutierrez-Clellen, 2012). Structured probes are contrived efforts made during the assessment in play and can be used to ascertain the presence or absence of certain linguistic skills.

In addition, dynamic assessment procedures that include efforts made during assessment to change the rate of input in order to note differences in performance can yield information on the level of cueing that is needed to induce change in both languages (Gutierrez-Clellen, 2012; Kohnert, 2012). This can also be applied to assessments of a child's narrative skills, tasks that aim to determine the child's comprehension, and collections of the child's language samples in both languages.

Overall, when the professional administers assessment on children with hearing loss who are CLD, a variety of formal and informal assessment procedures should be used relative to the child's hearing and intervention experience in order to thoroughly describe the individual's speech and language skills while detailing what language was tested under what conditions (Goldstein, 2012; Pena & Kester, 2012). Observations of the child interacting with his or her parents or siblings in familiar contexts and parent report of family history of speech and language difficulties will also be important components to include during assessment. When speech-language pathologists administer these measures in both languages and use them together with the caregiver's concerns they are likely to increase the accuracy of their diagnoses (Restrepo & Gutierrez-Clellen, 2012).

INTERPRETING ASSESSMENT

When assessment results are interpreted, the distinction must be made between a communication impairment and a dialectical, cultural, or language difference. As defined in IDEA, a determination of impairment cannot be due to limited English proficiency. Additionally, determination of communication impairment cannot be made on the basis of a single measure but requires data from a variety of assessment tools and strategies (IDEA, 2004). Therefore, sufficient evidence must be gathered in the assessment to allow the clinician to clearly document the presence or absence of communication impairment (Austin et al., 2005). Information gathered from the case history (e.g., family goals, child's medical and neuropsychological history) combined with dynamic assessment and structured probing results are considered to develop recommendations for therapy frequency, program placement, and modifications necessary to facilitate success.

To distinguish between communication impairment and a dialectical, cultural, or language difference in a child with a hearing impairment, the clinician must consider the results from

- formal and informal assessments in the context of developing listening and spoken language for children withhearing loss,
- bilingual issues,
- bilingual development in children with hearing loss, and the
- potential for adequate benefit from services.

Each of these is discussed in the following sections.

Interpreting Formal and Informal Language Assessment

Audiology information will often serve as the driving force towards a child's needs and capabilities (Chute & Nevins, 2002). If a child cannot perceive the full range of speech sounds of a language, the chances of learning spoken language intelligibly are remote. Furthermore, in order for children with hearing loss to hear the millions of words needed to communicate well enough to learn in the rigorous pace of academic situations, they must be able to learn the language incidentally (Kohnert & Derr, 2004; McKonkey-Robbins, 2007). This requires all children with hearing loss in spoken language programs, regardless of their linguistic background, to have access to soft conversational speech (35 dB HL or less) across all frequencies on the speech spectrum (Cole & Flexer, 2007; McKonkey-Robbins, 2007; Waltzman et al., 2003). Knowledge about what the child can or cannot distinguish auditorily will help the clinician understand the child's responses and learning potential during assessment (Cole & Flexer, 2007; MacLver-Lux, 2005). This information is necessary to help support or determine the effectiveness of the child's current hearing technology and should be communicated to the audiologist.

Regardless of the presence of other languages, HA is compared with IA and/or LA to determine reasonable amounts of progress (Douglas, 2011). Because children with hearing loss do not start listening like typically children with hearing until they receive their amplification and subsequent auditory-based intervention, interpreting baseline information or progress results simply by comparing a child with hearing loss to their chronological-age peers will give the child with hearing loss a significant disadvantage (Dorman et al., 2007). HA is compared with LA for children who received intervention immediately after their hearing aid fitting or cochlear implant activation. Minimal expectations of progress are considered to be met if the LA is congruent with the HA.

To determine appropriate progress with children who have language impairment or a period of time with no intervention immediately after their hearing aid fitting or cochlear implant activation, IA can be calculated then compared to their LA. In both cases, minimal expectations are considered to be met if LA is equal to IA and celebrated when LA is higher than their IA (time in intervention; Figure 13–1 and Figure 13–2).

An example would be a child with hearing loss who has a chronological age of 36 months and experienced activation of his or her cochlear implant at the age of 24 months. Although the child is behind CA peers, the HA and IA of 12 months

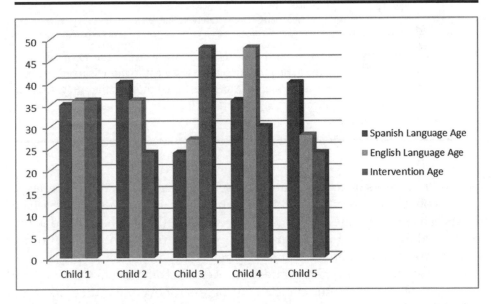

Figure 13–1. For children who have language impairment or a period of amplification without intervention, standard scores will not be as helpful as raw score comparisons (e.g., age-equivalencies). In some situations, by comparing language ages to intervention age, examiners can determine whether minimal expectations are being met and/or determine the amount of continued support needed in one or both languages. In the figure above, the language ages and intervention age of child one are relatively the same. The examiner could reasonably assume that the child is making minimal expectations of progress for his or her time in intervention and that intervention should continue in both languages. For child two, the language ages are higher than the intervention age, indicating that the child is making more than the minimal expectations for progress and that intervention should continue in both languages. Child three appears to be making slow progress relative to the intervention age, indicating the need for further assessment or a comparison of attained objectives between pre- and postintervention. (See Figure 13–2.) Child four and five are also making higher than the minimal expectations, but child four may need more support in Spanish and child five may need more support in English (Douglas, 2014).

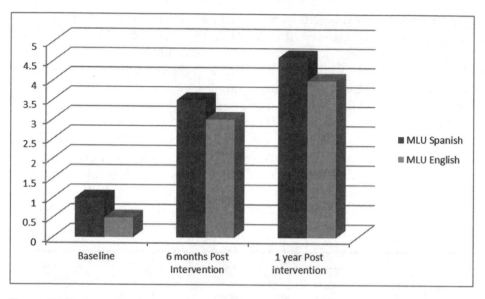

Figure 13–2. In cases where no change in raw score performance is made, examiners can compare skills that were observed during the baseline assessment to those learned by post-intervention measurement intervals. Progress is demonstrated through the comparison of a child's Spanish and English mean length of utterance (MLU) between baseline, 6-months and 1-year post intervention.

are not good indicators of actual abilities. Clinicians would not expect the child to display speech and language behaviors of a 12-month old. If that child were to have a re-evaluation after 12 months of intervention in which he or she demonstrated a language age of 20 months, the clinician could reasonably report that the child is responding well to the intervention.

Knowledge of the progress of children with hearing loss in spoken language programs will also guide judgments related to appropriate progress. Children with hearing loss in spoken language programs with no other disabilities may demonstrate: at a minimum, a month of progress for every month of intervention; steady rates of progress similar to their normal hearing peers; or the ability to close the gap between CA and LA after a period of four years of intervention (Buhler et al.,

2007; Dorman et al., 2007; Rhoades & Chisolm, 2000; Rhoades et al., 2008). It should be reiterated here that in order to close gaps in learning, children who demonstrate skills below the average range need to demonstrate faster than a month of progress for every month of intervention.

In cases where judgments based on rate of learning appear tenuous, such as concerns about the level of exposure to each language or those with additional disabilities who show no change in raw score performance on formal assessments, clinicians should compare lists of attained skills achieved between pre- and post-informal assessments in all the languages the child speaks. In some situations, development benchmarks, such as the one for expectations after cochlear implantation, can also be compared to the child's postassessment results while considering issues related to bilingual development (Moog-Brooks, 2001; see Appendix 13–B). It will be the responsibility of each examiner to make the most appropriate interpretation of assessment results based on the profile of each individual child.

Considering Bilingual Issues When Interpreting Assessment Results

Children with hearing loss who are monolingual in spoken language programs with corrected hearing in the mild range of hearing loss are typically compared to children with typical hearing. Likewise, comparing children with hearing loss who are CLD with their normal hearing CLD counterparts is a reasonable practice and should be done during analysis of assessment results (Buhler et al., 2007; Douglas, 2011). The following represents examples of our knowledge about children with typical hearing who are bilingual from Spanish-English learners. This list is not exhaustive and the reader is referred to the resource list in this chapter for further information.

- In developing bilinguals, vocabulary samples should be combined between the languages to get a true picture of their vocabulary size. One point is given for each concept (luna, arbol, ball = 3 points) whereas Spanish-English equivalents are given one point (leche/milk, elephant/elefante = 2 points) (Patterson & Pearson, 2012; Pena Kester & Sheng, 2012).
- Language samples should be scored within each language versus across languages to help determine the child's knowledge of each one, whereas phonological samples

should be combined and separated to understand true errors from dialect (Goldstein & Gildersleeve-Neumann, 2012; Patterson & Pearson, 2012).

- Transfer occurs when a language structure is common between two languages (Gutierrez & Clellen, 2012). Analysis of code-mixing or transfer of languages between each other can provide a window into the child's ability to apply linguistic knowledge from one language to another and should not be considered a deficit. For example, children learning English in the context of Spanish suppression may show cross-linguistic transfer from English into Spanish (Gutierrez-Clellen, 2012).
- Discrepancies between languages and even speech perception scores should be considered a reflection of children's amount of exposure to that language versus an inability to learn the language (Genesee & Nicolas, 2005; Gutierrez-Clellen, 2012; Patterson & Pearson, 2012; Roseberry-McKibbin, 2002).
- A typically developing bilingual child may demonstrate better performance on certain comprehension tests in one language and higher expressive skills on language tests in the other language (Kohnert & Derr, 2012).
- Morpho-syntax development tends to emerge with structures that are easier to hear in each language. For example, regular past tense camino (he or she walked) is easier to hear in Spanish versus English (walked), because the final phoneme in Spanish is stressed. Therefore, regular verbs in Spanish tend to

develop first while irregular verbs in English tend to develop first (Jackson-Maldonado, 2012).

- In cases where the comparison between language age and intervention age seem tenuous, the range of language structures exhibited in the child's language is probably more useful and reliable than information about rate (Bedore, 2012).

- Overall better comprehension with grammatical errors in one language is predictive of language loss, but code-mixing is not (Anderson, 2012; Guiberson et al., 2006).

- Grammatical errors in both languages increase a child's risk for speech and language difficulties (Restrepo & Gutierrez-Clellen, 2012).

- Bilingual children with language disorders have deficits with narratives and comprehension and limited syntax complexity in both languages (Gutierrez-Clellen, 2012).

- Determination of articulation impairment cannot be based only on the phonology of the majority language. If the individual's articulation skills are within normal limits in the minority language, then impairment does not exist. Dialectical variations cannot be considered as articulation errors (Austin et al., 2005).

- Slowed phonological development is also a typical, yet short-lived symptom of bilingual children acquiring the phonological system of two languages (Goldstein & Gildersleeve-Neumann, 2012).

- For children who develop bilingual skills in a typical manner, accuracy for shared phonemes will be higher than unshared phonemes (Goldstein & Gildersleeve-Neumann, 2012).

- Children with phonological disorders who are bilingual will show a continued use of processes beyond the expected age in both languages (Goldstein & Gildersleeve-Neumann, 2012).

Considering Bilingual Development in Children With Hearing Loss

The bilingual development of children with hearing loss from minority-language-speaking homes immersed in English-speaking preschools has not yet been widely investigated. Such information is necessary to form a legitimate basis for assessment and to design appropriate intervention in this growing population (Douglas, 2011; Gildersleeve-Neumann, Kester, Davis, & Pena, 2008). In the meantime, videotape and progress note documentation for children with hearing loss from minority-language-speaking homes who received bilingual support can be considered (Douglas, 2011). According to Douglas (2011), bilingual children with hearing loss tend to show the following milestones during their bilingual language development that are consistent with the bilingual language learning of children with typical hearing (Comeau et al., 2001; Deuchar & Quay, 2000; Paradis, Nicoladis, & Genesee, 2000):

- A transition from a silent or listening period that lasts about 4 to 6 months to single words for concepts by 12 to 13 months of intervention.

- As single words develop, children begin to understand a one-to-one concept such as if the children hear milk, they say *leche* in response.

- Between the first and second year, bilingual children with hearing loss appear very echolalic in both languages.
- Ultimately, they are able to engage in code switching and start to separate the two languages as they become more conversationally fluent. This may happen sometime after their second year of intervention.
- The children seem to demonstrate a steady increase in vocabulary, phrases, and morpho-syntax in both languages over the years.

It is important to consider when developing conclusions about type and frequency of intervention that the timing of acquisition of words and syntax in each language will be congruent with the amount of intelligible exposure and practice in each language (Douglas, 2011).

DETERMINING PROGNOSIS AND MAKING RECOMMENDATIONS

The complexity of hearing loss and second-language issues requires the ability of examiners to integrate and comprehend enough data to determine the child's potential to benefit from services. According to the ASHA Code of Ethics (2010) services should be provided only when professional judgment indicates that benefits can reasonably be expected (ASHA Principles of Ethics, 2010 Rule I). Therefore, clinicians must collect enough data to make a reasonable judgment on the future success of the child with hearing loss who is CLD.

Positive prognostic indicators for the development of more than one spoken language include:

- early identification and hearing aid fitting;
- early, auditory-based intervention;
- early implantation, especially before the age of 2;
- excellent speech perception (range of 60–100% with a mean of 89%);
- absence of additional disabilities;
- intact first language;
- good family involvement and familial motivation for multilanguage learning;
- exposure to rich and complex language models in both languages; and
- opportunities to practice each language meaningfully (Cole & Flexor, 2007; Easterbrooks, O'Rourke, & Todd, 2000; Geers & Brenner, 2003; Kohnert & Derr, 2012; McKonkey-Robbins, 2007; Rhoades et al., 2008; Sharma et al., 2002; Svirsky et al., 2004; Waltzman et al., 2003; Wie Falkenberg, Tvete, & Tomblin, 2007; Wu & Brown, 2000).

Dynamic assessment procedures that result in immediate to no change in learning behavior may be a window into a child's memory abilities and may also contribute to the prognosis (Gutierrez-Clellen, 2012). Information gained during the assessment that considers bilingual issues along with prognostic indicators for each individual case should be shared with the family before determining the child's ability to make reasonable progress and respond to speech therapy services (ASHA Principles of Ethics I, Rule H; McKonkey-Robbins, 2007).

Concerns should be discussed with the family about factors that can change, and depending on the severity, the areas that may simply slow the rate of or prevent the child's progress. In severe cases where multiple disabilities are present, it will be up to the examining clinician to design the most appropriate treatment plan based on the child's language profile, giving careful consideration to the amount of resources and time that will be needed to help the child communicate (Rhoades et al., 2008). Once this information is considered, either intervention, a referral to a more appropriate professional, a period of trial therapy, or a combination of these options can be recommended.

CASE EXAMPLE

Case History: Joe, Chronological Age 3.5 Years

Joe's medical history was unremarkable. His developmental history was only remarkable for delays in speech and language development. Joe was identified at birth with a bilateral profound sensory-neural hearing loss. He received hearing aids at 7 months that he didn't use consistently. Joe received speech therapy, and auditory training services in Spanish through his state's early intervention program since his 8th month of life. Joe received a cochlear implant on his right ear at 13 months of life. He did not wear the cochlear implant or opposite hearing aid consistently until his 15th month of life when he started to attend speech therapy with a bilingual certified auditory-verbal therapist. At 18 months, Joe was enrolled at an auditory-oral preschool for children with hearing loss where he currently receives instruction in English for 35 hours a week and Spanish instruction with active parent involvement once time a week for 50 minutes. According to a home language survey, the primary language spoken at home is Spanish. The parents report that Joe uses and understands two-word combinations in Spanish. His teachers report that he speaks and understands two-word combinations in English. The parents report they do not speak English well and prefer to receive instruction in and speak in Spanish.

Impressions of Case History and Assessment Plan

According to the home language survey, the primary language use at home indicates a language other than the majority language of English. Joe also attends an auditory-oral preschool where he is exposed to English 35 hours a week. Using the home language log (see Appendix 13–B), it was determined that Joe hears Spanish 56 hours a week. According to an interview to determine language dominance, Joe did not demonstrate a stronger language; therefore, assessment was conducted in both languages using a bilingual speech-language pathologist fluent in the languages being tested. Simple sentence type assessments were chosen with analysis of language samples and dynamic assessment to determine his stimulability for expanded sentence lengths.

Joe: Administerd Assessment: Formal, Informal, Review of Existing Data

Audition:

  Hearing age, according to his consistent use of technology, is 24 months

  Sound field cochlear implant pure tone average (PTA) were 25 dB HL in both ears

  Speech Awareness Thresholds (SAT) were 20 dB HL in both ears, and

  Speech recognition using the NuChips in English was 72% in both ears

Technology: Listening check using the Ling Six-Sounds revealed detection of all sounds

Language:

  PLS-4 in Spanish revealed age equivalency of 2-6 months with standard scores of 82

  PLS-4 in English revealed age equivalency of 2-8 months with standard scores of 80

  Uses single words and 2-word combinations. Stimulable for 3-word combinations in both languages with teaching.

Vocabulary: McArthur-Bates (English): 123 words. McArthur-Bates (Spanish): 184 words. McArthur-Bates: 287 concepts and 20 Spanish/English cognates.

Speech: Intelligible with careful listening; Joe met the requirements for his age on the PLS-4 Spanish articulation screener

Intellectual: Not assessed, not a concern

Behavioral/Emotional: Very outgoing personality; no behavioral issues

Medical: Healthy, no other disabilities

Education: English Auditory-oral preschool, speech therapy weekly in Spanish interpreting assessment data:

Test results indicate that Joe presents with below-average language skills in both languages. Joe appears to demonstrate relatively equal development/abilities/deficiencies in Spanish and English. Analysis of his speech, vocabulary, and language test results, while considering points in the "Bilingual Issues" and "Bilingual Development" section, indicates typical bilingual development. Considering his hearing loss and intervention age, he is making good progress with his current intervention environment. Based on his suspected intellect, age of implantation, personality, dynamic assessment (ability to learn how to use three words in an utterance instead of two) and progress made thus far, he shows good prognosis for continued improvement. Taking into account his family language use, the language used at school, opportunities for practice in both languages, and the lack of a dominant language, the therapist considers recommending that the intervention team continue the same bilingual intervention with regular monitoring to ensure improvements are being made in both languages.

CONCLUSION

With the goal of providing a better understanding of basic procedures that must be used when conducting and interpreting evaluations, the guidelines and points described in this chapter are a starting point for consideration when performing assessments on children with hearing loss who are culturally and linguistically diverse (CLD). Professionals who understand the expected course of both monolingual and bilingual language acquisition as well as factors that contribute to the variability in children's language skills will be better prepared to analyze pertinent data crucial for facilitating each individual child's success (Douglas, 2011). In order to do this responsibly and competently when developing programs, conducting assessments, and designing effective intervention plans, professionals will need to integrate our continuously developing knowledge of hearing loss with our growing knowledge of bilingual acquisition and assessment issues.

RESOURCES

Douglas, M. (2014). *Facilitating dual-language learning for children with hearing loss: assessment, intervention and program development.* Innsbruck, Austria: MED-EL.

Goldstein, B. A. (2012). *Bilingual language development and disorders in Spanish–English speakers* (2nd ed.). Baltimore, MD: Brookes.

Gutierrez-Clellen, V. F., & Kreiter, J. (2003). Understanding bilingual acquisition using parent and teacher reports. *Applied Psycholinguistics, 24,* 267–288.

Haywood, C. H., & Lidz, C. S. (2007). *Dynamic assessment in practice: Clinical and educational applications.* New York, NY: Cambridge University Press.

Langdon, H. (2002). *Interpreters and translators in communication disorders: A practitioner's handbook.* Eau Claire, WI: Thinking Publications.

Linguistically diverse populations: Considerations and resources for assessment and intervention. Retrieved from http://www.txsha.org/Diversity_Issues/index.asp

The Minnesota Speech-Language Hearing Association. (2014). *Talk with Me Manual, Revised.* Retrieved from http://msha.net/displaycommon.cfm?an=1&subarticlenbr=86

Moog-Brooks, B. (2001). *My baby and me: A book about teaching your child to talk.* St. Louis, MO: Moog Center for Deaf Education.

Other bilingual assessment tools are available at http://www.asha.org and Academic Communication Associates at http://www.acadcom.com

REFERENCES

American Speech-Language-Hearing Association (ASHA). (2004). *Knowledge and skills needed by speech-language pathologists and audiologists to provide culturally and linguistically appropriate services* [Knowledge and skills]. Retrieved from http://www.asha.org/policy

American Speech-Language-Hearing Association (ASHA). (2010). *Code of ethics* [Ethics]. Available from http://www.asha.org/policy

American Speech-Language-Hearing Association (ASHA). (2014). *Self-assessment for cultural competence.* Retrieved from http://www.asha.org/practice/multicultural/self/

Anderson, R.T. (2012). First language loss and implications for clinical practice. In B. Goldstein (Ed.), *Bilingual language development and disorders in Spanish-English speakers* (2nd ed., pp.193–212). Baltimore, MD: Paul H. Brookes.

Austin, L., Glover, G., Aoyama, K., Stubbe Kester, E., Cárdenas, N., . . . Lopez, J. (2005). Linguistically diverse populations: Considerations and resources for assessment and intervention. Retrieved from http://www.txsha.org/Diversity_Issues/index.asp

Baker, C. (2006). *Foundations of bilingual education and bilingualism* (4th ed.). Bristol, UK: Multilingual Matters.

Bedore, L. M., Cooperson, S. J., & Boerger, K. M. (2012). Morphosyntactic development. In B. Goldstein (Ed.), *Bilingual language development and disorders in Spanish-English speakers* (2nd ed., pp. 175–192). Baltimore, MD: Paul H. Brookes.

Buhler, H. C., DeThomasis, B., Chute, P., & Decora, A. (2007). An analysis of phonological process use in young children with cochlear implants. *Volta Review, 107*, 55–74.

Bunta, F., & Douglas, M. (2013). The effects of dual language support on the English language skills of bilingual children with cochlear implants and hearing aids as compared to monolingual peers. *Language, Speech, and Hearing Services in Schools, 44*, 281–290.

Carrow-Woolfolk, E. (1995). *Oral and written language scales.* Circle Pines, MN: American Guidance Service.

Chin, B. C., & Lento Kaiser, M. S. (2002). Measurement of articulation in pediatric users of cochlear implants [Monograph]. *The Volta Review, 102*, 144–156.

Chute, P. M., & Nevins, M. E. (2002). *The parents' guide to cochlear implants.* Washington, DC: Gallaudet University Press.

Cole, E., & Flexor, C. (2007). *Children with hearing loss: Developing listening and talking–birth to six.* San Diego, CA: Plural.

Comeau, L., & Genesee, F. (2001). Bilingual children's repair strategies during dydadic communication. In J. Cenoz & F. Genessee (Eds.), *Trends in bilingual acquisition* (pp. 231–256). Amsterdam, the Netherlands: John Benjamins.

Department of Justice. (2014). *Policy guidance on the prohibition against national origin discrimination as it affects persons with limited English proficiency. Civil Rights Act of 1964, Title VI.* Retrieved from http://www.justice.gov/crt/about/edu/types.php

Deuchar, M., & Quay, S. (2000). *Bilingual acquisition: Theoretical implications of a case study.* Oxford, UK: Oxford University Press.

Dorman, D., Hickson, L., Murdoch, B., & Houston, T. (2007). Outcomes of an auditory-verbal program for children with hearing loss: A comparative study with a matched group of children with normal hearing. *Volta Review, 107*(1), 37–54.

Douglas, M. (2011). Spoken language assessment considerations for children with hearing impairment when the home language is not English. *Perspectives on childhood hearing and hearing disorders, 21*, 4–19.

Easterbrooks, S. R., O'Rourke, C. M., & Todd, N. W. (2000). Child and family factors associated with deaf children's success in auditory-verbal therapy. *The American Journal of Otology, 21*, 341–344.

Geers, A., & Brenner, C. (2003). Background and educational characteristics of prelingually deaf children implanted by five years of age. *Ear and Hearing, 24*(1), S2–S13.

Genesee, F. (2003). Bilingualism and language impairment. In R. Kent (Ed.), *MIT Encyclopedia of communication disorders*. Cambridge, Mass: MIT Press.

Genesee, F., & Nicoladis, E. (2005). *Bilingual first language acquisition.* Montreal, Québec, Canada: McGill University. Retrieved from http://www.psych.mcgill.ca/perpg/fac/genesee/HDBK%20BFLA%20FINAL.pdf

Gildersleeve-Neumann, C. E., Kester, E. S., Davis, B. L., & Pena, E. D. (2008). English speech sound development in preschool-aged children from bilingual English-Spanish environments. *Language, Speech, and Hearing Services in Schools, 39*, 314–328.

Goldstein, B. A. (2012). *Bilingual language development and disorders in Spanish-English speakers* (2nd ed.). Baltimore, MD: Paul H. Brookes.

Goldstein, B. A., & Gildersleeve-Neumann, C. (2012). Phonological development and disorders. In B. Goldstein (Ed.), *Bilingual language development and disorders in Spanish-English speakers* (2nd ed., pp. 285–310). Baltimore, MD: Paul H. Brookes.

Guiberson, M., Barrett, K. C., Janosek, E. G., & Yoshinag- Itano, C. (2006). Language maintenance and loss in preschool-age children of Mexican immigrants: Longitudinal study. *Communications Disorders Quarterly, 28*(1), 4–17.

Gutierrez-Clellen, V. F. (2012). Narrative development and disorders in bilingual children. In B. Goldstein (Ed.), *Bilingual language development and disorders in Spanish-English speakers* (2nd ed., pp. 233–250). Baltimore, MD: Paul H. Brookes.

Gutierrez-Clellen, V. F., & Kreiter, J. (2003). Understanding bilingual acquisition using parent and teacher reports. *Applied Psycholinguistics, 24*, 267–288.

Hammer, C. S., Miccio, A. W., & Rodriguez, B. L. (2012). Bilingual language acquisition and the child socialization process. In B. Goldstein (Ed.), *Bilingual language development and disorders in Spanish-English speakers* (2nd ed., pp. 31–46). Baltimore, MD: Paul H. Brookes.

Iglesias, A., & Rojas, R. (2012). Bilingual language development of English language learners: Modeling the growth of two languages. In B. Goldstein (Ed.), *Bilingual language development and disorders in Spanish-English speakers* (2nd ed., pp. 3–30). Baltimore, MD: Paul H. Brookes.

Individuals with Disabilities Education Act (IDEA). (2004). *Federal Register, 71* (156) Part V, Department of Education, 34 CFR part 300.

Jackson-Maldonado, D. (2012). Verbal morphology and vocabulary in monolinguals, emerging bilinguals, and monolingual children with primary language impairment. In B. Goldstein (Ed.), *Bilingual language development and disorders in Spanish-English speakers* (2nd ed., pp. 153–174). Baltimore, MD: Paul H. Brookes.

Kohnert, K. (2012). Processing skills in early sequential bilinguals. In B. Goldstein (Ed.), *Bilingual language development and disorders in Spanish-English speakers* (2nd ed., pp. 95–112). Baltimore, MD: Paul H. Brookes.

Kohnert, K., & Derr, A. (2012). Language intervention with bilingual children. In B. Goldstein (Ed.), *Bilingual language development and disorders in Spanish-English speakers* (2nd ed., pp. 337–356). Baltimore, MD: Paul H. Brookes.

Kühn-Inacker, H., Weichbold, V., Tsiakpini, L., Coninx, S., & D'Haese, P. (2003). *Little Ears: Auditory questionnaire.* Innsbruck, Austria: MED-EL.

Langdon, H. (2002). *Interpreters and translators in communication disorders: A practitioner's handbook.* Eau Claire, WI: Thinking Publications.

MacLver-Lux, K. (2005). Predicting auditory potential in auditory-verbal therapy: A partnership of audiologist, auditory-verbal therapist, and parent. *The Listener,* Summer (special edition), 49–60.

McClatchie, A., & Therres, M. (2003). *AuSpLan: Auditory speech and language. A manual for professionals working with children who have cochlear implants or amplification.* Oakland, CA: Children's Hospital and Research Center at Oakland.

McConkey-Robbins, A. (2007) Clinical management of bilingual families and children with cochlear implants. *Loud and Clear. Loud & Clear, 1,* 1–12. Retrieved from http://www.bionic ear.com

McConkey-Robbins, A., Green, J. E., & Waltzman, S. B. (2004). Bilingual oral language proficiency in children with cochlear implants. *Archives of Otolaryngology-Head & Neck Surgery, 130*(5), 644–647.

Moog, J. S., & Geers, A. E. (2010). Early educational placement and later language outcomes for children with cochlear implants. *Otology & Neurotology, 31,* 1315–1319.

Nicholas J. G., & Geers, A. E. (2008). Expected test scores for preschoolers with a cochlear implant who use spoken language. *American Journal of Speech-Language Pathology, 17,* 121–138.

Niparko, J. K. (2000) *Cochlear implants: Principles and practices.* Philadelphia, PA: Lippincott Williams & Williams.

Paradis, J., Nicoladis, E., & Genesee, F. (2000). Early emergence of structural constraints on code-mixing: Evidence from French-English bilingual children. *Bilingual Language and Cognition, 3,* 348–352.

Patterson, J. L., & Pearson, B. (2012). Bilingual lexical development, assessment and intervention. In B. Goldstein (Ed.), *Bilingual language development and disorders in Spanish-English speakers* (2nd ed., pp. 113–130). Baltimore, MD: Paul H. Brookes.

Pearson, B. Z. (2008). *Raising a bilingual child.* New York, NY: Random House.

Pena, E. D., Kester, E. S., & Sheng, L. (2012). Semantic development in Spanish-English bilinguals: Theory, assessment, and intervention. In B. Goldstein (Ed.), *Bilingual language development and disorders in Spanish-English speakers* (2nd ed., pp. 105–130). Baltimore, MD: Paul H. Brookes.

Restrepo, M. A., & Gutierrez-Clellen, V. F. (2012). Grammatical impairments in Spanish-English bilingual children. In B. Goldstein (Ed.), *Bilingual language development and disorders in Spanish-English speakers* (2nd ed., pp. 213–232). Baltimore, MD: Paul H. Brookes.

Rhoades, E. A. (2006). *Auditory-based therapy when the home language is not English (HOPE).* Retrieved November 30, 2006, from http://www.audiologyonline.com

Rhoades, E. A. (2008) Working with multicultural and multilingual families of young children. In C. Flexor & J. Madell (Eds.), *Pediatric audiology* (pp. 264–270). New York, NY: Thieme Medical.

Rhoades, E. A., & Chisolm, T. H. (2000). Global language progress with an auditory-verbal approach for children who are deaf or hard of hearing. *The Volta Review, 102*(1), 5–24.

Rhoades, E. A., Perusse, M., Douglas, W. M., & Zarate, C. M. (2008). Auditory based bilingual children in North America: Differences and choices. *Volta Voices, September/October Issue,* 20–22.

Roseberry-McKibbin, C. (2002). *Multicultural students with special language needs* (2nd ed.). Oceanside, CA: Academic Communication Associates.

Roseberry-McKibbin, C., & Brice, A. (2005). *Acquiring English as a second language: What's "normal," what's not.* Retrieved from http://www .asha.org/public/speech/development/easl/

Ryan, C. (2013). *Language use in the United States 2011: American community survey reports.* Retrieved from https://www.census.gov/ prod/2013pubs/acs-22.pdf

Sharma, A., Dorman, M. F., & Spahr, A. J. (2002). A sensitive period for the development of the central auditory system in children with cochlear implants: Implications for age at implantation. *Ear and Hearing, 23*(6), 532–539.

Shipley, K. G., & McAfee, J. G. (2009). *Assessment in speech-language pathology: A resource manual* (4th ed.). New York, NY: Delmar Cengage Learning.

Svirsky, M. A., Teoh, S. W., & Neuburger, H. (2004). Development of language and speech perception in congenitally, profoundly deaf children as a function of age at cochlear implantation. *Audiology & Neurotology, 9*(4), 224–233.

Teschendorf, M., Janeschik, S., Bagus, H., Lang, S., & Arweiler-Harbeck, D. (2011). Speech development after cochlear implantation in children from bilingual homes. *Otology & Neurotology, 32,* 229–235.

Thomas, E., El-Kashlan, H., & Zwolan, T. A. (2008). Children with cochlear implants who live in monolingual and bilingual homes. *Otology & Neurotology, 29,* 230–234.

U.S. Census Bureau. (2008). *An older and more diverse nation by midcentury.* Retrieved from https://www.census.gov/newsroom/re leases/archives/population/cb08-123.html

Waltzman, S. B., Robbins, A. M., Green, J., & Cohen, N. (2003). Second oral language capabilities in children with cochlear implants. *Otology & Neurotology, 24*(5), 757–763.

Wie, O., Falkenberg, E., Tvete, O., & Tomblin, B. (2007). Children with a cochlear implant: Characteristics and determinants of speech recognition, speech-recognition growth rate, and speech production. *International Journal of Audiology, 46*(5), 32–243.

Wu, C. D., & Brown, P. M. (2004). Parents' and teachers' expectations of auditory-verbal therapy. *The Volta Review, 99,* 107–119.

Yoshinaga-Itano, C. (May, 2008) Presentation to Widex International Pediatric Congress, Amsterdam, Netherlands.

Zimmerman, F. J., Gilkerson, J. R., Christakis, D. A., Xu, D., Gray, S. M., & Yapanel, U. (2009). Teaching by listening: The importance of adult-child conversations to language development. *Pediatrics, 124,* 342–349.

Home Language Survey

Where was your child born? Country _____ State _____

Which dialect of **English** does the child speak (ex. Southern, northern, Midwest)?

_____

Who is the primary caregiver of the child and what is her or his relationship to the child (e.g., mother, father, grandmother, etc.)? _____

Mother's native language _____ and native country _____

If the mother is **<u>NOT</u>** the primary caregiver, list the primary caregiver's native language _____ and native country _____

Father's native language _____ and native country _____

What was the child's date of arrival to the US? Estimate if precise date is not available. DATE: _____

What is the child's native language or languages? You can list more than one if the child learned more languages from birth.

_____

What languages does your child speak? Please list all of them.

_____

If your child speaks **Spanish,** which dialect of **Spanish** does the child speak? (Island, European, Mexican, etc.) _____

If the child speaks a **Spanish** dialect from **Mexico**, please list which region.

_____

If there is anything else that you feel is interesting or important about your child's language background or language use, please comment below.

_____

_____

_____

_____

_____

Home Language Log

Interview

1. How many hours is your child awake each day? _____

2. What languages does your child hear? _____

Tell us about your day

Daily Activity	Time (i.e., 8:30 am to 12:00 = 4 hrs)	Language Used	By Whom
Morning Routine	____ to ____ = ___ hrs		
Other	____ to ____ = ___ hrs		
School/Day Routine	____ to ____ = ___ hrs		
Other	____ to ____ = ___ hrs		
Afternoon Routine	____ to ____ = ___ hrs		
Other	____ to ____ = ___ hrs		
Weekends at home	____ to ____ = ___ hrs		

Total Exposure:

Language: _____ Total Daily Hours ____ Total Hours Awake (Total/Awake) ____%

Language: _____ Total Daily Hours ____ Total Hours Awake (Total/Awake) ____%

Language: _____ Total Daily Hours ____ Total Hours Awake (Total/Awake) ____%

continues

Language Dominance Questionnaire

Language Use at Home

1. Which language does your child seem to know better?

   _____ , _____ or both

2. Which language do you usually speak to your child?

   If another language other than _____ , in what language does your child respond?

   _____ , _____ or both

3. Which language does your child usually speak to you?

   _____ , _____ or both

4. Does your child mix languages together in the same word or sentence?

   Yes   No

5. Does your child have brothers or sisters who speak _____ ?

   If YES, what language does your child usually speak to his or her siblings?

   _____ , _____ or both

6. Does your child play and speak with other children?

   If YES, which language does your child use to speak to his or her friends when not in school?

   _____ , _____ or both

7. In which language are the television programs your child usually watches?

   _____ , _____ or both

Language Use at School

1. Which language does his or her teacher usually use in the classroom?

   _____ , _____ or both

2. Which language does he or she usually use to speak to his or her friends at school?

   _____ , _____ or both

3. Which language is read to him or her?

   _____ , _____ or both

4. In which language does he or she usually read?

   _____ , _____ or both

For Examiner:

Based on your familiarity with the child and your discussion with the family about the child's presence or absence of language dominance, classify the degree of bilingualism into one of four categories below. Then indicate the language that will be used for presenting instructions during test administration.

- Uses _____ A/B _____ exclusively at home and in school with minimal knowledge of _____ B/A _____

- Speaks mostly _____ A _____ but also knows some _____ B _____

- Speaks both _____ A _____ and _____ B _____ with equal ease

- Speaks mostly _____ B _____ but also knows some _____ A _____

CHAPTER 14

From Assessment to Intervention

K. Todd Houston, Tamala S. Bradham, and Andrea Bell

KEY POINTS

- Children with hearing loss are being identified as newborns and require appropriate fitting of hearing technology and enrollment in family-centered early intervention with well-trained and knowledgeable professionals.
- Intervention starts with comprehensive assessments that provide data about the child's current levels of performance; in turn, the professional can devise an intervention plan that leads to positive behavior change and skill development in the child and family.
- Increasingly, parents of young children with hearing loss are choosing listening and spoken language outcomes, and professionals must have the knowledge and skills to successfully facilitate these outcomes.
- Data-driven decisions ensures that professionals are delivering appropriate services that meet the developmental, communicative, and learning needs of the child as well as the parents and caregivers.

INTRODUCTION

For professionals working with children with hearing loss—or any population of children suspected of having delays in development or communication—the assessment results should frame the intervention process. Research continues to demonstrate that early identified children with hearing loss can experience positive speech, language, and social-emotional outcomes (Calderon & Naidu, 2000; Dornan et al., 2010; Moeller, 2000; Yoshinaga-Itano, 2003; Yoshinaga-Itano & Gravel, 2001). For these results to occur, professionals must rely on their own knowledge, the intervention approach—such as listening and spoken language—and their skills for planning, delivering, and evaluating the intervention. Furthermore, while the assessment of the child's developmental, communicative and other functional domains yields data on which to make decisions about the intervention plan, the professionals must also consider the desires and expected outcomes of the child's parents and family. Through the establishment of a strong professional-parent partnership, a family-centered early intervention plan can be formulated and implemented that meets the needs of the child as well as the family.

THE NEED FOR EARLY INTERVENTION

When children have the opportunity to master developmental processes such as language, cognition, and motor functions as close to the time that they are biologically wired to do so, the result is developmental synchrony (Robbins et al., 2004). Since the late 1950s, a "critical period" hypothesis (Penfield & Roberts, 1959) has been debated but remains generally accepted among most psycholinguists and cognitive scientists. Lenneberg (1967) further popularized the concept of critical periods when he theorized that language is an innate process and proposed that maturational (i.e., biological) constraints will limit the critical period when a child can learn language. Lenneberg described this critical period for language learning as a "window of opportunity."

For any infant or toddler who is acquiring language, the brain will organize itself based on the input that is received. Without adequate language stimulation during this window of opportunity, the child most likely will be language delayed. If this delay continues without adequate intervention, the child not only may experience a permanent language delay, but his or her language may also become disordered. For children with hearing loss, it is critical that the hearing loss is identified early, amplification fitted, and intervention begun—so that developmental synchrony can be maintained. Once the diagnosis is confirmed and amplification (i.e., digital hearing aids) is fitted, prompt implementation of appropriate family-centered early intervention services must occur.

If the child's parents have chosen a spoken language outcome, intensive and concentrated efforts must focus on building those auditory connections within the brain. Because these areas of the brain haven't been stimulated consistently prior to receiving amplification, the child's first responses may be minimal. However, through consistent exposure to auditory input and planned reinforcement of listening and spoken language, those neural connections will quickly form. The child will begin to respond. If the child has full access to the speech spectrum (i.e., low-, mid-, and high-frequency sounds), he or she will start to gain greater environmental awareness and begin to form speech sounds, combine those sounds through babbling, and produce first words. Through management of the hearing loss, with intense and consistent family-centered early intervention, and with high expectations for listening, most children with hearing loss can regain developmental synchrony and progress through these typical stages in the acquisition of spoken language. For children with severe and profound sensorineural hearing loss, cochlear implantation may be necessary, but parents should have the same expectations for developmental synchrony.

DEFINING THE INTERVENTION PROCESS

For children with hearing loss, the acquisition of listening and spoken language involves a range of perceptual, cognitive, and linguistic processes that are simultaneously independent and overlapping.

Children with hearing loss who are learning to listen, process, and use spoken language often experience success with both direct and indirect intervention that also include the active participation of their parents and/or caregivers. Through the intervention process, professionals model language facilitation activities and strategies and then coach the parents to integrate these targets into the child's daily routines. Over time, the parents, who are the child's first and best communication teachers, develop their skills and become more comfortable with language modeling and facilitation.

As Bray, Ross, and Todd (1999) affirm, intervention can be defined as the provision of a facilitative context in which the client (i.e., the child with hearing loss) and/or significant other(s) (i.e., the parents, caregivers, or family) can change in a positive direction. The change may be in understanding, the development or refinement of a skill, or the attainment of a new or different attitude. The context that the professional creates comes about through the interaction of knowledge, approaches (e.g., listening and spoken language), and skills (Bray, Ross, & Todd, 1999).

ASSESSMENT TO INTERVENTION OR TREATMENT PLAN

If done appropriately, the assessment should provide critical information about the child's skill acquisition across multiple developmental and communication domains, which leads the interventionist or clinician to a diagnosis, prognosis, and recommendations for intervention or treatment. Most importantly, the assessment will allow the opportunity for parent education about the typical course of

development and where their child falls within that framework (Capone, 2010). For the listening and spoken-language practitioner to be successful, he or she must have knowledge about typical development and the corresponding milestones in various domains of learning, such as language, listening, speech, cognition, and conversational competence. The formulation of an intervention plan will include goals that will address each of these learning domains.

Developing a Plan of Action

As Capone (2010) explains, the overarching goal of intervention is to facilitate development to age-expected or cognitively appropriate levels. Goals are the target behavior the clinician will facilitate in the intervention process. The target behaviors are those behaviors that the child must acquire next in development and/or the component skills necessary to reach a particular milestone (Capone, 2010). Thus, there are three types of goals that are developed: long-term, short-term, and session objectives. The following descriptions are adapted from Capone (2010).

- Long-term goals relate to the broadest areas of development or the end product of therapy or intervention (i.e., listening and spoken language, or auditory-verbal therapy). For example, a long-term goal could be, " . . . the child will demonstrate appropriate expressive language at home and in other social contexts." The judgment as to whether the child is experiencing success and moving toward the long-term goal does not generally include a percentage of accuracy measure, but rather tends to be measured within the functional context of daily living.

■ Short-term goals are the smaller steps taken to achieve the long-term goal. Short-term goals are meant to be accomplished within weeks to months of setting them. For example, the short-term goal may be, " . . . the child will produce present progressive verbs (e.g., is verbing) in two- or three-word phrases within play-based activities at least 80% of the time."

■ Goals set for a particular intervention or therapy session are known as session objectives. A session objective is the smallest step taken to achieve the short-term goal. A session objective may be " . . . the child will produce present progressive verbs (e.g., is verbing) when provided an immediate model and an auditory cue by the clinician in 80% of trials." In this example, the clinician uses scaffolding (a model and a cue) to provide the child the best opportunity to learn the target behavior. As the child gains increased mastery producing present progressive verbs, the clinician can reduce the scaffolding as the child's language use expands and he or she becomes a more independent communicator.

Developing Appropriate and SMART Goals

Developing appropriate goals for intervention are often described as SMART. The following descriptions are adapted from Wright and Wright (2011):

■ S = Specific
■ M = Measurable
■ A = Action Words
■ R = Realistic and relevant
■ T = Time-limited

SMART intervention and treatment plans have *specific* goals and objectives. Specific goals target areas of development and functional performance. They include clear descriptions of the knowledge and skills that will be taught and how the child's progress will be measured. For example, consider these two goals. Which one is more *specific*?

■ Johnnie will expand his expressive language.
■ Johnnie will use two-word (noun + verb, descriptor + noun) combinations during structured activities 80% of the time as judged by the clinician.

SMART intervention and treatment plans have *measurable* goals and objectives. Measurable means something can be counted or observed. Measurable goals allow parents and interventionists or clinicians to know how much progress the child has made since the performance was last measured. With measurable goals, the professional will know when the child reaches the goal.

For example, consider the following two goals. Which one is more *measurable*?

■ Johnnie will increase his vocabulary.
■ Johnnie will spontaneously use 20 new vocabulary words per week from the following preschool categories—body parts, household items, and transportation—in at least three different settings.

SMART goals in intervention or treatment plans should include three components that must be stated in measureable terms:

a. Direction of behavior (i.e., increase, decrease, maintain),
b. Area of need (i.e., receptive language, expressive language, listening, speech, conversational competence, cognition, etc.), and
c. Level of attainment (i.e., to age level, without assistance, in conversations, etc.).

These SMART goals should contain *action words* to ensure that the direction of behavior, area of need, and level of attainment are are specific and measurable. For example, consider the following two goals. Which one is *specific, measurable,* and includes *action words*?

■ Johnnie will increase his auditory memory.
■ Johnnie will increase his auditory memory by recalling three critical elements (noun+ noun + noun, action verb + descriptor + noun) during play-based activities in 9 out of 10 trials.

SMART intervention and treatment plans have *realistic* and *relevant* goals and objectives that address the child's unique needs that result from the hearing loss. SMART goals are based on the results of formal and informal assessment and observations. Which one is *specific, measurable,* and *realistic*?

■ Johnnie will improve his articulation.
■ Johnnie will produce the /s/ in the initial position of words at the conversational level with 80% accuracy as judged by the clinician.

SMART intervention and treatment plans are *time-limited*. What does the child need to know and be able to do after 3 months, 6 months or 1 year—depending on how the intervention or treatment plan is organized. What is the starting point for each of the child's needs (i.e., present developmental levels and functional performance)? Time-limited goals and objectives enable the professional to monitor progress at regular intervals. For the child with hearing loss who is learning to listen and use spoken language, ongoing tracking of skill development is essential. Many of these children are striving to achieve typical developmental milestones and functioning as compared to their hearing peers. Careful monitoring of their skill acquisition through direct observation, tracking, and parental reporting will ensure that the intervention or therapy has been appropriately tailored to meet the specific individualized developmental and communicative needs of the child.

Determining the Frequency and Duration of the Intervention

Once a comprehensive assessment has been completed and the child's present level of functioning has been determined, the frequency and duration of the intervention or treatment must be decided. Typically, for most infants and toddlers with hearing loss who are learning to listen and use spoken language, weekly therapy or intervention sessions, which can be in the home or at center with well-trained practitioners, are recommended.

The reason for weekly sessions is based on research by Hart and Risley (1995) where they found that typical developing children will hear on average between 616 to 2,153 words per hour depending on the social economic background. From these measures, Hart and Risley (1995) were able to demonstrate that the number of words heard at age 3 years predicted language skills at ages 9 to 10 years; the greater the word exposure, the higher their language scores on the Peabody Picture Vocabulary Test and the Test of Language Development-Intermediate (Hart & Risley, 1995). Now, imagine a child with hearing loss with a hearing age of 12 months (Figure 14–1). Not only has the child missed a year of listening opportunities, he or she

now has to close the language gap which can only be achieved through diagnostic therapy carefully monitoring the child's progress on a weekly basis. Other families may benefit from telepractice service delivery models (Houston, 2014). These sessions will focus on parent training and coaching while facilitating listening and spoken language in the child. If the child is older or late identified with hearing loss, the same scenario can be followed or the child could be placed a self-contained program or educational setting that will focus on listening and spoken language throughout the day. The younger the child starts the intervention process—as an infant or toddler—the more developmental the approach to intervention can

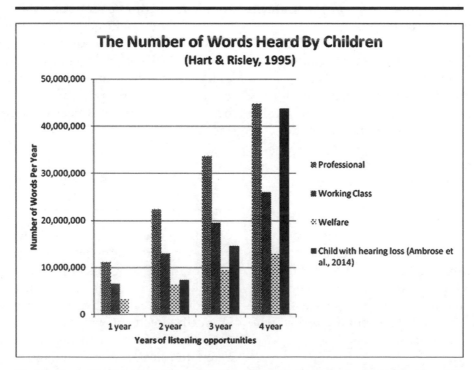

Figure 14–1. The number of words heard by children by income groups compared to children with hearing loss. Children with hearing loss can close the gap with intense coaching intervention. Data from *Meaningful Differences in the Everyday Experience of Young American Children*, by B. Hart and T. R. Risley, 1995, Baltimore, MD: Paul H. Brookes Publishing.

be; however, the older the child is when he or she starts to focus on listening and spoken language, the more likely the approach will involve remediation, and possibly, a highly structured educational environment.

Multiple factors that affect the child's learning and prognosis should be considered in order to determine the frequency and duration of listening and spoken language intervention or therapy. While not an exhaustive list, the following set of factors should be considered when determining whether the child needs weekly 1-hour sessions, more frequent therapy sessions, or placement in a structured educational program that has a concentration on listening and spoken language. Those factors may include:

- Degree of hearing loss;
- Age at identification of hearing loss;
- Age at enrollment in early intervention;
- Intensity of early intervention services that facilitate listening and spoken language with well-trained providers;
- Length of time using appropriate fit and maintained hearing technology;
- Child's learning style; and
- Level of parent engagement in listening and spoken language facilitation.

As the long-term goal for most children with hearing loss is to achieve spoken language outcomes that are comparable to their same-age hearing peers, the duration of their intervention or therapy should depend on the child's rate of progress. Those children who are identified as newborns with hearing loss, are fitted appropriate hearing technology, and receive well-coordinated early inter-

vention services with parent coaching may obtain developmental synchrony by the time they are preschoolers—if not sooner. Other children may require a longer period of intervention or treatment to achieve similar outcomes. Regardless of the service delivery model or educational placement implemented, parent engagement should be an ongoing expectation.

PARENT ENGAGEMENT IN INTERVENTION AND TREATMENT: INCREASING POSITIVE OUTCOMES

Almost without exception, parents want their children to have more successful lives than themselves. Whether it is academically, socially, or career-related, parents want what is best for their children. Determining what is "best" is a complicated process. Parents must use their own familial experiences, cultural perspectives, belief systems, and knowledge to make decisions that will affect the developmental, communicative, and academic success of their children.

Although early identification of hearing loss and use of hearing technology are critical first steps, obtaining auditory access does not automatically result in improved language abilities, especially spoken language. There is growing evidence that family-centered early intervention services that facilitate parent engagement in the child's intervention often result in improved language acquisition (DesJardin & Eisenberg, 2007; Moeller, 2000; Zaidman-Zait & Young, 2007). The important role that parents and caregivers—and by extension, families—have in the intervention of children with hearing loss—regardless of the child's degree of hearing loss or the type of technology employed (e.g., hearing aids, cochlear implants, or FM systems)—cannot be overemphasized.

When parents learn that their infant or toddler has hearing loss, communication may become even more strained. For more than forty years, concerns have been raised about parents speaking less to their child after a hearing loss is diagnosed (Gross, 1970). Furthermore, as Easterbrooks and Estes (2007) point out, parents may feel distanced from their infant with hearing loss when he or she is noncommunicative and may become frustrated with the intervention or habilitation process. Conversely, when parents actively participate in the child's habilitation, they assume the natural role of the child's first and primary language models. Learning proper strategies that facilitate language and communication allows parents to integrate goals for language expansion during regularly occurring routines throughout the day, or when the family is together. Receiving this level of support can replace feelings of frustration with observable progress in the child's communication development. For parents to achieve this level of engagement, however, early interventionists and other service providers must have the knowledge and skills to encourage, facilitate, and include parents in the child's habilitation.

Fleming, Sawyer, and Campbell (2011, p. 234) describe a model of parent participation as "providers directly teach[ing] caregivers how to embed learning strategies within a family's naturally occurring activities and routines by maximizing already existing learning opportunities or creating individualized learning opportunities, including using adaptations and assistive technology. In participation-based services, the provider takes on a role of caregiver educator by teaching and supporting the caregiver to interact with the child using strategies to promote learning."

Reluctance to Engage Parents

Despite research that supports parents' engagement and participation in providing intervention to their child, few professionals actually structure their intervention with the goal of involving the parents or other members of the family. Several studies demonstrate that early interventionists continue to spend a majority of their time delivering traditional child-centered services, and focus less on the involvement or participation of parents in the activities (Campbell & Sawyer, 2007; Peterson et al., 2007). Fleming, Sawyer, and Campbell (2007) review several internal barriers related to providers that may prevent greater parent participation, including limited confidence or experience working with families, lack of formal training, and varying beliefs about the importance of caregiver involvement. Therefore, parents should seek those professionals and related services, such as auditory-verbal therapy or auditory-verbal education, that support their participation in their child's learning.

Engaging Parents to Foster Success

Practitioners who are providing listening and spoken language intervention to young children with hearing loss and their families must learn to embrace parent participation as a key element of their service delivery. Unfortunately, practitioners may have less experience with this model of intervention, and failure to recognize the crucial role of parents could affect the child's potential for communication success. Child-centered approaches, which support only passive involvement by the parents, are no longer considered adequate. To increase the communicative success of the child, parents must become the primary consumers of the intervention. After parents are given opportunities to participate in the intervention sessions, they should practice the language-facilitating activities and strategies with their child under the observation and guidance of well-trained practitioners.

SUPPORTING AND FACILITATING LISTENING AND SPOKEN LANGUAGE OUTCOMES

For professionals, there is a range of knowledge and skills that support and facilitate positive listening and spoken language outcomes for children with hearing loss and their families. Regardless of the professional preparation, background or experience, practitioners serving this population should obtain the content knowledge and skills for listening and spoken language facilitation, implement family-centered early intervention that incorporates parent engagement and parent coaching as core elements, understand and apply the principles of auditory-verbal therapy and/or auditory-verbal education, and possess the experience and skills to carefully plan, evaluate, and deliver their intervention or therapy sessions.

Professional Knowledge for Listening and Spoken Language Facilitation

The Alexander Graham Bell Academy for Listening and Spoken Language (AGBA) has a well established international certifi-

cation program for Listening and Spoken Language Specialists (LSLS) as Certified Auditory-Verbal Educators (Cert. AVEd) and Certified Auditory-Verbal Therapists (Cert. AVTs). These professionals may be teachers of the deaf and hard of hearing, speech-language pathologists, audiologists, or others from related disciplines who complete this comprehensive certification process. (For more information about the LSLS certification process, please visit the AGBA at http://www.listeningandspokenlanguage.org/AGBellAcademy/)

For the listening and spoken language specialists (LSLS), the AGBA has defined the knowledge that the practitioner should process prior to certification. These domains of knowledge span a range of disciplines, including—but not limited to—medicine, psychology, social sciences, linguistics, audiology, speech-language pathology, early intervention, early childhood education, and education of the deaf and hard of hearing. More specifically, the practicing LSLS must integrate these knowledge domains into his or her intervention when working with children with hearing loss and their families:

- Hearing and hearing technology (i.e., digital hearing aids, cochlear implants, and assistive listening devices);
- Auditory functioning;
- Spoken language communication;
- Child development;
- Parent guidance, education, and support;
- Strategies for listening and spoken language development;
- Education (i.e., supporting the child with hearing loss in the general education curriculum); and
- Emergent literacy.

The knowledge domains on which the certification is based continues to evolve and be refined as new research, public policy, and clinical outcomes shape the practice of LSLS professionals and their delivery of services.

Family–Centered Early Intervention

Children with special needs and their families need access to appropriate family-centered early intervention services that are delivered by professionals who are well-trained and experienced in the use of current evidence-based practices. Unfortunately, a lack of qualified practitioners, especially in remote and rural communities, in addition to limited funding, can affect the quality of services that some children receive. The program outlined in Part C of the Individuals with Disabilities Education Act (IDEA) of 1997 (PL 105-17) requires the implementation of family-centered intervention in a natural learning environment (Rush & Shelden, 2011). Family-centered early intervention is a service delivery model that is critical for infants and toddlers who have developmental and communication delays, especially those with hearing loss. For children and their families who qualify under this legislation, early intervention services are designed to enhance the quality of their lives by facilitating the parent's capacity to promote the development of skills in their infants and toddlers (Cason, 2011). That is, during family-centered intervention, the professional focuses on enhancing the parent's ability, through coaching, to promote the growth and development of their infant or toddler during every day learning opportunities (Campbell & Sawyer, 2007; McWilliams, 2010; Rush & Shelden, 2011; Spagnola & Fiese, 2007; Trivette,

Dunst, & Hamby, 2004). When parents follow their children's lead by supporting their interests and participation, there is a positive effect on the child's development and learning (Dunst, Bruder, Trivette, & Hamby, 2006). Families are viewed as having existing capabilities, the ability to make informed decisions, the power to act on their decisions to strengthen family competence and improve family functioning, and the capacity to become increasingly competent (Trivette, Dunst, & Hamby, 1996).

The Listening and Spoken Language Approach: Lessons Learned from Auditory–Verbal Therapy and Auditory–Verbal Education

Ninety-two percent of parents of children with hearing loss have typical hearing themselves (Mitchell & Karchmer, 2004) and trends indicate that many parents are choosing spoken language as the primary mode of communication for their children 90% of the time (Brown, 2006; Cole & Flexer, 2011), especially when they know spoken language is a viable outcome for their child. And these parents typically select listening and spoken language approaches without initiating visual communication systems. These parents, therefore, often choose auditory-verbal therapy or auditory-verbal education as the approach used to facilitate listening and spoken language in their child with hearing loss.

Auditory-verbal practice is defined as the application and management of hearing technology, in conjunction with specific strategies, techniques, and conditions, which promote optimal acquisition of spoken language primarily through listening for children who are deaf and hard of hearing. The children learn to listen to the sounds of their own voices, the voices of others, and all sounds of life (Esta-brooks, 2006). Listening and spoken language become a major force in nurturing the development of the child's personal, social, and academic life. When auditory-verbal practice is carried out with the necessary thoughtfulness, expertise, guidance and love, most of our children develop excellent conversational competence (Esta-brooks, 2006).

The principles of LSLS auditory-verbal practice are well established (AGBA, 2007) and have been defined for the both the certified auditory-verbal therapist (Cert. AVT) and the certified auditory-verbal educator (Cert. AVEd). The following describes auditory-verbal practice (adapted from Estabrooks, Houston, & MacIver-Lux, 2014).

- Auditory-verbal practice promotes:
  - Early detection and diagnosis of hearing loss in the child, ideally as a newborn;
  - Consistent use (i.e., wearing during all waking hours) of two hearing aids and/or cochlear implants, and other assistive listening devices for the maximum detection of all sounds and the understanding of speech; and
  - Individualized therapy/ education and learning environments where listening and spoken language are the expected modes of communication.
- Auditory-verbal practice helps parents:
  - To develop skills that will enable their child to learn through listening and communicate through spoken language;

- To become the primary models for listening, speech, and language development; and
- To understand the impact of deafness on the entire family.
- Auditory-verbal practice encourages:
  - The child to realize his or her auditory potential by maximizing the use of bilateral hearing technology;
  - Involvement of parents through observations, discussions, counselling and active participation in all therapy sessions and educational environments; and
  - Aggressive audiological management of hearing loss, use of hearing technology, and technical support.
- Auditory-verbal practice celebrates:
  - The whole child through the development of skills in hearing, listening, speech, language; cognition and communication;
  - The inclusion of children who are deaf or hard hearing in regular education environments with support services; and
  - Full family engagement at every stage of the child's development.

Practitioner Skills That Support Successful Intervention

In addition to mastering the auditory-verbal techniques and strategies (Esta-brooks, 2006, 2012; Pollack, Goldberg, & Caleffe-Schenck, 1997) that facilitate listening and spoken language, professionals must maintain the skills to carefully plan, evaluate, and deliver their intervention sessions. The following skills, while not exhaustive, are adapted from Bray, Ross, and Todd (1999).

- Skills involved with planning intervention or therapy include:
  - Writing goals and objectives for intervention plan, including session goals that target the child, parents/caregivers, and family;
  - Planning appropriate activities that include materials, explanations, procedures, and the type of cues, feedback, and rewards;
  - Planning modifications that may be necessary to the tasks depending on the response from the child, parent, or family member;
  - Planning how a skill in listening, speech, or language will generalize;
  - Planning a balanced and motivating—to both the child and parent or caregiver;
  - Identifying opportunities and making arrangements for involving, advising, and collaborating with other professionals who are serving the child and family;
  - Planning appropriate ways in which the child and parent or caregiver can be involved in all aspects of intervention (e.g., negotiating goals and objectives, joint planning of activities, tasks, and rewards); and
  - Planning how to formally and informally evaluate the intervention plan and the outcomes of each session.
- Skills involved with the delivery of intervention include:
  - Establishing and maintaining a positive relationship with the child and strong rapport with the parents, caregivers, and family;
  - Valuing and showing appreciation for the knowledge, experience, and contributions of the child and parents, caregivers, and family;
  - Using active listening skills;
  - Using appropriate counseling skills and techniques;
  - Using effective explanation skills with the child and parents, caregivers, and family;
  - Applying specific auditory-verbal techniques and strategies that facilitate listening and spoken language;
  - Observing the child's and the parent's response to a task and making immediate alterations to the level of difficulty;
  - Giving feedback and/or rewards to the child and parent during the session;
  - Adding or removing cues as necessary during a specific activity or within a session;
  - Giving feedback at the end of an activity or session to both the child and the parents;
  - Answering questions in a professional and coherent manner;
  - Using and/or troubleshooting equipment, hearing technology, and other materials (e.g., assessment protocols and instruments, therapy protocols, toys, other items);
  - Organizing materials during the session;
  - Recording child and parent or family outcomes during the session;
  - Structuring and appropriately pacing the session; and

- Adapting communication style, interactions and activities within the session based on the child's and parents' learning needs.
- Skills involved in the evaluation of intervention include:
  - Self-reflection;
  - Eliciting and using appropriate feedback from relevant sources (e.g., the child, parents, caregivers, and family);
  - Using and evaluating formal and informal outcome measures;
  - Revising hypotheses (i.e., prognoses, long-term goals, and outcomes); and
  - Revising the intervention or therapy plan.

DATA-DRIVEN DECISION MAKING

Early interventionists and speech-language pathologists are constantly making decisions and providing recommendations for further intervention or treatment. These decisions must be made using data collected from the early intervention or treatment sessions, which provide insight into how the child is functioning on a defined set of tasks or activities that support the session objectives. Each session provides the professional with ample opportunities to gather critical information (i.e., data). As Groark (2011) explains, a five-step process is suggested to guide providers in making **data-driven decisions**, which includes gathering information, documenting, summarizing, analyzing, and interpreting data.

While formal assessments are used to measure the child's current level of performance when services are initiated as well as at specific intervals (i.e., every

6 months, annually, etc.), professionals should view each intervention or treatment session as being diagnostic in nature.

The professional should keenly observe how the child is performing on each activity within every session. Likewise, the professional also should monitor how the parents or caregivers are progressing in their skills at facilitating listening and spoken language.

When planning intervention for the child, the professional should ensure that the activities that occur in the session are designed to target knowledge and skills just above where the child is currently functioning. Building on the work of Vygotsky (1962), the clinician should focus intervention within a zone of proximal development for the child, which is defined as the distance between the child's actual developmental level and the level of his or her potential development (Kaufman, 2004).

Through consistent and careful data collection, the clinician can track the child's listening and spoken language acquisition. By observing the child's behavior during each session and documenting progress on session objectives, the clinician will be able to summarize the child's performance and offer a regular analysis of his or her progress. The goal is to close the gap between the child's current developmental level and the potential level of functioning. Over time, with appropriate intervention, use of hearing technology, and parental engagement, most children with hearing loss will be successful at closing that developmental gap and achieve spoken language outcomes that rival their hearing peers.

For some children, however, their progress may be slowed or they may fail to reach the goals established in the intervention plan. For those children, a careful review of the factors that may be impacting the child's progress would be warranted. For example, has the child's hearing loss worsened? Is the hearing technology functioning correctly and well maintained? Are the parents or caregivers engaged in the child's intervention or therapy? Some of these factors can be easily managed while others may require collaboration with other service providers. Regardless of the reasons, if a child is failing to make adequate progress, the practitioner must ascertain why this is occurring. Because the sessions are diagnostic in nature and the practitioners are constantly gathering data, professionals may be able to modify the intervention or treatment plan to better meet the learning needs of the child. These changes should occur in a timely manner—within one or two therapy sessions—rather than allowing the child to struggle without making appropriate progress.

As Estabrooks (2006) describes, auditory-verbal sessions are diagnostic in design and execution and used to evaluate the progress of the child and the parents. Because each child and family is unique, professionals must manage—or at least understand—a host of variables that may impact the child's progress. Those variables include (adapted from Estabrooks, 2006):

- Age at diagnosis of hearing loss;
- Cause of hearing loss;
- Degree of hearing loss;
- Effectiveness of the hearing technology (hearing aids, cochlear implants, assistive listening devices);
- Effectiveness of the child's audiology;
- Child's accessibility to hearing all the sounds of spoken language;

- Health of the child;
- Emotional state of the family;
- Quality of family engagement;
- Skills of the practitioner;
- Skills of the parents or caregiver;
- Child's learning style;
- Parent's learning style; and the
- Child's intelligence.

While this appears to be a daunting task, professionals can successfully manage these variables and/or understand how they impact the child's progress. This may require more flexibility in the planning of and delivery of services to the child or family, the need for additional training, skill development, and mentoring, and additional coordination and collaboration with other disciplines or services. With a commitment to data-driven intervention and therapy, professionals can ensure that each child and family receives appropriate services that meet their ongoing learning and communication needs.

CONCLUSION

Professionals delivering listening and spoken language intervention or therapy to children with hearing loss and their families must tie those services to comprehensive assessment. Although baseline assessments are completed when services are initiated and periodically thereafter, the professional's mindset should view each session as diagnostic in nature—an opportunity to observe the child's performance and collect data on the child's and family's progress. With a steadfast commitment to meeting the child's learning needs when he or she has the potential to master the content, professionals can ensure that each intervention session is designed to meet the child's skill acquisition in listening, speech, language, cognition, and conversational competence. Similarly, the practitioner should closely monitor the parents' or caregivers' ability to facilitate language and communication and feel comfortable providing the necessary modeling and coaching to finely tune parent-child interactions to maximize learning. When assessment facilitates data-driven decision making, more ethical, evidence-based and appropriate services can be rendered. For the children and families that we serve, they deserve nothing less.

REFERENCES

A.G. Bell Academy for Listening and Spoken Language (AGBA). (2007). *Principles of LSLS auditory-verbal therapy.* Retrieved from http://www.listeningandspokenlanguage.org/uploadedFiles/Get_Certified/Getting_Certified/Principles%20of%20LSLS%20Cert.%20AVT%281%29.pdf

Ambrose, S. E., VanDam, M., & Moeller, M. P. (2014). Linguistice input, electronic media, and communication outcomes of toddlers with hearing loss. *Ear and Hearing, 35*(2), 139–147.

Bray, M., Ross, A., & Todd, C. (1999). *Speech and language: Clinical process and practice.* London, UK: Whurr.

Brown, C. (2006). *Early intervention: Strategies for public and private sector collaboration.* Paper presented at the 2006 Convention of the Alexander Graham Bell Association for the Deaf and Hard of Hearing, Pittsburgh, PA.

Calderon, R., & Naidu, S. (2000). Further support for the benefits of early identification and intervention for children with hearing loss. *The Volta Review, 100*(5), 53–84.

Campbell, P. H., & Sawyer, L. B. (2007). Supporting learning opportunities in natural settings through participation-based services. *Journal of Early Intervention, 29,* 287–305.

Capone, N. C. (2010). Language assessment and intervention: A developmental approach. In B. Shulman & N. C. Capone (Eds.), *Language development: Foundations, processes, and clinical applications.* Sudbury, MA: Jones & Bartlett.

Cason, J. (2011). Telerehabilitation: An adjunct service delivery model for early intervention services. *International Journal of Telerehabilitation, 3*(1), 19–28.

Cole, E., & Flexer, C. (2011). *Children with hearing loss: Developing listening and talking—birth to six* (2nd ed.). San Diego, CA: Plural.

DesJardin, J. L., & Eisenberg, L. S. (2007). Maternal contributions: Supporting language development in young children with cochlear implants. *Ear and Hearing, 28*(4), 456–469.

Dornan, D., Hickson, L., Murdoch, B., Houston, K. T., & Constantinescu, G. (2010). Is auditory-verbal therapy effective for children with hearing loss. *The Volta Review, 110*(3), 361–387.

Dunst, C. J., Bruder, M. B., Trivette, C. M., & Hamby, D. W. (2006). Everyday activity settings: Natural learning environments, and early intervention practices. *Journal of Policy and Practice in Intellectual Disabilities, 3,* 3–10.

Easterbrooks, S. R., & Estes, E. L. (2007). *Helping deaf and hard of hearing students to use spoken language.* Thousand Oaks, CA: Corwin Press.

Estabrooks, W. (Ed.). (2006). *Auditory-verbal therapy and practice.* Washington, DC: Alexander Graham Bell Association for the Deaf and Hard of Hearing.

Estabrooks, W. (Ed.). (2012). *101 frequently asked questions about auditory-verbal practice.* Washington, DC: Alexander Graham Bell Association for the Deaf and Hard of Hearing.

Estabrooks, W., Houston, K. T., & MacIver-Lux, K. (2014). Therapeutic approaches following cochlear implantation. In S. B. Waltzman & J. T. Roland (Eds.), *Cochlear implants* (3rd ed.). New York, NY: Thieme Medical.

Fleming, J. L., Sawyer, B. L., & Campbell, P. H. (2011). Early intervention providers' perspectives about implementing participation-based practices. *Topics in Early Childhood Special Education, 30*(4), 233–244.

Groark, C. (Ed.). (2011). *Early childhood intervention: Shaping the future for children with special needs and their families.* Santa Barbara, CA: Praeger.

Gross, R. (1970). Language used by mothers of deaf children and mothers of hearing children. *American Annals of the Deaf, 115,* 93–96.

Hart, B., & Risley, T. R. (1995). *Meaningful Differences in the everyday experience of young American children.* Baltimore, MD: Paul H. Brookes.

Kaufman, D. (2004). Constructivist issues in language learning and teaching. *Annual Review of Applied Linguistics, 24,* 303–319.

Lenneberg, E. H. (1967). *Biological foundations of language.* New York, NY: John Wiley & Sons.

McWilliam, R. A. (2010). *Working with families of young children with special needs.* New York, NY: Guilford Press.

Mitchell, R. E., & Karchmer, M. A. (2004). Chasing the mythical ten percent: Parental hearing status of deaf and hard of hearing students in the United States. *Sign Language Studies, 4,* 138–163.

Moeller, M. P. (2000). Early intervention and language development in children who are deaf and hard of hearing. *Pediatrics, 106,* E43.

Penfield, W., & Roberts, L. (1959). *Speech and brain mechanisms.* Princeton, NJ: Princeton University Press.

Peterson, C. A., Luze, G. J., Eshbaugh, E. M., Jeon, H. J., & Kantz, K. R. (2007). Enhancing parent-child interactions through home visiting: Promising practice or unfulfilled promise. *Journal of Early Intervention, 29,* 119–140.

Pollack, D., Goldberg, D., & Caleffe-Schenck, N. (1997). *Educational audiology for the limited-hearing infant and preschooler: An auditory-verbal program* (3rd ed.). Springfield, IL: Charles C. Thomas.

Robbins, A. M., Koch, D. B., Osberger, M. J., Zimmerman-Philips, S., & Kishon-Rabin, L. (2004). Effect of age at cochlear implantation on auditory skill development in infants and toddlers. *Archives of Otolaryngology-Head & Neck Surgery, 130*(5), 570–574.

Rush, D., & Shelden, M. (2011). *The early childhood coaching handbook.* Baltimore, MD: Brookes.

Spagnola, M., & Fiese, B. H. (2007). Family routines and rituals: A context for development in the lives of young children. *Infants and Young Children, 20*(4), 284–299.

Trivette, C. M., Dunst, C. J., & Hamby, D. (1996). Characteristics and consequences of helpgiving practices in contrasting human services programs. *American Journal of Community Psychology, 24*(2), 273–293.

Vygotsky, L. (1962). *Thought and language.* Cambridge, MA: MIT Press.

Wright, P., & Wright, P. (2011). *Wrightslaw: From emotions to advocacy—The special education survival guide* (2nd ed.). Hartfield, VA: Harbor House Law Press.

Yoshinaga-Itano, C. (2003). From screening to early identification and intervention: Discovering predictors to successful outcomes for children with significant hearing loss. *Journal of Deaf Studies and Deaf Education, 8*(2), 11–30.

Yoshinaga-Itano, C., & Gravel, J. S. (2001). The evidence for universal hearing screening. *American Journal of Audiology, 10*(2), 62–63.

Zaidman-Zait, A., & Young, R. A. (2007). Parental involvement in the habilitation process following children's cochlear implantation: An action theory perspective. *Journal of Deaf Studies and Deaf Education, 13*(2), 195–214.

APPENDIX A

OPTION*Schools:* Assessment Reference Guide (2014)

Vocabulary

Table A–1. Battelle Developmental Inventory, 2nd Edition (BDI-2)

Author	Jean Newbord
Publisher	Riverside Publishing
Contact Information	Riverside Publishing 3800 Golf Road, Suite 100 Rolling Meadows, IL 60008 Phone: 800.323.9540 630.467.7000 (outside US) Fax: 630.467.7192 RPC_Customer_Service@hmhpub.com
Cost	$1,232.70 for complete kit *(Price current as of April 2014)*
Purpose	Screening, diagnosis, and evaluation of early development.
Age Range	Birth to 7–11
Time	60 to 90 minutes—Full Assessment 10 to 30 minutes—Screening Test
Scores or Subtests	Self-Care, Personal Responsibility, Adaptive Total, Adult Interaction, Peer Interaction, Self-Concept and Social Role, Personal-Social Total, Receptive Communication, Expressive Communication, Communication Total, Gross Motor, Fine Motor, Perceptual Motor, Motor Total, Attention and Memory, Reasoning and Academic Skills, Perception and Concepts, Cognitive Total, Total.
Description	This test is designed to measure developmental strengths of children with and without disabilities, to screen children considered to be at risk for developmental delays, to assist with the development of individualized family service plans and individualized education plans, and to monitor short- and long-term progress.
Reliability	Internal consistency estimates are acceptable for each age level and subdomain, although certain subdomains at certain ages are problematic. For example, indices for the Attention and Memory subdomain drop below 0.8 after age 3½. Total test scores and screening test scores are adequately reliable. Test-retest reliability estimates are based on a sample of 252 children at 2 and 4 years of age over a 2- to 25-day retest interval. Problems are noted with stability for the Attention and Memory subdomain, as well as the Communication and Cognitive domains. Interscorer agreement was calculated only on 17 items that require examiners' interpretation, such as the Fine Motor and Perceptual Motor items in the student workbook, and these items appear to be reliable.
Validity	Evidence for content validity consists of judgments of professionals regarding coverage of important constructs, as well as empirical item analysis procedures including item-total correlations, age trends, and model-data-fit statistics. Items deemed unsatisfactory based on these procedures were deleted. Criterion-related evidence for validity was investigated by correlating BDI-2 scores with those of other measures of development, as well as measures of other constructs (e.g., phonological processing, intelligence, and academic achievement). Patterns of correlations generally support the BDI-2 constructs, but some of the samples were relatively small. Construct validity evidence is provided in the forms of factor analyses, age differentiation, and patterns of intercorrelations. These indices support the BDI-2 as a measure of development.

Table A–1. *continued*

Norms	The BDI-2 was standardized on a sample of 2,500 children in more than 30 states. The sample was stratified on the bases of age, sex, race/ethnicity, geographic region, and socioeconomic level. The sample very closely matches 2001 U.S. Census data, but children with disabilities were not included. Because the instrument is designed in part to measure the developmental skills of children with disabilities, such children should have been included in the norm sample at a rate reflective of national demographics.
Who Can Give the Test?	This test should be administered by a professional trained in standardized assessment of children, including but not limited to speech-language pathologists and teachers.
Strengths	Flexibility in administration procedures; Items' correspondence with early childhood curricula.
Concerns	Additional criterion-related evidence for validity is needed.

Table A–2. Bayley Scales of Infant and Toddler Development, 3rd Edition

Author	Nancy Bayley
Publisher	PsychCorp/Pearson
Contact Information	Pearson Attn: Inbound Sales & Customer Support 19500 Bulverde Road San Antonio, TX 78259-3701 Phone: 800.627.7271 Fax: 800.232.1223 ClinicalCustomerSupport@Pearson.com
Cost	$1,125 for complete kit *(Price current as of April 2014)*
Purpose	Designed to assess the developmental functioning of infants and young children.
Age Range	Ages 1 to 42 months
Time	30 to 90 minutes
Scores or Subtests	Cognitive, Language (Receptive Communication, Expressive Communication, Total), Motor (Fine Motor, Gross Motor, Total), Social-Emotional, Adaptive Behavior (Communication, Community Use, Functional Pre-Academics, Home Living, Health and Safety, Leisure, Self-Care, Self-Direction, Social, Motor, Total).
Description	The Bayley-III assesses young children's developmental functioning across five domains: Cognitive, Language (Receptive and Expressive), Motor (Fine and Gross), Social-Emotional, and Adaptive (Conceptual, Social, and Practical) Behavior. Its stated purposes are to identify children with developmental delay(s) and to provide data for intervention planning.
Reliability	The overall reliability coefficients, as calculated with Fisher's z transformation, ranged from .86 (Fine Motor) to .91 (Cognitive, Expressive Communication, and Gross Motor). The reliabilities of the Social-Emotional and Adaptive Behavior Scales were similarly strong (.83 to .94; .79 to .98, respectively). Taken together, these results suggest strong internal consistency for the measurement of functioning within these five domains. Test–retest reliability results indicate a strong consistency in responding over time (with a mean retest interval of 6 days). Discrepancies, when they occurred, were attributed to maturation and/or practice effects.
Validity	The Bayley-III manual provides comprehensive validity information including detailed descriptions of the content, concurrent, and construct validity of the instrument. The content validity information includes descriptions of the comprehensive literature searches and expert reviews conducted to ensure appropriate test items and test construction. The concurrent validity of the Bayley-III was established by examining the scale's relation to other instruments including the Bayley Scales of Infant Development, 2nd Edition (BSID-II), the Wechsler Preschool and Primary Scale of Intelligence, 3rd Edition (WPPSI-III), the Preschool Language Scale, 4th Edition (PLS-4), the Peabody Developmental Motor Scales, 2nd Edition (PDMS-2), and the Adaptive Behavioral Assessment System-Second Edition, Parent/Primary Caregiver Form (ABAS-II-P). In addition to these studies comparing Bayley-III scores with scores from these tests, further evidence to support the validity of the Bayley-III as a comprehensive diagnostic assessment tool was provided through several special group studies. The special groups in the studies included children with Down syndrome, pervasive developmental disorders, cerebral palsy, language impairment, and others.

Table A–2. *continued*

Norms	The normative sample for the Cognitive, Language, and Motor Scales of the Bayley-III consists of 1,700 children between the ages of 16 days and 43 months 15 days. The normative sample was stratified by race/ethnicity, age, sex, parent educational level, and geographic location. The norms for the Social-Emotional Scale were obtained from 456 children (.5 months to 42 months) who were included in the normative sample of the Greenspan Social-Emotional Growth Chart (Greenspan, 2004); similarly, the norms for the Adaptive Behavior Scale were obtained from 1,350 children (birth to 5 years 11 months) in the ABAS-II normative sample.
Who Can Give the Test?	This test should be administered by someone skilled in standardized assessment of children, including but not limited to speech-language pathologists and teachers.
Strengths	Easy to administer, well-designed.
Concerns	Large test kit; difficult to travel with.

Reference

Greenspan, S. I. (2004). *Greenspan Social-Emotional Growth Chart.* San Antonio, TX: PsychCorp, Pearson Education.

Table A–3. Developmental Assessment of Young Children (DAYC)

Author	Judith K. Voress and Taddy Maddox
Publisher	Pro-Ed, Inc.
Contact Information	Pro-Ed, Inc. 8700 Shoal Creek Boulevard Austin, Texas 78757-6897 Customer Service: Phone: 800.897.3202 Fax: 800.397.7633 Publishing Team: Phone: 800.897.3202 Fax: 800.397.7633 info@proedinc.com
Cost	$345.00 *(Price current as of April 2014)*
Purpose	Measures different developmental abilities in young children; used to identify children with developmental deficits at a young age in order to facilitate early intervention.
Age Range	Birth to 5;11
Time	10 to 20 minutes for each domain
Scores or Subtests	Subtests: Cognitive, Communication, Social-Emotional, Physical Development, Adaptive Behavior. Scores: standard scores, percentile ranks, and age equivalents for each subtest; General Development Quotient (GDC).
Description	The DAYC is designed to assess cognitive skills, communication skills, social-emotional skills, physical development, and adaptive behavior. The examiner completes each subtest by observing the child, interviewing the parents or caregivers, or testing the child.
Reliability	Coefficient alphas for the DAYC subtests across age range intervals range from .91 to .97; coefficient alphas for the DAYC subtests for seven subgroups (European American, African American, Hispanic, Males, Females, At-Risk, and Disabled) range from .98 to .99; test–retest reliability for the DAYC in two studies was Cognitive: .85–.93, Communication: .86–.92, Social-Emotional: .89–/95, Physical Development: .89–.95, Adaptive Behavior: .85–.95, and Composite: .86–.94.
Validity	Criterion-referenced validity, construct-validity, and content-description validity were evaluated. The group with identified disabilities scored approximately two standard deviations lower than the typically-developing group on each DAYC subtest; results of the t-tests indicate that these differences are large enough to be statistically significant.
Norms	1,269 children representative of the nation as a whole including 7 % who were determined to be "at risk" for a disability or having a disability; most frequently cited disabilities were learning disabilities, speech-language delays, and mental retardation.
Who Can Give the Test?	Those who have training in administering early childhood assessments; prior to administering the DAYC, examiners should consult local school policies and state regulations, especially in the case where the purpose is to diagnose disabling conditions or to qualify children for special programs.
Strengths	Fairly easy to administer and score; examines different areas of development and separates each into a subtest so one can examine each area separately.
Concerns	The Cognitive subtest includes many verbal items so it is not appropriate for very young deaf children who have limited verbal skills; GDQ may be deflated because the Cognitive score may be an underestimate of the child's learning potential.

Table A–4. Developmental Programming for Infants and Young Children

Author	Sally J. Rogers., Carol M. Donovan, Diane D'Eugenio, Sara L. Brown, Eleanor Lynch, Martha S. Moersch, and D. Sue Schafer
Publisher	University of Michigan Press
Contact Information	University of Michigan Press c/o Perseus Distribution 1094 Flex Dr. Jackson, TN 38301 Phone: 800.343.4499, ext. 154 Fax: 877.364.7062 731.935.7731 jamey.moon@perseusbooks.com
Cost	$27.95 (for volumes 1–3), $25.95 (for volumes 4 & 5), $2.50 each for profiles (Volumes 2 and 5: minimum order of 5 copies required) *(Prices current as of April 2014)*
Purpose	Assesses functional development of children in six areas: perceptual/fine motor, cognition, language, social-emotional, self-care, and gross motor.
Age Range	Ages 0 to 60 months (Volumes 1–3 are for 0–35 months, Volumes 4 & 5 are for ages 3:0–5:0)
Time	Not specified; likely to be highly variable
Scores or Subtests	Six areas are of development are evaluated: perceptual/fine motor, cognition, language, social/emotional, self-care, and gross motor.
Description	The Developmental Programming for Infants and Young Children is designed to give the test administrator information about a child's development. In addition, the test also bridges the assessment–program planning gap by giving information about objectives to form functional activities. The assessment is divided into five volumes, offering specific profiles for certain purposes and age groups: Volume 1: Assessment and Application Volume 2: Early Intervention Developmental Profile Volume 3: Stimulation Activities Volume 4: Preschool Assessment and Application Volume 5: Preschool Developmental Profile
Reliability	Interrater reliability is reported, ranging from 80% to 97% (89% average) agreement. This reliability information is based on nine raters scoring the same 100 profile items.
Validity	Concurrent validity is reported as a result of a study comparing performance across different assessments (i.e. Bayley Mental Scale, Bayley Motor Scale, and the REEL). These studies, however, used a small sample size (the most for an assessment was 14 individuals). The validity data reported is highly variable, with some subtests as low as .33 correlation coefficient to .96.
Norms	N/A
Who Can Give the Test?	The test manual specifies that the assessment "was designed to be administered by a multidisciplinary team which includes a psychologist or special educator, physical or occupational therapist, and a speech and language therapist."
Strengths	The test can be given to a wide range of ages, and it gives information about many aspects of development that can then be used to plan educational objectives and activities.
Concerns	This assessment is not standardized; it is criterion-referenced and therefore cannot be used to compare child performance to a normative sample. The test was published in 1981, and thus the test items and scales do not reflect more modern research. In addition, the test item graphics look extremely dated.

Table A–5. Hawaii Early Learning Profile (HELP)

Author	Setsu Furuno, Katherine A. O'Reilly, Carol M. Hosaka, Takayo T. Inatsuka, Barbara Zeisloft Falbey, and Toney Allman
Publisher	VORT Corporation
Contact Information	VORT Corporation Phone: 888.757.8678 P.O. Box 60132-W Fax: 650.327.0747 Palo Alto, CA 94306 custserv@vort.com
Cost	$158.40 (manual and parent handouts), $3.25 per assessment booklet (discounted price for ordering more at a time) *(Prices current as of April 2014)*
Purpose	Assesses developmental skills/behaviors.
Age Range	Ages birth to 3 years
Time	10 to 15 minutes
Scores or Subtests	Item scores only; six developmental areas: cognitive, language, gross motor, fine motor, social, self-help.
Description	The HELP Checklist (Hawaii Early Learning Profile) is not a formal psychometric instrument, but a list of developmental skills and behaviors that would be typical of infants from birth to 3 years of age. The Checklist structure includes 16 pages of items with approximately 45 items per page. These items are arranged by skill area (such as Cognitive) and ordered by age in months. The items typically are clauses describing infant behavior such as: 'Plays with paper' or 'Grasps crayon adaptively'. The user of the instrument records whether the skill was observed, reported by the parent, assessed but not observed, or is emerging, but not complete.
Reliability	N/A
Validity	N/A
Norms	N/A
Who Can Give the Test	This test should be given by a professional trained in assessment of children, including but not limited to speech-language pathologists and teachers.
Strengths	Larger than usual number of items could give a more reliable score.
Concerns	No norms or criterion-based scoring; Could take multiple administration attempts to complete entire test due to length.

Table A–6. Vineland Adaptive Behavior Scales, 2nd Edition

Author	Sara S. Sparrow, Domenic V. Cicchetti, and David A. Balla	
Publisher	Pearson	
Contact Information	Pearson Attn: Inbound Sales & Customer Support 19500 Bulverde Road San Antonio, TX 78259-3701	Phone: 800.627.7271 Fax: 800.232.1223 ClinicalCustomerSupport@Pearson.com
Cost	Price varies depending on the type of form used; basic starter kit (with Survey Interview Forms): $198.50 *(Price current as of October 15, 2014)*	
Purpose	Designed as an adaptive behavior assessment system that measures self-sufficiency across the life-span.	
Age Range	Birth to 90	
Time	20 to 65 minutes; 25 to 90 minutes for Expanded Interview Form	
Scores or Subtests	4 subject domains are tested and scored: Communication, Daily Living Skills, Socialization, and Motor Skills.	
Description	The Vineland-II is an individually administered measure of adaptive behavior with several different rating and interview forms for respondents (parents, caregivers, and teachers) who are very familiar with the individual.	
Reliability	Coefficient alphas for the Teacher Report Form and adjusted split-half Pearson correlations for the two other forms are consistently quite strong (mostly mid- to high .90s) for the Adaptive Behavior Composite. The one exception was the Survey Forms (Survey Interview Form and Parent/Caregiver Rating Form) for the ages 32–71, where scores tend to be the highest and therefore are less variable and reliable. The internal consistency reliability for the domain scores is also very good to excellent (mostly high .80s to mid- .90s), with the exception of the slightly lower reliability in the Motor Skills domain. The adjusted test-retest reliability coefficients for the Teacher Report Form (n = 135 students), Survey Forms (n = 414 respondents), and the Expanded Form (n = 220 respondents) are generally good to excellent for the Adaptive Behavior Composite (low .80s. to mid-.90s).	
Validity	In terms of test structure, comparisons between the subdomain, domain, and Adaptive Behavior Composite scores on all forms indicate moderately high correlations, which support the strong influence of overall adaptive behavior on the individual domains and subdomains. Correlations between the subdomains within a domain tend to be slightly stronger than with subdomains across domains. However, overall modest subdomain clustering illustrates the interrelatedness of the adaptive behaviors across domains. Confirmatory factor analysis results on the Teacher Report Form and Survey Forms indicate that a three- to four-factor model fits the data reasonably well. The adjusted correlations between each of the three Vineland-II forms and the corresponding Vineland Adaptive Behavior Scale form are moderately high, most in the .80s and .90s. Correlations between the different forms of the Vineland-II with each other were also calculated. The relationship between the two forms completed by parents/guardians (Survey Form and Expanded Form) was moderate (.68 to .80 for the Adaptive Behavior Composite). Weaker correlations were found between the TRF and the Survey Form (.32 to .48 for Adaptive Behavior Composite). However, this pattern of relationship between the teacher and parent forms of the Vineland-II is very similar to the early Vineland ABS and likely reflects the fact that the respondents observe the students' behavior in significantly different environments. Correlations between the Vineland and other similar measures were variable, ranging from .19 to .95.	

continues

Norms	A nationally representative sample of individuals, from birth through age 90 (broken down into 20 age groups), comprised the standardization sample for the Survey Interview Form and Parent/Caregiver Rating Form ($n = 3,695$) and the Expanded Interview Form ($n = 2,151$). A relatively higher proportion of the norm sample was clustered at birth through age 5 (about 30% for the Survey Interview Form; over 40% for the Expanded Interview Form). The TRF was administered to 2,570 teachers and day care providers (from a larger pool of over 19,000) for 15 age groups of children, ranging from age 3 to 17/18. In all versions of the Vineland-II, the samples were designed to be evenly split between males and females and to match the 2001 US Census data in the areas of race/ethnicity, SES, geographic region, community size, and special education placement.
Who Can Give the Test?	Professionals with a graduate degree and specific training in early childhood assessment and interpretation.
Strengths	Long history of effective use in identifying individuals with adaptive behavior deficits and intervention planning.
Concerns	Relatively weak inter-rater reliability; professionals who administer the Vineland should have training in semistructured interview format.

Table A-7. Vineland Social-Emotional Early Childhood Scales

Author	Sara S. Sparrow, David A. Balla, and Dominic V. Cicchietti
Publisher	Pearson
Contact Information	Pearson Phone: 800.627.7271 Attn: Inbound Sales & Customer Support Fax: 800.232.1223 19500 Bulverde Road ClinicalCustomerSupport@Pearson.com San Antonio, TX 78259-3701
Cost	$103 *(Price current as of April 2014)*
Purpose	Designed to assess the social and emotional functioning of young children.
Age Range	Birth to age 5:11
Time	15 to 25 minutes
Scores or Subtests	Four scores: Interpersonal Relationships, Play and Leisure Time, Coping Skills, Composite.
Description	Administered as a structured oral interview. The Vineland SEEC Scales are a subset of items from the Socialization Domain of the Vineland Adaptive Behavior Scales, Expanded Form.
Reliability	Internal consistency levels are adequate, with median values of the Interpersonal Relationships, Play and Leisure Time, and Coping Skills Scales ranging from .80 to .87. The internal reliability coefficients of the Scale Composite, across six age groups, range from .89 to .97 with a median value of .93. Test-retest reliability coefficients are also reported following re-administration of the scale after a 2- to 4-week interval (mean interval of 17 days). Adequate stability is also well documented with the vast majority of the component scale and composite score test-retest correlations falling between .71 and .79. Only the Coping Skills scale, for the age group 0-6 to 2-1, yielded an unacceptable stability coefficient ($r = .54$). Test-retest reliability drops substantially when the interviewer is different.
Validity	See information re: validity of the Vineland ABS. No separate validity measurements were made for the Vineland SEEC alone.
Norms	See information re: Vineland ABS above. From the total sample, 1200 children were birth-5:11 and 58% of these subjects aged 3:0 through 5:11 were enrolled in preschool or school programs, which matched Dept. of Education data from 1982. Norms are provided at 1-month intervals from birth to age 2, and at 2-month intervals from age 2 through 5 years, 11 months.
Who Can Give the Test?	Professionals with a graduate degree and specific training in early childhood assessment and interpretation.
Strengths	Assesses the social and emotional behaviors of young children; standardization process was comprehensive; easy to administer and score; concurrent and predictive validity with other developmental scales is acceptable.
Concerns	The norms for the Vineland SEEC are almost two decades old.

Table A–8. Arizona Articulation Proficiency Scale–3

Author	Janet Barker Fudala
Publisher	Western Psychological Services, 2003
Contact Information	Western Psychological Services 12031 Wilshire Blvd. Los Angeles, CA 90025-1251	Phone: 800.648.8857 Fax: 310.478.7838 customerservice@wpspublish.com
Cost	$176 *(Price current as of April 2014)*
Purpose	Provides speech-language pathologists (or another examiner trained in phonetic transcription) with a quick measure to assess articulation proficiency in children; assesses consonant and vowel sounds.
Age Range	1:6 to 18 years
Time	3 min. or less
Scores or Subtests	Optional assessment tasks: word reading administration, language screening task, and spontaneous speech task.
Description	Looks at articulation in multiple contexts to effectively evaluate ability and stimulability of different sounds. There are 42 target words (mostly monosyllabic).
Reliability	Internal consistency: range alpha score .078–0.96, median 0.925; inter-rater reliability: mean reliability coefficient 0.82; intrarater reliability: high accuracy rates in several studies over the last 30 years; test-retest reliability: median correlation 0.97.
Validity	The Arizona 3 has high correlations with other articulation tests (Templin-Darley Screening and Diagnostic Tests of Articulation, Photo Articulation Test, and Goldman-Fristoe Test of Articulation).
Norms	Data is standardized on a nationally representative sample of over 5,500 children and teenagers. It is gender specific up to age 6 years. The sample is representative of ethnicity, region, gender, and parental education.
Who Can Give the Test?	Speech-language pathologist or another professional who is trained in phonetic transcription.
Strengths	Easy and quick to administer; all major speech sounds assessed in less than 3 minutes; quantitative scoring rules.
Concerns	Pictures are black line drawings; some are old-fashioned and may be more difficult for examinees to identify.

Table A–9. Clinical Assessment of Articulation & Phonology (CAAP)

Author	Wayne A. Secord and JoAnn S. Donohue
Publisher	Super Duper Publications
Contact Information	Super Duper Publications P.O. Box 24997 Greenville, SC Phone: 800.277.8737 Fax: 800.978.7379 Outside the US: Phone: 001.864.288.3536 Fax: 001.864.288.3880 customerhelp@superduperinc.com
Cost	$229.00 *(Price current as of April 2014)*
Purpose	Designed to assess English articulation and phonology in preschool and school-aged children.
Age Range	Ages 2:6 to 8:11
Time	15 to 20 minutes
Scores or Subtests	Consonant Inventory Score, School Age Sentence Score, Final Consonant Deletion, Cluster Reduction, Syllable Reduction, Gliding, Vocalization, Fronting, Deaffrication, Stopping, Prevocalic Voicing, Postvocalic Devoicing.
Description	The Clinical Assessment of Articulation and Phonology (CAAP) is a norm-referenced test of Standard American English consonant articulation. The test has two parts, Consonant Inventory and School Age Sentences, that assess consonant production in single word and connected speech, respectively.
Reliability	Test-retest reliability was measured on the raw scores from 32 children. Comparing total raw scores, the correlation was .975. Comparing just the School Age Sentences raw score from children 5 to 9 years, the correlation was .865. Interexaminer reliability was computed on just four examiners. Analyses of variance performed on their scores from 56 protocols showed a reliability coefficient of .99.
Validity	According to the authors, face validity was established during test construction and preliminary testing. Concurrent validity (a.k.a., criterion-related validity) was established by comparing CAAP performance of 49 children with identified articulation and phonological problems to their concurrent performance on the Bankson-Bernthal Test of Phonology (Bernthal & Bankson, 1990). Pearson product-moment correlations for these comparisons ranged between .62 and .88, whereas Spearman rho correlations ranged between .56 and .84; all correlations were significant beyond $p <.01$.
Norms	The CAAP was standardized on a total sample of 1,707 American and Canadian children. The sample generally mirrors the demographic characteristics of the United States (2000 US Census data) with respect to region, gender, race, maternal education, and home language.
Who Can Give the Test?	This test should be administered by a professional trained and skilled in decoding the speech of children, such as a speech-language pathologist.
Strengths	Quick, efficient. Comes with puppets to use in story for younger children.
Concerns	Vowels are not sampled in the CAAP. More reliability and validity data are desired.

Reference

Bernthal, J. E., & Bankson, N. W. (1990). *BBTOP: Bankson-Bernthal Test of Phonology.* Austin, TX: Pro-Ed.

Table A–10. Goldman-Fristoe Test of Articulation–2 (GFTA-2)

Author	Ronald Goldman and Macalyne Fristoe
Publisher	Pearson
Contact Information	Pearson Phone: 800.627.7271 Attn: Inbound Sales & Customer Support Fax: 800.232.1223 19500 Bulverde Road ClinicalCustomerSupport@Pearson.com San Antonio, TX 78259-3701
Cost	$282.00 *(Price current as of April 2014)*
Purpose	Provides speech-language pathologists (or another examiner trained in phonetic transcription) with a measure to assess articulation proficiency in children; assesses consonant sounds; can be used for diagnostic potential to determine the level of articulation difficulty; growth of articulation skills over time can also be monitored.
Age Range	2 to 21:11 years
Time	5 to 15 minutes (Sounds-in-Words subtest)
Scores or Subtests	Subtests: Sounds-in-Words, Sounds-in-Sentences, Stimulability (imitation of speech sounds).
Description	Looks at articulation in multiple contexts to effectively evaluate ability and stimulability of different sounds. There are 77 target words.
Reliability	Internal reliability for females: 0.96; Median reliability for males: 0.94; median test-retest reliability 0.98 for initial, medial, and final sounds; inter-rater reliability median percentages of agreement for initial, medial, and final sounds are 93, 90, 90 respectively.
Validity	Content: 23 of 25 sounds recognized as Standard American English consonants were included on the test. Construct: Means and Standard Deviations for Standard Sample by Age: Age N Mean SD 2 200 36.2 16.1 3 200 22.8 15.0 4 250 14.3 12.9 5 250 8.6 10.3 6 250 5.9 8.3 7 200 3.3 7.3 8 200 2.4 5.5 9–10 200 2.5 6.1 11–12 200 1.2 3.8 13–14 200 1.6 5.5 15–21 200 0.8 4.0
Norms	Data from a representative sample of 2,350 subjects was used to develop the normative scores. There are age-based standard scores, percentiles, and test-age equivalents available. The sample controlled for age/gender, race, geographic region, SES/parent education, and included special populations (did not say what specific special populations).
Who Can Give the Test?	Speech-language pathologist or another professional who is trained in phonetic transcription.

Table A–10. *continued*

Strengths	Easy to administer; most widely used test of articulation; user-friendly color-coding for recording initial, medial, and final sounds as well as initial consonant blends; colorful, entertaining pictures to elicit responses.
Concerns	Limited sample size and cultural bias of standardization sample; developmental data given may be outdated; does not assess vowel production.

Table A–11. Identifying Early Phonological Needs in Children With Hearing Loss (IEPN; Paden-Brown)

Author	Elaine Paden and Carolyn Brown	
Publisher	Med-El Corporation (North America)	
Contact Information	Med-El Corporation 2511 Old Cornwallis Road, Suite 100 Durham, NC 27713	Phone: 888.633.3524 919.572.2222 Fax: 919.484.9229 usaeducators@medel.com
Cost	$35.00 *(Price current as of October 15, 2014)*	
Purpose	Designed to assess spontaneous use of first level phonological patterns in children with hearing loss.	
Age Range	Preschool to Adult	
Time	10 to 15 minutes	
Scores or Subtests	Mean percent correct for Word Patterns, Vowel Areas, Consonant Manner, Consonant Place, Consonant Voicing.	
Description	Children label 25 pictures; words include variety of vowels, diphthongs, and constants. Numerical scoring indicates whether child's skills are missing, emerging, or mastered.	
Reliability	N/A	
Validity	N/A	
Norms	N/A	
Who Can Give the Test?	Because phonetic transcription is a requirement of this test, a speech-language pathologist or other professional trained in phonetics should administer this test.	
Strengths	Comprehensive evaluation of phonology.	
Concerns	Must be administered by someone well-trained in phonetics.	

Table A–12. Auditory Perception Test for the Hearing Impaired Revised (APT-HI)

Author	Susan Allen	
Publisher	Plural Publishing, Inc.	
Contact Information	Plural Publishing, Inc. 5521 Ruffin Road San Diego, CA 92123	Phone: 866.758.7251 858.492.1555 Fax: 866.758.7255 858.492.1020 information@pluralpublishing.com
Cost	$249.95 *(Price current as of April 2014)*	
Purpose	Evaluates children's discrete auditory perception ability by profiling in 16 different skill areas; identifies specific auditory perception and processing deficits across the continuum of listening.	
Age Range	3:0 and older; can also be applied to adults in auditory rehabilitation	
Time	20 to 30 minutes	
Scores or Subtests	Organized into 8 subtests of auditory perception tasks: (a) auditory awareness; (b) duration, intensity, and pitch identification; (c) prosodic perception; (d) vowel perception; (e) consonant perception; (f) other segmental perception; (g) linguistic perception and (h) communicative comprehension (some categories have subtests of skills, i.e., consonant perception tasks broken into consonants differing in voice, manner, and place of production).	
Description	Measures speech perception capabilities in individuals with hearing loss ranging from mild to profound. Can be used to measure a student's progress in therapy over time, to relate speech production capabilities to auditory perception skills and to assist with identifying speech targets and discrete auditory tasks for training.	
Reliability	Reliability was determined using a Spearman-Brown test of split-half reliability, correlation was 0.99. Kuder-Richardson test was used to determine the homogeneity of items in the test and gave resulting correlation of 0.97. Test-retest reliability: 0.98.	
Validity	Correlations and Coefficients of Determination Between APT/HI Scores and Age and Degree of Hearing Loss 	Variable	r	r^2
Age	0.43	0.18
Pure Tone Avg—Unaided	−0.69	0.48
Pure Tone Avg—Aided	−0.77	0.58 | | Variable	R	R^2
Age & pure tone avg—Aided	0.84	0.71
Age & pure tone avg—Unaided	0.81	0.66
Aided & Unaided	0.86	0.74		
Norms	Piloted on 118 children with hearing loss; 55% male, 45% female; 72% European American, 13% African American, 14% Hispanic American, 1% other ethnic/racial backgrounds.	

Who Can Give the Test?	Should be administered by professionals experienced in working with children who have hearing loss. Typically, speech-language pathologists, audiologists, educational diagnosticians, or classroom teachers of children with hearing loss. Should have fundamental core knowledge about equipment, appropriate amplification, the **speech banana**, behavioral conditioning, chronological age vs. hearing age, etc.
Strengths	Specifically designed for children with hearing loss.
Concerns	Limited number of children in pilot study.

Table A–13. Contrasts for Auditory & Speech Training (CAST)

Author	David J. Ertmer	
Publisher	LinguiSystems	
Contact Information	LinguiSystems 3100 4th Avenue East Moline, IL 61244	Phone: 800.776.4332 Fax: 800.577.4555 service@linguisystems.com
Cost	$49.95 *(Price current as of April 2014)*	
Purpose	To determine speech perception ability prior to, during, and after auditory training; To be used in conjunction with the CAST system.	
Age Range	Ages 3 to 12; Grades PreK to 7	
Time	10 minutes	
Scores or Subtests	Percent Correct for Levels 1 to 7.	
Description	The tester produces the target stimuli in random order a total of five times while the child points to the word he or she heard. The examiner calculates percent correct for each level. There are seven levels of this pretest, and cards 1–28 are used.	
Reliability	N/A	
Validity	N/A	
Norms	N/A	
Who Can Give the Test?	A professional trained in phonetics and auditory training who will be providing training services to the child should administer this pretest.	
Strengths	Quick, easy measure of auditory discrimination. Easily translates to therapy activities and goals.	
Concerns	Not a standardized measure of ability.	

Table A–14. Early Speech Perception Test (ESP)

Author	Jean S. Moog and Anne E. Geers
Publisher	Central Institute for the Deaf, St. Louis, MO
Contact Information	Central Institute for the Deaf 825 South Taylor Ave. St. Louis, Missouri 63110 Phone: 877.444.4574 314.977.0132 Fax: 314.977.0023 TTY: 314.977.0037 http://www.cidedu.com
Cost	$250.00 *(Price current as of April 2014)*
Purpose	Assesses speech discrimination skills of children with profound hearing loss.
Age Range	Starting at 3 to 12 years
Time	15 to 20 minutes
Scores or Subtests	Standard Version: Pattern Perception, Spondee ID, Monosyllable ID, Total. Low-verbal Version: Pattern Perception, Word ID (Spondee and Monosyllable), Total.
Description	Assesses aspects of listening skills of children with profound hearing losses. The test focuses on the hierarchy of speech perception skills observed in children with hearing loss. It can be used to formulate goals/objectives for auditory training and to test progress in speech perception ability over time. It can also provide information on how the child is performing with amplification. Speech Perception Categories for profoundly hearing-impaired children: (1) No pattern perception; (2) Pattern perception; (3) Some word identification; (4) Consistent word identification.
Reliability	Test-Retest Reliability Correlation Coefficients: Standard Version: Pattern perception raw score: 0.78, Spondee and monosyllabic combined raw score: 0.89, Category placement: 0.94. Low-Verbal Version: Pattern perception raw score: 0.75, Monosyllable and spondee combined raw score: 0.77, Category placement: 0.89.
Validity	Standard Version: correlation with the WIPI, validity correlation coefficient of 0.87. Other validity data in charts in manual.
Norms	49 children (17 female, 32 male), ranging in age from 4 to 15 years, who attended classes at Central Institute for the Deaf. All children had better ear pure tone threshold averages (at 500, 1000, and 2000 Hz) equal to or greater than 90 dB HL and displayed nonverbal intelligence quotients in the normal range. All children were also familiar with the vocabulary and tested only when wearing appropriate amplification.
Who Can Give the Test?	Should be administered by professionals experienced in working with children who have hearing loss. Typically, speech-language pathologists, audiologists, educational diagnosticians, or classroom teachers of children with hearing loss.
Strengths	Specifically for children with hearing loss; easy to administer.
Concerns	Only examines listening skills in four discrete categories; limited data on test-retest reliability and validity.

Table A–15. Infant-Toddler Meaningful Auditory Integration Scale (IT-MAIS)

Author	Susan Zimmerman-Phillips, Mary Joe Osberger, and Amy McConkey Robbins
Publisher	Advanced Bionics Corporation
Contact Information	Advanced Bionics, LLC 28515 Westinghouse Place Valencia, CA 91355 Phone: 877.829.0026 661.362.1400 Fax: 661.362.1503 TTY: 800.678.3575 CustomerService@advancedbionics.com
Cost	Free; download from website: http://www.advancedbionics.com *(Price current as of April 2014)*
Purpose	Modification of MAIS, structured interview schedule designed to assess the child's spontaneous responses to sound in his or her everyday environment. Consists of 10 probes which assess vocalization behavior, alerting to sounds, and deriving meaning from sound.
Age Range	Birth to 3 years
Time	Less than 10 minutes
Scores or Subtests	Total score only.
Description	Parent does not directly fill out. Examiner uses probes to elicit child's spontaneous behavior and can ask parent questions to elicit further information. Combination of parent report and clinical observation. Ask parent to give as many examples as possible to make more accurate.
Reliability	N/A
Validity	N/A
Norms	N/A
Who Can Give the Test?	Audiologists, speech-language pathologists, and/or teachers experienced in working with children who have hearing loss.
Strengths	Fast administration time; provides information regarding parent's perception of child's response to sound in the natural environment.
Concerns	Parent responses may be biased; may not reflect actual behavior of the child.

Table A–16. LittlEARS Auditory Questionnaire

Author	L. Tsiakpini, V. Weichbold, H. Kuehn-Inacker, F. Coninx, P. D'Haese, and S. Almadin
Publisher	Med-El Corporation (North America)
Contact Information	Med-El Corporation 2511 Old Cornwallis Road, Suite 100 Durham, NC 27713 Phone: 888.633.3524 919.572.2222 Fax: 919.484.9229 usaeducators@medel.com
Cost	$40.00 *(Price current as of May 26, 2011)*
Purpose	Parent questionnaire that evaluates all types of auditory behaviors which are observable as a reaction to acoustic stimuli; follows auditory development of children after newborn hearing screening from birth to 24 mos; can also follow children with cochlear implants or hearing aids with a hearing age of 0 to 24 months.
Age Range	Birth to 24 months/children with hearing loss with hearing age of 0 to 24 mos.
Time	10 minutes
Scores or Subtests	Total score only.
Description	There are 35 questions which give expected values and minimal values for individual comparison. Also LittlEARS Diary, which provides a guided documentation and observation of the development of the child over half a year after device fitting.
Reliability	Scale analysis showed Pearson's: r −0.91, r >0.6. Split-half: r = 0.88, criterion r >0.7. Guttman's lambda = 0.93, criterion >0.7. Homogeneous, Cronbach's alpha = 0.96, criterion >0.7. Proved reliable to record preverbal-auditory development within first 2 years of hearing.
Validity	Proved valid to record preverbal-auditory development within first 2 years of hearing. Also validation study of use of LEAQ in CI-children.
Norms	Standardization on 218 normal hearing children aged 0–24 mos. and currently being evaluated on children with cochlear implants.
Who Can Give the Test?	Parent Questionnaire.
Strengths	Can assess preverbal auditory development in very young children; only takes about 10 min. for parents to complete; Spanish version available.
Concerns	Parent responses may be biased; may not reflect actual behavior of the child.

Table A–17. Meaningful Auditory Integration Scale (MAIS)

Author	Amy M. Robbins
Publisher	Indiana University School of Medicine
Contact Information	Indiana University School of Medicine Department of Otolaryngology Head and Neck Surgery DeVault Otologic Research Laboratory 699 Riley Hospital Dr. RR044 Indianapolis, IN 46202-5119 Phone: 317.274.4915 Fax: 317.274.4949 devinfo@iupui.edu
Cost	Free; download from website: http://medicine.iu.edu/oto/research/devaultlab/testing/ (Price current as of June 1, 2011)
Purpose	Parent report scale to assess a child's responses to sound in his or her everyday environment;10 probes that include assessment of device bonding, alerting to sound, and deriving meaning from sound; designed for children with hearing loss who are aurally rehabilitated.
Age Range	3 to 4 years and up
Time	Less than 10 minutes
Scores or Subtests	Device Usage Raw Score, Alerting to Sound Raw Score, Deriving Meaning Raw Score; Total Score out of a possible 40 points.
Description	10 probes: (1) Does the child ask to have his device put on, or put it on himself or herself, WITHOUT being told? (2) Does the child report and/or appear upset if the device is nonfunctioning for any reason? (3) Does the child spontaneously respond to his or her name in quiet when called auditorally only with no visual cue? (4) Does the child spontaneously respond to his or her name in the presence of background noise when called auditorally only with no visual cues? (5) Does the child spontaneously alert to environmental sounds (doorbell, telephone) in the home without being prompted or told to listen? (6) Does the child alert to auditory signals spontaneously when in new environments . . . ? (7) Does the child spontaneously recognize auditory signals that are part of his or her everyday routines? (8) Does the child show the ability to discriminate spontaneously among two speakers, using audition alone . . . ? (9) Does the child spontaneously know the difference between speech and nonspeech stimuli when listening alone . . . ? (10) Does the child spontaneously associate vocal tone (anger, excitement, anxiety) with its meaning, based on hearing only?
Reliability	N/A
Validity	N/A
Norms	N/A
Who Can Give the Test?	Parent Questionnaire.
Strengths	Provides information regarding parent's perception of child's response to sound in natural environment; quick and easy to administer.
Concerns	Parent responses may be biased; may not reflect actual behavior of the child.

Table A–18. Test for Auditory Comprehension of Language, 3rd Edition (TACL-3)

Author	Elizabeth Carrow Woolfolk
Publisher	Pro-Ed

Contact Information	Pro-Ed, Inc.
	8700 Shoal Creek Boulevard
	Austin, Texas 78757-6897
	
	Customer Service:
	  Phone: 800.897.3202
	  Fax: 800.397.7633
	Publishing Team:
	  Phone: 800.897.3202
	  Fax: 800.397.7633
	  info@proedinc.com

Cost	$328.00 *(Price current as of April 2014)*
Purpose	Designed as a measure of receptive spoken vocabulary, grammar, and syntax.
Age Range	Ages 3:0 through 9:11, Grades K to 4
Time	15 to 25 minutes
Scores or Subtests	4: Vocabulary, Grammatical Morphemes, Elaborated Phrases and Sentences, Total.
Description	The Test for Auditory Comprehension of Language, 3rd ed. (TACL-3) was developed by the same author as its preceding versions. Therefore, the TACL-3 is very similar to their standardization and test structure, but with better all- around improvement in psychometric properties and layout. The test consists of 139 items grouped into three subtests (vocabulary, syntax, and grammar). Vocabulary measures the meanings of word classes; Syntax measures understanding of grammatical morphemes; and Elaborated Phrases and Sentences tests understanding of syntactically based word relations.
Reliability	Internal consistencies are reported for the Quotient and each of the three subtests by age; all are within the .90s except Vocabulary at ages 5 and 9 years (.89 and .84, respectively). Furthermore, the test shows consistency across various subgroups including gender, ethnicity, and disability. Some positive evidence is provided for stability; however, the sample is small and limited to 2nd and 3rd graders in an elementary school in Austin, Texas. Efforts were also directed at establishing inter-rater reliability for each of the subtests and the Quotient. Surprisingly, reliabilities for two of the subtests fell below .90; it is difficult to imagine how this might have occurred because the format of the test (multiple choice) leaves little room for judgment as to the accuracy of the response. Nevertheless, the Quotient is a robust index across age, gender, ethnicity, disability, time, and scorers.
Validity	Support for the validity of the test came from factor analysis (which demonstrated a single factor) and subtest intercorrelations (which showed that the subtests were related but not so strongly that each was not measuring a different aspect of comprehension). In addition, the Vocabulary subtest from the TACL-3 was shown to correlate more highly with the Receptive than the Expressive Vocabulary subtest of the Comprehensive Receptive and Expressive Vocabulary Test. There were no current studies to support the claim that the TACL-3 is useful in predicting success in the early grades, although there were two studies reported using the 1973 version of the test that showed correlations with reading and other achievement measures.

Norms	The normative sample (1,102) is stratified by age and generally represents the 1997 US Census with the exception of fewer numbers from urban areas (55% vs. 75%) and more from rural areas (47% vs. 25%), which is most notable across the 5 to 9–year age span. Children with speech-language disorders and children with learning disabilities were included in the sample.
Who Can Give the Test?	The TACL-3 should be given to children by someone trained in the speech and language development of children, as proper speech and decoding are essential for administering and scoring this test.
Strengths	Easy to administer and score; addition of color pictures adds to its appeal.
Concerns	The TACL-3 should be used in conjunction with other tests for making decisions regarding placement and to get a full picture of a child's abilities.

Table A–19. Test of Auditory Processing Skills, 3rd Edition (TAPS-3)

Author	Nancy A. Martin and Rick Brownell
Publisher	Academic Therapy Publications
Contact Information	Academic Therapy Publications Phone: 800.422.7249 20 Commercial Blvd. Fax: 888.287.9975 Novato, CA 94949 sales@academictherapy.com
Cost	$160.00 *(Price current as of April 2014)*
Purpose	To measure a child's functioning in various areas of auditory perception.
Age Range	Ages 4 to 0 through 18 to 11
Time	60 minutes
Scores or Subtests	Word Discrimination, Phonological Segmentation, Phonological Blending, Number Memory Forward, Number Memory Reversed, Word Memory, Sentence Memory, Auditory Comprehension, Auditory Reasoning.
Description	The TAPS-3 focuses specifically on skills used in developing, using, and understanding spoken language. The TAPS-3 is composed of nine core subtests and an optional Auditory Figure-Ground Screening measure that can be used to initiate the test session. The test is presented on CD and is useful in screening for hearing loss and/or attention problems but should not, the test authors caution, act as a tool to diagnose attention disorders.
Reliability	Estimates of internal consistency are reported to range from ".49 to .97 for the various age groups, with medians of .69 to .94 across all ages" (manual, p. 52). Test-retest reliability is reported to range from .64 to .93.
Validity	The TAPS-3 examiner's manual reports several investigative validity studies that in the aggregate do a fair job convincing users that the instrument would be appropriate for its intended purpose. Evidence is provided to suggest that the TAPS-3 may be useful in discriminating between children with and without auditory processing skill deficits. Children with a previous diagnosis of auditory processing difficulties ($N = 56$) were found to score significantly (both statistically and materially) below typically developing students ($N = 244$) on TAPS-3 measures.
Norms	The standardization sample for the TAPS-3 was composed of approximately 2,000 children evaluated at over 182 testing sites throughout the United States. The sample was closely stratified in accordance with 2000 U.S. Census data on the variables of gender, race/ethnicity, parent education level, residence, and geographic region. In addition, children were well represented across the intended age range of use, with nearly 100 children represented at each 1-year interval through age 11, and multiyear intervals in later years through age 18.
Who Can Give the Test?	Speech-language pathologists, audiologists, teachers, and other clinicians trained to assess the spectrum of student auditory skills.
Strengths	Can be used with a wide range of children; appears to do a good job of discriminating between children with and without auditory processing difficulties.
Concerns	Should not be used to diagnose attention disorders. There is little discussion in the test manual that cross-contamination of other skills was minimized in the test authors' focus on measuring auditory skills.

Table A–20. The Listening Comprehension Test 2

Author	Rosemary Huisingh, Linda Bowers, and Carolyn LoGiudice
Publisher	LinguiSystems
Contact Information	LinguiSystems 3100 4th Avenue East Moline, IL 61244	Phone: 800.776.4332 Fax: 800.577.4555 service@linguisystems.com
Cost	$159.95 *(Price current as of April 2014)*
Purpose	To assess auditory processing and listening comprehension skills in children.
Age Range	Ages 6 to 11, Grades 1 to 6
Time	40 minutes
Scores or Subtests	5 Subtests: Main Idea, Details, Reasoning, Vocabulary, Understanding Messages.
Description	The Listening Comprehension Test 2 assesses listening through natural classroom situations rather than evaluating listening through simple repetition or discrimination subtests. The tasks reveal students' strengths and weaknesses in integrated language problem solving, reasoning, and comprehension of material presented auditorily.
Reliability	Reliability Studies: – SEM – Inter-Rater Reliability – Test-Retest – Reliability Based on Item Homogeneity (KR20)
Validity	Validity Studies: – Contrast Groups (t-values): Test discriminates between subjects with normal language development and subjects with language disorders. – Biserial Correlations. – Subtest Intercorrelations. – Correlations Between Subtests and Total Test.
Norms	This test was normed on 1,504 subjects. Demographics reflect the national school population demographics from the 2000 National Census. Test performances reflect typically achieving students as well as those in subgroups found in the school population. Subjects included in the study: regular education; special education; regular education with IEPs for special services; all socioeconomic levels; White, Black, Hispanic or Latino, Asian, Pacific Islander, and Native American groups; 49 states. Subjects excluded from the study: not able to use English proficiently at school; nonverbal; degree of hearing loss; reside or attend school outside of the United States.
Who Can Give the Test?	The test should only be administered by a trained professional familiar with language disorders (e.g., speech-language pathologist, psychologist).
Strengths	Easy to administer.
Concerns	Little available research/reviews on this test.

Table A–21. Clinical Evaluation of Language Fundamentals, Preschool–2 (CELF P-2)

Author	Elisabeth Wiig, Wayne Secord, and Eleanor Semel
Publisher	The Psychological Corporation
Contact Information	Pearson Attn: Inbound Sales & Customer Support 19500 Bulverde Road San Antonio, TX 78259-3701 Phone: 800.627.7271 Fax: 800.232.1223 ClinicalCustomerSupport@Pearson.com
Cost	$389.00 *(Price current as of April 2014)*
Purpose	Measures a broad range of expressive and receptive language skills in preschool-aged children.
Age Range	3:0 to 6:11
Time	Test administration varies in time depending on the child but on average it usually takes 30 to 45 minutes
Scores or Subtests	Subtests: Sentence Structure, Word Structure, Expressive Vocabulary, Concepts & Following Directions, Basic Concepts, Recalling Sentences, Word Classes–Receptive, Word Classes–Expressive, Word Classes–Total. Scores: Core Language, Receptive Language, Expressive Language, Language Content, and Language Structure; standard scores, percentile ranks, age equivalents, and growth scores.
Description	The CELF–Preschool 2 is designed to assess performance in aspects of language that are fundamental to the development of effective communication skills. These are defined as receptive and expressive language abilities in the areas of word meanings (semantics), word and sentence structure (morphology and syntax), and recall of spoken language (auditory memory). There are six subtests, and the results can be used to identify language disorders, determine eligibility for treatment or special services programs, and analyze relative strengths and weaknesses in language.
Reliability	Test-retest reliabilities ranged from .94 for Expressive Vocabulary (5:0–5:11) to a low of .75 for Sentence Structure (6:0–6:11). Correlations across all ages ranged from a high of .90 for Expressive Vocabulary and Recalling Sentences to a low of .78 for Sentence Structure. Time between test and retest was 2–24 days. Internal consistency: average alpha coefficients across all ages ranged from high of .95 (Pre-Literacy Rating Scale and Descriptive Pragmatics Profile) to low of .77 (Basic Concepts). Some coefficients low (Basic Concepts .59 for 5:0–5:6 and .61 for 5:6–5:11).
Validity	Content validity: subtests and composite scores linked to research. Construct validity-moderate to high subtest intercorrelations. Concurrent validity between test and CELF-4 and PLS-4 moderate to high.
Norms	800 children representative of preschool population in US: gender, age, race-ethnicity, geographic region, mother's education level.
Who Can Give the Test?	Professionals with a graduate degree and specific training in language assessment and interpretation.
Strengths	Colorful, appealing pictures; item analysis; fairly easy to administer and score; available in English and Spanish.
Concerns	Lower than acceptable reliability for some subtests/age groups (particularly Expressive Vocabulary).

Table A–22. Clinical Evaluation of Language Fundamentals–4 (CELF-4)

Author	Eleanor Semel, Elisabeth Wiig, and Wayne Secord
Publisher	PsychCorp, Harcourt Assessment
Contact Information	Pearson Attn: Inbound Sales & Customer Support 19500 Bulverde Road San Antonio, TX 78259-3701 Phone: 800.627.7271 Fax: 800.232.1223 ClinicalCustomerSupport@Pearson.com
Cost	$535.00 *(Price current as of April 2014)*
Purpose	Measures a broad range of expressive and receptive language skills in school-aged children, adolescents, and young adults.
Age Range	5 to 21 years
Time	Test administration varies in time depending on the child but on average it usually takes 30 to 60 minutes
Scores or Subtests	Subtests: Concepts and Following Directions, Core Language, Expressive Language, Expressive Vocabulary, Familiar Sequences 1 and 2, Formulated Sentences, Language Content, Language Memory, Language Structure, Number Repetition 1 and 2, Phonological Awareness, Rapid Automatic Naming, Recalling Sentences, Receptive Language, Semantic Relationships, Sentence Assembly, Sentence Structure, Understanding Spoken Paragraphs, Word Associations, Word Classes 1 and 2 Receptive, Expressive, and Total, Word Definitions, Word Structure. Scores: Core Language Receptive Language, Expressive Language, Language Content, Language Memory, and Working Memory; standard scores, percentile ranks, age equivalents, and growth scores.
Description	Developed to identify, diagnose, and provide follow-up evaluation of language and communication disorders in children, adolescents, and young adults. Like the CELF–Preschool 2, the test assesses language content and form in both expressive and receptive language modalities; CELF-4 includes a subtest for the assessment of pragmatics.
Reliability	The authors evaluated the reliability of the CELF-4 with measures of test-retest, internal consistency, and interscorer reliability. Results of test-retest reliability with 320 students yielded high correlations for all age groups' composite scores (.90+). However, test-retest reliability coefficients for each subtest and each age group range from poor (.60) to excellent (.90+) with an average administration interval of 16 days. Measures of internal consistency revealed higher reliability for the composite scores than for individual subtest scores. Reliability alpha coefficients range from .89 to .95 for the former and from .70 to .91 for the latter.
Validity	The authors provide evidence of content validity by indicating that they conducted a thorough review of the literature on the development of language skills of 5- to 21-year-old students. As a result, the language skills sampled (e.g., morphology, syntax, semantics) reflect well-documented language constructs. The authors show response process validity by showing that the verbal responses and behaviors required of the examinees to accomplish the tasks measured language skills by providing a sound rationale for the selection of subtest tasks in terms of language components and their rules (e.g., semantics, syntax), language modalities (receptive, expressive), and cognitive skills (e.g., working memory). The internal structure of the test was assessed by factor analysis, which yielded high correlations between the Core Language score and the other language indexes. In addition, Expressive and Receptive Language were highly correlated at all age levels and their respective indexes showed moderate-to-high correlation with other indexes and composite scores.

continues

Table A–22. *continued*

Norms	Standardized on 2,650 students; 5- to 17-year-olds included 200 examinees at each age level, 17- to 21-year-olds included 50 students for each age year. The sample represented the US population with respect to age, gender, race/ethnicity, geographic region, and parent education level. In contrast to earlier versions of the test, which included only normally developing children, about 9% of children in the CELF-4 normative sample were receiving special services and 7% were diagnosed with speech and/or language disorders. These numbers are consistent with those reported by the National Dissemination Center for Children with Disabilities (2003) and the US Office of Education Program (n.d.a, n.d.b) for children in special education.
Who Can Give the Test?	Professionals with a graduate degree and specific training in language assessment and interpretation.
Strengths	Evaluates multiple aspects of language, pragmatics, and memory; available in English and Spanish.
Concerns	If all subtests are administered, administration time can be lengthy and fatigue of the child may influence scoring.

Table A–23. Comprehensive Assessment of Spoken Language (CASL)

Author	Elizabeth Carrow-Woolfolk	
Publisher	Pearson Assessments, PsychCorp	
Contact Information	Pearson Attn: Inbound Sales & Customer Support 19500 Bulverde Road San Antonio, TX 78259-3701	Phone: 800.627.7271 Fax: 800.232.1223 ClinicalCustomerSupport@Pearson.com
Cost	$460.00 *(Price current as of April 2014)*	
Purpose	Designed to measure the processes of comprehension, expression, and retrieval in oral language; assesses lexical and syntactic as well as pragmatic and supralinguistic language skills.	
Age Range	3 to 21 years old	
Time	30 to 45 minutes for core battery	
Scores or Subtests	Consists of 15 subtests in 4 language structure categories **Lexical/semantic tests:** Comprehension of Basic Concepts (age 3:0–4:11, Core Test: age 5:0–6:11, Supplemental Test) Antonyms (age 5–12, Core Test, age 13–21, Supplemental Test), Synonyms (age 7–12, Supplemental Test; age 13–21 Core Test), Sentence Completion (age 3–21, Supplemental Test), and Idiomatic Language (age 11–21, Supplemental Test) **Syntactic Components:** Syntax Construction (age 3–10, Core Test, age 11–21 Supplemental Test), Paragraph Comprehension of Syntax (age 5–10, Core Test; ages 3–4 and 11–12, Supplemental Test), Grammatical Morphemes (age 11–12 Core Test; ages 7–10 and 13–21 Supplemental Test), Sentence Comprehension of Syntax (age 11–12, Core Test; age 13–21, Supplemental Test), and Grammaticality Judgment (age 7–12, Supplemental Test; age 13–21 Core Test) **Supralinguistic component tests:** Nonliteral Language, Meaning from Context, Inference, and Ambiguous Sentences **Pragmatic test:** Pragmatic Judgment	

Description	Developmentally based battery of oral language tests. It uses a purely linguistic orientation, so the subject does need to know how to read or write-only pointing, single word, or open-ended verbal responses required. Subtests designed to assess auditory comprehension, receptive, and expressive spoken English language competence. Provides an in-depth evaluation of oral language processing systems, knowledge and use of words and grammatical structures of language, ability to use language to assist higher level cognitive functions, and the contextual/communicative use of language (pragmatics).
Reliability	Test-retest reliabilities ranged from .65 to .95 for the Core Battery scores and .88 to .96 for the Indices. Split-half reliability yielded reliabilities of .80 to .90. Split-half reliability yielded reliabilities of .80 to .90.
Validity	The intercorrelation coefficients among CASL tests range from .30 to .79, low enough to support the interpretation that each test is measuring something unique but high enough to support their combination to produce the Core Composite and Index scores. (See Chapter 8 in manual for complete reporting of intercorrelation coefficients.) Correlations with other measures of language: The CASL was correlated with the following: TACL-R (35 examinees aged 5:0 to 5:11), OWLS LC and OE (50 examinees aged 7:10 to 10:11), PPVT-III (45 examinees aged 7:1 to 10:11) EVT (45 examinees aged 7:1 to 10:11) (See Chapter 8 in manual for complete reporting of these correlations.) Correlations with measures of cognitive ability: The CASL was correlated with the following: K-BIT (52 examinees aged 14:0 to 17:9) (See Chapter 8 in manual for complete reporting of these correlations.) Construct: Developmental progression of scores, intercorrelations of tests, and factor structures of the Indexes show construct validity. (See Chapter 8 in manual for construct validity data.) Clinical Sample: Differences between means of clinical and control group in Core Composite scores in the following areas: Speech Impairment: 1.5 Language Delay: 12.4* Language Impairment: 15.6* Mental Retardation: 32.2* Learning Disability (Reading): 9.9* (ages 8–11); 14.5* (ages 12–18) Learning Disability (Undifferentiated): 20.3* Emotional Disturbance: 9.9* Hearing Impairment: 26.2 * = significant at .001 level
Norms	Normed on nationwide standardization sample of 1,700 examinees, stratified to match US census data on gender, race/ethnicity, region, and maternal education.
Who Can Give the Test?	Professionals with a graduate degree and specific training in language assessment and interpretation.
Strengths	Easy to administer.
Concerns	Black-and-white drawings; occasional scoring inconsistencies; not always clear about when to administer supplemental tests.

Table A–24. Cottage Acquisition Scales for Listening, Language, and Speech (CASLLS)

Author	Elizabeth M. Wilkes
Publisher	Sunshine Cottage School for Deaf Children
Contact Information	Sunshine Cottage School for Deaf Children Phone: 210.824.0579 603 E. Hildebrand Ave. Fax: 210.826.0436 San Antonio, TX 78212 info@sunshinecottage.org
Cost	$170.00 *(Price current as of April 2014)*
Purpose	Designed to promote child language acquisition through assessment, selection of objectives, instruction planning, and progress monitoring.
Age Range	0 to 8 years, listening age
Time	Varies; intended to be an ongoing assessment, to be used in classroom teaching and progress monitoring.
Scores or Subtests	Forms are available for use with different language development levels: Pre-Verbal, Pre-Sentence, Simple Sentence, or Complex Sentence. The other form, Sounds & Speech, can be used at the same time as the language assessment. (Individual skills within each form are marked as achieved, mastered in some contexts, or generalized to many contexts.)
Description	This assessment gives parents and professionals a descriptive method for capturing the degree and speed of a child's language progress. Once the examiner chooses the correct assessment form for the child being assessed, this same form is used over time to monitor changes in the child's language. Each language feature is divided by age ranges based on general knowledge of child language development (not based on normative information gathered for this assessment).
Reliability	N/A
Validity	N/A
Norms	N/A
Who Can Give the Test?	Professionals trained in child language acquisition and the speech and language of children with hearing loss should administer this test.
Strengths	Combines listening, speech, and language measures into one tool. The CASLLS includes pragmatics as a component of language and can thus be assessed.
Concerns	This assessment is not norm-referenced. The CASLLS is an ongoing assessment based on continuous language sampling and cannot, therefore, give a quick snapshot of a child's language skills. (There is a time-thoroughness relationship that should be considered.)

Table A–25. Illinois Test of Psycholinguistic Abilities–3 (ITPA–3)

Author	Donald Hammill, Nancy Mather, and Rhia Roberts
Publisher	Pro-Ed

Contact Information	Pro-Ed, Inc.
	8700 Shoal Creek Boulevard
	Austin, Texas 78757-6897
	
	Customer Service:
	  Phone: 800.897.3202
	  Fax: 800.397.7633
	  Publishing Team:
	  Phone: 800.897.3202
	  Fax: 800.397.7633
	  info@proedinc.com

Cost	$213.00 *(Price current as of April 2014)*
Purpose	Measures children's spoken and written language skills; subtests assess oral language, writing, reading, and spelling.
Age Range	5:0 to 12:11
Time	45 to 60 minutes
Scores or Subtests	12 subtests: Spoken Analogies, Spoken Vocabulary, Morphological Closure, Syntactic Sentences, Sound Deletion, Rhyming Sequences, Sentence Sequences, Written Vocabulary, Sight Decoding, Sound Decoding, Sight Spelling, Sound Spelling.
Description	Based on Charles Osgood's original communication model and adaptations of that model made by Samuel Kirk, James McCarthy, and Winifred Kirk. Underlying assumptions: 1. Language is an important part of a child's development. 2. The essential components of language are measurable. 3. These language components can be improved through instruction. 4. Instruction in language is relevant to success in basic school subjects, particularly reading and writing. Helps determine children's specific strengths and weaknesses among linguistic abilities and differentiate between children with poor phonological coding and/or poor orthographic coding.
Reliability	Correlations between subtests. Average coefficients for individual and subtest composites are at 0.90 or greater, except for Rhyming Sequences, 0.79. Time sampling error measured using test-retest, correlations ranged from 0.86–0.99, mean correlation across the test 0.95 (2 weeks in between). Interscorer correlations ranged from 0.95–0.99.
Validity	Content-description: Authors provide rationales for format and items. Psychometric and demographic support is given for 4 clinical groups. Evidence present to validate content is in agreement with Osgood's (1957) model. Conventional item analysis data presented and differential item functioning analysis was done to identify items with bias. Criterion-prediction: Strong, correlation data comparing ITPA-3 to same child's performance on either Woodcock-Johnson Psycho-ed. Battery-Revised, Comprehensive Scales of Student Abilities, Comprehensive Test of Phonological Processing, Test of Language Development-Intermediate: Third ed. All but one subtest demonstrated correlation coefficients of at least 0.75. Construct-identification validity: data showing test correlates as well with child's age, differentiating between children with different language levels, subtest score inter-correlations, relationship to school achievement, relationship to intelligence, confirmatory factor analysis, and subtests correlation to total test performance.

continues

Table A–25. *continued*

Norms	1,522 children aged 5–12, from 27 states. Selected to reflect nation based on geographic region, gender, race, rural or urban residence, ethnicity, family income, educational attainment of parents, and disability status.
Who Can Give the Test?	Professionals with a graduate degree and specific training in language assessment and interpretation.
Strengths	Psychometrically sound measure of children's psycholinguistic abilities; easy to administer and score.
Concerns	Interpretation requires knowledge and competence in language development and psycholinguistics.

Table A–26. MacArthur-Bates Communicative Development Inventories

Author	Larry Fenson, Philip S. Dale, Steven J. Reznick, Donna Thal, Elizabeth Bates, Jeffery P. Hartung, Steve Pethick, and Judy S. Reilly
Publisher	Brookes
Contact Information	Customer Service Department Brookes Publishing Co. P.O. Box 10624 Baltimore, MD 21285-0624 — Phone: 800.638.3775 410.337.9580 Fax: 410.337.8539 http://www.brookespublishing.com
Cost	$121.95 *(Price current as of April 2014)*
Purpose	Evaluates young children's communication skills with norm-referenced parent checklists.
Age Range	8 to 37 months
Time	20 to 30 minutes
Scores or Subtests	Consists of two forms/subtests: Words and Gestures (8–16 months) and Words and Sentences (16–30 months).
Description	The infant inventory generates scores for vocabulary comprehension, vocabulary production, and use of gestures. The toddler inventory yields scores for vocabulary production and various aspects of grammatical development. The inventories are completed by parents and rely on a recognition format rather than requiring parents to recall information.
Reliability	All three vocabulary scales and the sentence complexity scales demonstrate high internal consistency with alpha values of .95 or greater. Test-retest reliability: .8–.9+.
Validity	Good face/content validity. Concurrent validity was examined by comparing results to child performance on associated laboratory measures, such as the OWEVT, PLS-4, and Bayley Expressive Language Scale. These correlations were in the .53 to .73 range. It would not be expected that correlations would be higher since the inventories assess a broader vocabulary range than in possible in a picture identification task.
Norms	Normative data are based on 671 infants and 1,142 toddlers from New Haven, Seattle, and San Diego. 77% of the norming population had at least some college education, indicating a lack of representativeness of the norming population.
Who Can Give the Test?	Parent/caregiver inventory.
Strengths	Can be used to document a child's present language level, to develop intervention goals for vocabulary development, and to document vocabulary changes over time; particularly useful for a family-centered early intervention approach.
Concerns	Inventories should not be used to identify infants or toddlers as language delayed, due to the lack of representativeness in the normative sample.

Table A–27. Oral and Written Language Scales (OWLS)

Author	Elizabeth Carrow-Woolfolk
Publisher	Pearson
Contact Information	Pearson Attn: Inbound Sales & Customer Support 19500 Bulverde Road San Antonio, TX 78259-3701	Phone: 800.627.7271 Fax: 800.232.1223 ClinicalCustomerSupport@Pearson.com
Cost	$409.00 *(Price current as of April 2014)*
Purpose	Designed to assess receptive and expressive language.
Age Range	3:0 to 21:11
Time	15 to 40 minutes
Scores or Subtests	3 scores: Listening Comprehension, Oral Expression, Oral Composite.
Description	Listening Comprehension: measured by asking the examinee to select one of four pictures that best depicts a statement. Oral Expression: assessed by asking the examinee to look at one or more line drawings and respond verbally to a statement by the examiner (i.e. tell me what is happening here and how the mother feels . . .). Tests not typical of classroom tasks. Examiner can conduct a descriptive analysis of correct and incorrect responses on the Oral Expression subtest, different classifications of error types. Computer scoring and interpretation available. Test provides opportunity to capture pragmatic and supralinguistic structures of language, connected language.
Reliability	**Reliability type** LC OE Oral comp. Internal Consistency .84 .87 .91 Test-retest .76 .81 .85 Interrater — .95 —
Validity	**Content Validity:** Detailed construct definitions and descriptions of the scales are provided. **Construct Validity:** Developmental Progression of Scores: Listening Comp. and Oral Expression Scales, steady increases in mean raw scores throughout the age range with greater increases in early years and more gradual changes in later years. **Intercorrelations of the Scales:** Moderate intercorrelations between Listening Comp. Scale and Oral Expression Scale, coefficients range from .54 to .77 (mean = .70); Low enough to support that each scale measures something unique but high enough to support combination to produce Oral Composite **Criterion–Related Validity:** Administered OWLS to group of individuals with mild-to-moderate hearing impairment.
Norms	1,795 subjects ranging in age from 3–21 years. Grouped by 6-month age intervals. Sample representative of the U.S. population for gender, geographical region, race/ethnicity, and SES. Norms established by age level.
Who Can Give the Test?	This test should be administered by a professional trained in standardized assessment of children, including but not limited to speech-language pathologists.
Strengths	Both Listening Comprehension and Oral Expression subtests constructed on a basis of a strong theoretical foundation; the test is fairly easy to administer.
Concerns	Because there are no subtests, it does not help identify a child's language strengths and weaknesses.

Table A–28. Preschool Language Assessment Instrument–2 (PLAI-2)

Author	Marion Blank, Susan A. Rose, and Laura J. Berlin
Publisher	Pro-Ed

Contact Information	Pro-Ed, Inc.
	8700 Shoal Creek Boulevard
	Austin, Texas 78757-6897 Customer Service:
	    Phone: 800.897.3202
	    Fax: 800.397.7633
	
	    Publishing Team:
	    Phone: 800.897.3202
	    Fax: 800.397.7633
	
	    info@proedinc.com

Cost	$236.00 *(Price current as of April 2014)*
Purpose	Developed to test a preschool child's discourse skills across 4 different levels of abstraction and two modes of response.
Age Range	3:0 to 5:11
Time	30 minutes
Scores or Subtests	Subtests: matching, selective analysis, reordering and reasoning. Scores: scaled scores, percentile rank, age equivalent, and discourse ability standard score (calculated from two modes of response: expressive and receptive).
Description	Assesses how effectively a child integrates cognitive, linguistic and pragmatic components to deal with student-to-teacher verbal exchanges. Looks at how a child understands and answers different levels of abstract questions.
Reliability	Reliability coefficients of .80 and above were obtained for the Receptive and Expressive Subtests and the Discourse Ability Score across content and time sampling.
Validity	Based on information from the examiner's manual, the PLAI-2 is a valid measure of children's discourse skills.
Norms	Normed on a sample of 463 children in 16 states. Data were collected between spring 1999 and fall 2000. The characteristics of the sample with regard to geographic region, gender, race, ethnicity, family income, educational attainment of parents and disability were compared to those reported in the *Statistical Abstract of the United States* (1999) for the preschool-age population. The comparison demonstrates that the PLAI-2 sample is representative.
Who Can Give the Test?	Anyone who is reasonably competent in the administration of tests in education, language, and psychology.
Strengths	Questions are based off what may be seen in the classroom; includes a nonstandardized assessment which provides diagnostic information about two pragmatic aspects of a child's communication: adequacy of response and selected interfering behavior.
Concerns	Does not give detailed language information. (Should be used in conjunction with another language test such as the PLS-4 or CELF-Preschool 2.)

Table A–29. Preschool Language Scale–4 (PLS-4)

Author	Irla Lee Zimmerman, Violette G. Steiner, and Roberta Evatt Pond
Publisher	Harcourt Assessment Inc.
Contact Information	Pearson Attn: Inbound Sales & Customer Support 19500 Bulverde Road San Antonio, TX 78259-3701 Phone: 800.627.7271 Fax: 800.232.1223 ClinicalCustomerSupport@Pearson.com
Cost	Kit with Manipulatives: $438.25 *(Prices current as of April 2014)*
Purpose	Designed to identify children who have a language disorder or delay.
Age Range	Birth to 6:11
Time	20 to 45 minutes
Scores or Subtests	Consists of 2 core subscales, Auditory Comprehension subscale (AC) and Expressive Communication subscale (EC); Supplemental Instruments-Language Sample Checklist, Articulation Screener, and Caregiver Questionnaire. 3 scores: AC, EC, and Total Lang (TL).
Description	Manipulatives needed for test: medium-sized ball, 5 blocks, 2 small bowls, box with lid, bubbles, 2 small toy cars, a cloth, crackers, 3 small cups, 3 keys on a key ring, paper sandwich bag, 3 plastic spoons, rattle, squeaky toy, teddy bear, several age-appropriate books/toys, watch with a second hand, and a windup toy.
Reliability	Test-retest subscale stability coefficients 0.82-0.95. Cronbach's alpha ranged 0.81–0.91 for TL score. Standard error of measurement reliability coefficient ranged 0.66–0.97, with means of 0.86 on AC, 0.91 on EC, and 0.93 for TL. Inter-rater reliability at 99% (only scores on open-ended tasks used, don't know which tasks considered open-ended). Large differences in amount of time taken to administer and score the test. Possible inconsistencies in administration.
Validity	Elicits similar responses, scoring, and interpretation as the Denver II, which assesses language development level in children. Correlation between PLS-3 and PLS-4 0.65 (AC) and 0.79 (EC). Extensive expert checks throughout instrument development.
Norms	2,400 children who could speak and understand English. Data were collected at 357 sites in 48 states. Age and gender represented equally. Sample stratified based on 2000 Census data by ethnicity, SES, and geography. 13.2% participants identified with conditions/diagnoses.
Who Can Give the Test?	The core subscales (AC and EC) should be administered and scored by qualified users who might include speech-language pathologists, early childhood specialists, psychologists, educational diagnosticians, and others with training in assessment.
Strengths	Child friendly; colorful, appealing pictures and toys; item analysis; available in English and Spanish.
Concerns	Concerns over consistency of administration and scoring; some concern that scores may be inflated when compared to other language tests.

Table A–30. Preschool Language Scale, 5th Edition (PLS-5)

Author	Irla Lee Zimmerman, Violette G. Steiner, and Roberta Evatt Pond
Publisher	Harcourt Assessment Inc.
Contact Information	Pearson Attn: Inbound Sales & Customer Support 19500 Bulverde Road San Antonio, TX 78259-3701 Phone: 800.627.7271 Fax: 800.232.1223 ClinicalCustomerSupport@Pearson.com
Cost	Kit with Manipulatives: $350.00 *(Prices current as of April 2014)*
Purpose	Designed to identify children who have a language disorder or delay. PLS-5 revised most of the questions (25% of the questions are new, 50% are modified from PLS-4, and only 25% of the questions remained unchanged). These new and changed test items are supposedly easier to administer and score.
Age Range	Birth to 7:11
Time	45 to 60 minutes
Scores or Subtests	Total language, auditory comprehension, expressive communication standard scores, growth scores, percentile ranks, language age equivalents.
Description	Manipulatives needed for test: medium-sized ball, 8 blocks, 2 small bowls, bubbles, 2 small toy cars, a washcloth, crackers, 3 small cups, 3 keys on a key ring, 3 plastic spoons, 2 rattle, squeaky duck, plastic teddy bear, comb, paper, pitcher, opaque box with lid, sealable plastic bag, several age-appropriate books/toys, watch with a second hand, and a windup toy.
Reliability	Split half reliabilities range from .80 to .97. Sensitivity for the Total Language score is .83; specificity is .80.
Validity	NA
Norms	Norms are reported for 3-month intervals for children birth to 11 months and 6-month intervals for ages 12 months through 7 years, 11 months. Normed on 1,400 children who could speak and understand English. Data were collected in over 45 states. Sample stratified based on 2008 census data by ethnicity/race, region, and level of caregiver education. Included participants identified with conditions/diagnoses.
Who Can Give the Test?	The core subscales (AC and EC) should be administered and scored by qualified users who might include speech-language pathologists, early childhood specialists, psychologists, educational diagnosticians, and others with training in assessment.
Strengths	Child friendly; colorful, appealing pictures and toys; item analysis; available in English and Spanish.
Concerns	Concerns over consistency of administration and scoring; some concern that scores may be inflated when compared to other language tests.

Table A–31. Receptive-Expressive Emergent Language Test, 3rd Edition (REEL-3)

Author	Kenneth R. Bzoch, Richard League, and Virginia L. Brown
Publisher	Pro-Ed
Contact Information	Pro-Ed, Inc. 8700 Shoal Creek Boulevard Austin, Texas 78757-6897 Customer Service: Phone: 800.897.3202 Fax: 800.397.7633 Publishing Team: Phone: 800.897.3202 Fax: 800.397.7633 info@proedinc.com
Cost	$116.00 *(Price current as of May 23, 2011)*
Purpose	Designed to identify babies or young children with delayed language acquisition, to determine discrepancy between receptive and expressive processes of emergent language, and to document intervention effects.
Age Range	Ages 0 to 36 months
Time	20 to 30 minutes
Scores or Subtests	Receptive Language Ability, Expressive Language Ability, Language Ability.
Description	The Receptive-Expressive Emergent Language Test, 3rd Edition (REEL-3) is a test designed to assess the receptive and expressive emerging language abilities of children from birth to 36 months of age. The REEL-3 assesses two components of emergent language: receptive and expressive language. The REEL-3 also includes a vocabulary inventory and supplementary questions, the purpose of which is to further probe the informant's understanding of the infant's or young child's emergent language abilities. The REEL-3 uses structured questions presented to parents, guardians, or caregivers who are very familiar with the child's language behaviors (i.e., informants). The REEL-3 has 66 questions to be answered by the informant regarding expressive language and 66 questions to be answered by the informant regarding receptive language.
Reliability	Reliability was assessed with internal consistency, test-retest reliability, and inter-rater reliability coefficients. Coefficient alphas ranged from .71 (for 3-month-olds on the Expressive Language subtest) to .98 (for 36-month-olds on the Expressive Language subtest and the Language Ability Composite score) with a mean of .92, .93, and .93 for the Receptive and Expressive Language subtests, and the Language Ability Composite score, respectively. Test-retest reliability was evaluated by assessing 44 infants and toddlers aged 0 to 36 months of age. The correlation coefficients for the Time 1 and Time 2 administrations of the Receptive and Expressive Language subtests and the Language Ability Composite were .89, .78, and .80, respectively. Inter-rater reliability was assessed utilizing Cohen's kappa. The kappa values ranged between .69 and 1.00 (mean of .99), and .79 and 1.00 (mean of .99) for the Receptive and Expressive Language subtests. The mean kappa score for the Language Ability Composite was .99.
Validity	Validity was assessed with content validity (including item rationale, conventional item analysis, and differential item functioning analysis), criterion-related validity, and construct validity. Content validity was demonstrated by comparing test questions to items on other similar measures. Criterion-related validity was examined by comparing the REEL-3 with the DAYC. The correlation coefficients between the standard score on the DAYC Communication subtest and the standard scores from the Receptive and Expressive subtests, and the Language Ability Composite score were .55, .62, and .57, respectively. Construct validity was demonstrated using both age and group differentiation.

Table A–31. *continued*

Norms	The REEL-3 was standardized with a norming group of 1,112 infants and young children from 32 states with 91% of the sample having no disability, 2% having language disabilities, and 7% having 'other' disabilities. The normative sample was very similar to the demographic characteristics of the population of the United States.
Who Can Give the Test?	This test should be administered by a professional trained in standardized assessment of children with hearing loss, including but not limited to speech-language pathologists and teachers.
Strengths	Cost-effective evaluative and diagnostic tool for measuring early receptive and expressive language development.
Concerns	Because this tool is an informant questionnaire, responses may be biased, and not indicative of true performance.

Table A–32. The New Reynell Developmental Language Scales (NRDLS)

Author	Joan K. Reynell and Christian P. Gruber	
Publisher	Western Psychological Services	
Contact Information	Western Psychological Services 12031 Wilshire Blvd. Los Angeles, CA 90025-1251	Phone: 800.648.8857 Fax: 310.478.7838
Cost	$1,320 complete kit *(Price current as of April 2014)*	
Purpose	Developed to measure verbal comprehension and expressive language skills.	
Age Range	2 to 7:6	
Time	30 minutes	
Scores or Subtests	Verbal comprehension and expressive language scores.	
Description	There are 134 test items (67 Verbal Comprehension, 67 Expressive Language). Objects are arranged in a series of scenes or vignettes. There are no basal or ceiling rules. This test is useful in evaluation language processes in children who show delayed development, or physical or psychological disabilities. It identifies the nature and extent of each child's language disability.	
Reliability	Internal consistency reliability coefficients: Verbal Comprehension and Expressive Language scales: 0.90, some 0.80s, for children 3–6 to 4–11 coefficients in the 0.80s, coefficients for children 5–0 to 6–11 below 0.80.	
Validity	Criterion-related validity evidence (concurrent and predictive) was weak. Comes from study with New Zealand children over a decade ago. Limited applicability for American children.	
Norms	Standardized on a sample of 619 children aged 1–0 through 6–11. Children were selected (nonrandomly) by geographic region, ethnicity, parent education level, and sex.	
Who Can Give the Test?	Individuals experienced in language development and assessment.	
Strengths	Engaging stimulus materials; most reliability at youngest age levels.	
Concerns	Technical inadequacies; limited validity and data to support adequacy of test as a diagnostic tool.	

Table A–33. Rossetti Infant-Toddler Scale

Author	Louis Rossetti
Publisher	LinguiSystems
Contact Information	LinguiSystems, Inc. 3100 4th Avenue East Moline, IL 61244 USA	Phone: 800.776.4332 Fax: 800.577.4555 service@linguisystems.com
Cost	$109.95 *(Price current as of April 2014)*
Purpose	Assess communication in the birth to three population through direct observation, elicited behavior, or caregiver's report. Assesses preverbal and verbal areas of: interaction-attachment, pragmatics, gesture, play, language comprehension, & language expression; includes parent questionnaire.
Age Range	Birth to 3/Birth to preK
Time	About 45 minutes
Scores or Subtests	Areas assessed: Interaction-Attachment, Pragmatics, Gesture, Play, Language Comprehension, Language Expression.
Description	Assesses preverbal and verbal areas of communication and interaction, provides an overview of the child's development; monitors early language development. Allows clinician to gather information by: direct observation of the behavior, elicit the desired behavior, and parent reporting of the behavior.
Reliability	N/A
Validity	N/A
Norms	N/A
Who Can Give the Test?	This test should be administered by a professional trained in assessment of child language, including but not limited to speech-language pathologists.
Strengths	Can assess preverbal and verbal aspects of infants' and toddlers' communication development; available in English and Spanish.
Concerns	Parent responses may be biased; may not reflect actual behavior of the child.

Table A–34. Structured Photographic Expressive Language Test, 3rd Edition (SPELT-3)

Author	Janet I. Dawson, Connie E. Stout, and Julia A. Eyer
Publisher	Janelle Publications
Contact Information	Janelle Publications Phone: 800.888.8834 P.O. Box 811 Fax: 815.756.4799 DeKalb, IL 60115 info@janellepublications.com
Cost	$199.00 *(Price current as of April 2014)*
Purpose	Designed to examine expressive use of morphology and syntax.
Age Range	Ages 4 to 9:11
Time	20 minutes
Scores or Subtests	Total score only.
Description	The Structured Photographic Expressive Language Test, 3rd Edition (SPELT-3) is an individually administered 53-item assessment tool that measures a child's generation of specific morphological and syntactic structures. It is designed to elicit responses from children through the use of structured familiar visually and auditorily presented stimuli. The SPELT-3 is intended for use in identifying children whose performance is substantially below their age-equivalent peers in morphosyntactic structures, to note strengths and weaknesses in individual children, and for use in assessing morphosyntax development of children who may speak an African American English dialect.
Reliability	Evidence of score consistency is represented in test-retest, interjudge (i.e., rater) reliability, and internal consistency. Test-retest reliability with a median interval of 11 days was .94. Inter-rater reliability was achieved by having two judges independently score a sample of 85 females and 101 males from eight states. Inter-rater correlations ranged from .97 to .99. Internal consistency estimates on the standardization sample ranged from .76 to .92, with a median reliability estimate of .86.
Validity	Validity for the SPELT-3 was established using content, construct, and concurrent validity. Content validity relied on reviewing existing research on children's development of morphological and syntactical processes relative to the SPELT-II items. One means of evaluating the content was to compare items in the SPELT-3 to items in the Index of Productive Syntax (Scarborough, 1990), a widely used instrument used to analyze spontaneous language in clinical and research settings. The authors reported relevant overlap as evidence of content validity. Because the SPELT-3 is developmental in nature, the authors posited that an increase in age could be expected to parallel an increase in scores: evidence of construct validity. As expected, on the SPELT-3 test scores increased with age. Concurrent validity was established by using the Comprehensive Assessment of Spoken Language (CASL; Carrow-Woolfolk, 1999) as the criterion measure. The correlation between the two measures was .78, indicating substantial overlap between the measures.
Norms	The SPELT-3 was normed on 1,580 children 4 through 9 years of age from 20 states representing four major geographic areas of the United States: West, South, Northeast, and Midwest. Demographically, the distribution of the norming sample reflected closely African American and White children but underrepresented Hispanics. Approximately 7% of the sample was identified as Language Impaired.

continues

Who Can Give the Test?	Examiners using the SPELT-3 are expected to have a thorough grasp of child language development, in particular, a strong emphasis on morphology and syntax, training in evaluation and testing, as well as understanding of test administration, scoring, and test interpretation.
Strengths	Good measurement instrument of morphosyntax structures in children.
Concerns	Lack of sufficient construct validity and limited concurrent validity.

Table A–35. Teacher Assessment of Spoken Language (TASL)

Author	Jean Sachar Moog and Julia J. Biedenstein
Publisher	The Moog Center for Deaf Education
Contact Information	The Moog Center for Deaf Education Phone: 314.692.7172 12300 South Forty Drive Fax: 314.692.8544 St. Louis, MO 63141 publication@moogcenter.org
Cost	$26.95 (manual), $10.00 (package of 10 rating and reference forms) *(Prices current as of April 2014)*
Purpose	Designed to document the development of sentence structure in children with hearing loss.
Age Range	Not specified (but intended for use in school setting)
Time	Varies; ideally, completed over a span of several days/weeks.
Scores or Subtests	Scores given within 5 levels of development: Level 1 (Single Words and Word Combinations), Level 2 (Simple Sentences of Three or More Words), Level 3 (Simple and Complex Sentences of 6 or More Words), Level 4 (Complex Sentences of 8 or More Words, containing 2 verb forms), Level 5 (Very Complex Sentences of 10 or More Words, containing 3 verb forms).
Description	The test includes the TASL Rating Form and the TASL Syntactic Elements Reference Form. The teacher uses the Rating Form to evaluate the child's current level of sentence production as well as set goals for the year. The developers intend the Rating Form to be completed and updated three times per year: once in the beginning of the school year, once in the middle, and once at the end. To administer the TASL, the teacher determines the child's development level based on child's spontaneous use of sentence structure within a language sample. (Note: the language sample is not intended to be brief, but rather a continuous sample taken over time in order to capture the structures a child uses within a variety of communication situations.) The teacher then marks the elements under the level as emerging (used in 50% of obligatory contexts) or acquired (used consistently). Using his or her own understanding of what progress should be expected for the child, the teacher then sets goals for acquisition for the rest of the school year, either within the same developmental level or one above. The accompanying Syntactic Elements Reference Form contains a list of examples for each element and can be used either as a tool for developing lesson plans or as a way to record a child's progress.
Reliability	N/A
Validity	N/A
Norms	N/A
Who Can Give the Test?	The test is designed to be given by the child's classroom teacher; teacher should be comfortable in analyzing grammatical features of child language.
Strengths	This test allows for capturing a child's usage of varied syntactic elements, monitoring change over time, and setting individual goals.
Concerns	Normative information is not available. Therefore, teachers cannot select objectives for a child based on a normative sample. Also, the test can take a long time to administer. While the test account for use of complex syntax at its higher levels, it does not differentiate different types of clauses; in terms of language development, this classification of complex syntax only offers limited information.

Table A–36. Test of Early Language Development, 3rd Edition (TELD-3)

Author	Wayne P. Hresko, D. Kim Reid, and Donald D. Hammill
Publisher	Pro-Ed

Contact Information	Pro-Ed, Inc.
	8700 Shoal Creek Boulevard
	Austin, Texas 78757-6897
	
	Customer Service:
	  Phone: 800.897.3202
	  Fax: 800.397.7633
	Publishing Team:
	  Phone: 800.897.3202
	  Fax: 800.397.7633
	info@proedinc.com

Cost	$341.00 *(Price current as of April 2014)*
Purpose	• Identify candidates for early intervention. • Identify strengths and weaknesses of individual children. • Document children's progress as a consequence of early language intervention program. • Serve as research tool for language development in young children. • Accompany other assessments.
Age Range	2:0 to 7:11
Time	15 to 45 minutes
Scores or Subtests	Receptive Language, Expressive Language, Spoken Language Quotient.
Description	Designed to measure the early development of spoken language in the areas of receptive and expressive language, syntax, and semantics.
Reliability	Extensive studies of test reliability (coefficient alpha, test/retest, immediate test/retest with equivalent forms, and interscorer) support the use of the TELD-3 with individual students.
Validity	Content-description validity was established through careful selection of items, controlled vocabulary, construct review by a panel of language experts, conventional item analysis, differential item functioning analysis, and form equivalence. Criterion-prediction validity was established by correlating TELD-3 standard scores with a variety of widely recognized measures of language ability (i.e., CELF Preschool, EOWPVT, PLS-3, PPVT-Revised, ROWPVT, and TOLDP-3). Construct-identification validity was established by studying (a) the relationship of the TELD-3 standardized scores with age, IQ, and academic achievement and (b) the ability of the TELD-3's standard scores to differentiate groups with known language problems from those without such problems.
Norms	Normed on 2,217 children during 1990–1991 and 1996–1997 from four regions of US, 35 states. Organized by geographic area, gender, race, urban/rural, ethnicity, income, parental educational background, disability status, and age.
Who Can Give the Test?	Examiner should have knowledge of test statistics, administration of standardized measures, test scoring, and score interpretation.
Strengths	Clear test materials, manual easy to follow, later versions revised some reviewers' prior concerns, relatively short test time, flexibility in administration.
Concerns	Some reviewers feel that test does not provide extensive evidence to support purposes (i.e., appropriate refers for early identification).

Table A–37. Test of Language Development–Intermediate: 3 (TOLD-I:3)

Author	Donald D. Hammill and Phyllis L. Newcomer
Publisher	Pro-Ed

Contact Information	Pro-Ed, Inc.
	8700 Shoal Creek Boulevard
	Austin, Texas 78757-6897
	
	Customer Service:
	  Phone: 800.897.3202
	  Fax: 800.397.7633
	
	Publishing Team:
	  Phone: 800.897.3202
	  Fax: 800.397.7633
	
	  info@proedinc.com

Cost	$239.00 *(Price current as of April 2014)*
Purpose	To determine strengths and weaknesses in language skills.
Age Range	Ages 8 to 17:11
Time	30 to 60 minutes
Scores or Subtests	12: General Intelligence/Aptitude Quotient, Spoken Language Quotient (SLQ), Listening Quotient (LiQ), Speaking Quotient (SpA), Semantics Quotient (SeQ), Syntax Quotient (SyQ), Sentence Combining (SC), Picture Vocabulary (PV), Word Ordering (WO), Generals (GL), Grammatic Comprehension (GC), Malapropism (MP).
Description	The TOLD-I was originally developed to bridge the age gap between the Test of Language Development-Primary (TOLD-P), intended to examine the language development of children between the ages of 4:0 and 8:11 years, and the Test of Adolescent Language (TOAL), intended to examine the language development of children between the ages of 12:0 and 18:5 years. The TOLD-I:3 includes a new subtest, Picture Vocabulary, that replaced the Vocabulary subtest. The other subtests remain the same. The TOLD-I:3 assesses overall spoken language, semantics, syntax, listening, and speaking.
Reliability	Reliability was examined with internal consistency and test-retest correlation coefficients. Cronbach's coefficient alphas for 8-, 9-, 10-, 11-, and 12-year-old participants ranged from .80 to .97 for the subtests (*Mdn* = .88). The coefficient alphas for the composites were considerably larger ranging from .92 to .96 (*Mdn* = .94). Coefficient alphas were generated for the subgroups within gender, ethnicity, and disability status which resulted in coefficients ranging from .70 to .97 for the subtests and .90 to .97 for the composites. Test-retest reliability coefficients ranged between .83 to .93 for the subtests and .94 and .96 for the composites.
Validity	Validity was examined using content, criterion-related, and construct validity. Content validity was demonstrated by having professionals rate the test items. Criterion-related validity was assessed by correlating the subtest and composite scores on the TOLD-I:3 and the TOAL-3. The coefficients ranged from .58 to .86 for the subtests and .74 and .88 for the composites. The correlation coefficient between the Spoken Language Quotients for the TOLD-I:3 and the TOAL-3 was quite large (.85). Construct validity was evaluated in multiple ways. Subtest scores were shown to increase with age, disability groups were shown to be differentiated from non-disability groups, and subtest correlation coefficients ranged from .38 to .63 showing that the subtests are measuring a similar construct (language ability).
Norms	The TOLD-I:3 was normed with 779 children from 23 states. The norming sample closely approximated the US Bureau of the Census information with regard to geographic area, gender, race, residence (urban vs. rural), ethnicity, family income, parents' educational attainment, age, and disability status (i.e., no disability, learning disability, speech-language disorder, mental retardation, other).

continues

Table A–37. *continued*

Who Can Give the Test?	This test should be given by a professional trained in standardized assessment of children, including but not limited to speech-language pathologists and audiologists.
Strengths	Carefully constructed test of language ability.
Concerns	Can be lengthy to administer.

Table A–38. Test of Language Development–Primary: 3 (TOLD-P:3)

Author	Phyllis L. Newcomer and Donald D. Hammill
Publisher	Pro-Ed
Contact Information	Pro-Ed, Inc. 8700 Shoal Creek Boulevard Austin, Texas 78757-6897 Customer Service: Phone: 800.897.3202 Fax: 800.397.7633 Publishing Team: Phone: 800.897.3202 Fax: 800.397.7633 info@proedinc.com
Cost	$68.00 (set of 25 record forms; new test version available, therefore this version cannot be purchased). *(Price current as of May 24, 2011)*
Purpose	To determine children's specific strengths and weaknesses in language skills.
Age Range	Ages 4:0 to 8:11
Time	60 minutes
Scores or Subtests	15: Subtests (Picture Vocabulary, Relational Vocabulary, Oral Vocabulary, Grammatic Understanding, Sentence Imitation, Grammatic Completion, Word Discrimination [Optional], Phonemic Analysis [Optional], Word Articulation [Optional]); Composites (Listening, Organizing, Speaking, Semantics, Syntax, Spoken Language).
Description	This test measures receptive and expressive language skills of children in major linguistic areas (semantics, syntax, and phonology).
Reliability	The internal consistency of the subtests is in the .80 to low .90 range, whereas composite data are in the low .90 range. The overall Spoken Language Composite internal consistency is .95 or higher across all ages. The test-retest reliability estimates for the TOLD-P:3 over a 4-month interval are somewhat lower, but acceptable, ranging from .81 to .92. Inter-rater reliability is reported to be uniformly high (.99) across all scales.
Validity	Content validity was investigated qualitatively, through item reviews, as well as quantitatively by using classical item analysis and differential item functioning analysis. Generally, the results support a high degree of content validity, although there is limited item difficulty at ages 4 and 5. Criterion-related validity was examined by correlating scores from the TOLD-P:3 with those from the Bankson Language Test, 2nd Edition, for 30 primary age students. Uniformly high correlations were found supporting convergent validity. Construct validity was investigated through documentation of age differentiation, group differentiation, subtest interrelationships, factor analysis, and item validity.
Norms	The TOLD-P:3 was standardized on 1,000 children between the ages of 4 and 8, with all data collected in the spring of 1996. The normative sample closely approximates the 1990 US Census data on most demographic variables, including geographic region, gender, race, rural versus urban status, ethnicity, educational attainment of parents, and disability status. There was a slight overrepresentation of lower income families.
Who Can Give the Test?	This test should be administered by a professional trained in standardized assessment of childhood language, including but not limited to speech-language pathologists and teachers.
Strengths	Full-color pictures make test more appealing.
Concerns	Does not address all aspects of language, such as pragmatics.

Table A–39. Test of Semantic Skills Primary (TOSS-P)

Author	Linda Bowers, Rosemary Huisingh, Carolyn LoGiudice, and Jane Orman
Publisher	LinguiSystems
Contact Information	LinguiSystems, Inc. 3100 4th Avenue East Moline, IL 61244 USA — Phone: 800.776.4332, Fax: 800.577.4555, service@linguisystems.com
Cost	$169.95 *(Price current as of April 2014)*
Purpose	Analyze the receptive and expressive semantic skills that are crucial for conversation, reading comprehension, and academic achievement.
Age Range	Ages 4 to 8; Grades PreK to 3
Time	25 to30 minutes
Scores or Subtests	Identifying Labels; Identifying Categories; Identifying Attributes; Identifying Functions; Identifying Definitions; Stating Labels; Stating Categories; Stating Attributes; Stating Functions; Stating Definitions.
Description	The TOSS-P assesses a child's semantic skills with five receptive and five expressive tasks. The parallel subtests allow for analysis and comparison of verbal and nonverbal performance. Children respond to 20 picture scenes designed to represent aspects of everyday life that are familiar and important. Test items also emphasize vocabulary that is meaningful and relevant to the experiences of children. The multiple question types in the TOSS-P give subjects ample opportunities to demonstrate the flexibility, diversity, and richness of their language.
Reliability	Reliability Studies: – SEM – Test-Retest – Reliability Based on Item Homogeneity (KR20)
Validity	Validity Studies: – Contrast Groups (t-values): Test discriminates between subjects with normal language develoment and subjects with language disorders. – Point Biserial Correlations – Subtest Intercorrelations – Correlations Between Subtests and Total Test
Norms	This test was normed on 1,510 subjects randomly selected with consideration for race, gender, age, and regional geographic representation. Subjects included in the study: regular education; all socioeconomic levels; White, Black, Hispanic or Latino, Asian, and other groups.
Who Can Give the Test?	The test should only be administered by a trained professional familiar with children's language disorders (e.g., speech-language pathologist, psychologist, teacher of students with learning disabilities, special education consultant, etc.).
Strengths	Easy to use/administer.
Concerns	Limited review/research on this test.

Table A–40. The WORD Test 2: Elementary

Author	Linda Bowers, Rosemary Huisingh, Carolyn LoGiudice, and Jane Orman
Publisher	LinguiSystems
Contact Information	LinguiSystems, Inc. Phone: 800.776.4332 3100 4th Avenue Fax: 800.577.4555 East Moline, IL 61244 USA service@linguisystems.com
Cost	$159.95 *(Price current as of April 2014)*
Purpose	Designed to assess expressive vocabulary and semantics.
Age Range	Grades 1 to 6; Ages 6:0 to 11:11
Time	30 minutes
Scores or Subtests	Associations; Synonyms; Semantic Absurdities; Antonyms; Definitions; Multiple Definitions; Total.
Description	The WORD Test 2 Elementary is a diagnostic test of expressive vocabulary and semantics. It assesses students' grasp of the semantic relationship among words and how effectively students store, recall, and use vocabulary. Categorizing, defining, verbal reasoning, and choosing appropriate words are all indicative of a subject's grasp of semantic attributes. The specific tasks of The WORD Test 2 Elementary are constructed to yield information about these areas of expressive language and to assist the professional in identifying areas of strength and weakness in a child's language.
Reliability	Test-retest reliability coefficients and SEMs for each task and the total test at 6-month age intervals are reported. However, the time interval between the two testings is not mentioned. The lowest test-retest reliability coefficient is .37 in the Flexible Word Use task for the 11 years to 11 years, 5 months age group. The manual explains that several reliability indexes may be low because of the restricted scoring range of the group. On the other hand, test users should keep in mind that reliability indexes might be high for the young age groups. The KR20 estimates of internal consistency reliability for each task are also presented, ranging from .63 to .84. The manual reports 97.8% agreement in scoring six protocols among nine speech-language pathologists.
Validity	Correlations among the tasks average greater than .90, indicating that the different tasks may not necessarily test different language functions. Contrasted-groups validity information was obtained by comparing a sample of students from the normative population with a 'matched sample' of language-disordered students receiving special services.
Norms	This test was normed on 1,940 subjects. Demographics reflect the national school population demographics from the 2000 National Census. Test performances reflect typically-achieving students as well as those in subgroups found in the school population. Subjects included in the study: regular education; special education; language disorders; White, Black, Hispanic or Latino, Asian, Pacific Islander, and Native American groups. Subjects excluded from the study: ESL students with limited English proficiency; degree of hearing loss.
Who Can Give the Test?	The test should only be administered by a trained professional familiar with language disorders (e.g., speech-language pathologist, psychologist, teacher of the learning disabled, special education consultant).
Strengths	Easy to administer/record.
Concerns	Some feel that there should be ceiling rules in scoring this test, especially in certain subtests which may be more difficult for younger or delayed children.

Table A–41. Test of Early Reading Abilities–3 (TERA-3)

Author	D. Kim Reid, Wayne P. Hresko, and Donald D. Hammill
Publisher	Pearson Assessments
Contact Information	Pearson Attn: Inbound Sales & Customer Support 19500 Bulverde Road San Antonio, TX 78259-3701	Phone: 800.627.7271 Fax: 800.232.1223 ClinicalCustomerSupport@Pearson.com
Cost	$316.00 *(Price current as of April 2014)*
Purpose	Assesses mastery of early developing reading skills; five identified purposes: (a) identify children who are below peers in reading development; (b) identify strengths and weaknesses of individual children; (c) document progress as a result of early reading intervention; (d) serve as a measure in reading research; (e) serve as one component of a comprehensive assessment.
Age Range	3:6 to 8:6
Time	30 minutes
Scores or Subtests	Raw scores, age and grade equivalents, percentile scores, standard scores, and confidence scores for three subtests: Alphabet, Conventions, and Meaning. Overall Reading Quotient also calculated.
Description	Assesses the mastery of emergent literacy skills in young children.
Reliability	Test-retest reliability (interval of 2 weeks) resulted in correlation coefficients near .88, most comparisons near .92. Interscorer reliability near .99. Content sampling, Subtest II, Conventions, demonstrates lower reliability (.83) compared to other subtests (about .90) and Reading Composite (.95).
Validity	Content validity established using reviewing research, comparing lists of emerging reading behaviors, subjecting items for expert examination, employing a conventional item analysis, and a differential item functioning analysis. All supported that items on TERA-3 represent behaviors consistent with those expected for emerging readers and without bias.
Norms	Relatively small norm sample, $n = 875$. Matched to the general school- age population (gender, race, ethnicity, SES, disability, and urban/rural). Representative of regions across the US.
Who Can Give the Test?	Nonclinical staff can administer, but authors recommend formal training in assessment with a basic understanding of testing statistics, and general procedures regarding test administration, scoring, and interpretation.
Strengths	Accomplishes stated purposes; useful to combine with other assessments; easy to administer and score; based on modern reading theory.
Concerns	Validity depends on specific use in a given situation.

Table A–42. Test of Preschool Early Literacy (TOPEL)

Author	Ronald A. Madle
Publisher	Pro-Ed

Contact Information	Pro-Ed, Inc.
	8700 Shoal Creek Boulevard
	Austin, Texas 78757-6897
	
	Customer Service:
	  Phone: 800.897.3202
	  Fax: 800.397.7633
	Publishing Team:
	  Phone: 800.897.3202
	  Fax: 800.397.7633
	  info@proedinc.com

Cost	$247.00 *(Price current as of April 2014)*
Purpose	Designed to identify preschoolers who are at risk for literacy problems, allowing early intervention.
Age Range	3:0 to 5:11
Time	25 to 30 minutes
Scores or Subtests	Print Knowledge, Definitional Vocabulary, Phonological Awareness; three subtests are combined to form a measure of emergent literacy skills: the Early Literacy Index (ELI).
Description	Measures abilities associated with early literacy. Identifies children at risk for literacy problems, assists with documenting progress in literacy intervention programs, and provides a research measure of early literacy skills.
Reliability	ELI internal consistency coefficient of .96 (.95 to .96). Phonological Awareness coefficient (.87) is lower but still acceptable. Test-retest for the ELI over 2 weeks was .91, with a mean increase of 3 standard score points. The subtests showed 0–8-point increases on retesting with coefficients from .81 to .89. Interscorer agreement ranged from .96 for Print Knowledge to .98 for the ELI.
Validity	Authors provide review of professional literature on emergent literacy, demonstrating a consensus that skills in the areas of oral language, phonological awareness, and print knowledge serve as the cornerstones for learning to read and write. Authors provide rationale for selection of subtests, formats, and item content, citing both theory and empirical research. Conventional item analyses conducted. Criterion-prediction validity: all subtests and composite had large to very large (.59–.77) relationships with the other measures. Construct validity demonstrated by correlating subtest scores with age and by comparing performance of children from bilingual homes to Hispanic children from homes where only English is spoken.
Norms	Standardization sample of 842 children recruited from 12 states in the 4 major US geographic regions. Sample stratified on age then examined by geographic area, gender, race/ethnicity, Hispanic ethnicity, family income, educational attainment of parents, and exceptionality status.
Who Can Give the Test?	Trained professionals: early childhood educators, special educators, psychologists, or diagnosticians can administer the test after studying the manual and giving a recommended five trial administrations.
Strengths	Quick and easy to administer; well constructed standardization sample with high internal consistency and test-retest reliabilities.
Concerns	Lack of adequate floors and ceilings across the ages covered; subtests cannot obtain suitably low or high scores at a number of ages; the test is heavily loaded on oral language below age 5.

Table A–43. Boehm Test of Basic Concepts–3rd Edition

Author	Ann Boehm
Publisher	PsychCorp, Harcourt Assessment
Contact Information	Pearson — Attn: Inbound Sales & Customer Support — 19500 Bulverde Road — San Antonio, TX 78259-3701 — Phone: 800.627.7271 — Fax: 800.232.1223 — ClinicalCustomerSupport@Pearson.com
Cost	$162.25 complete kit *(Price current as of April 2014)*
Purpose	Designed to assess school readiness or to identify students who may be at risk for learning difficulty.
Age Range	Grades K to 2 (age 5:0 to 7:11)
Time	30 to 45 min. if administered in 1 session; 45 to 60 min. if administered in 2 sessions.
Scores or Subtests	Fifty items are administered in either Form E or F. There is a total score only.
Description	Assesses students' understanding of concepts related to school success. Defines basic concepts as words that describe qualities of people or objects, spatial relationships, time, and quantity.
Reliability	Internal consistency coefficients 0.80–0.91. Standard error measurement ranged from 1.14–2.43, indicating overall low variability. Test-retest reliability coefficients ranged from 0.80–0.89.
Validity	Correlation between Boehm-3 and Boehm-R ranged from 0.61–0.96. Correlation between Boehm-3 and Metropolitan Achievement Tests, 8th ed: 0.58–0.88. Boehm-3 and Metropolitan Readiness Test, 6th ed: 0.48–0.63. Correlation between Boehm-3 and Otis-Lennon School Ability Test, 7th ed: 0.45–0.68. Correlation between Forms E and F on Boehm-3, fall to spring long. study (273 K students) was 0.78.
Norms	Fall and spring standardization samples, fall over 6.000 students in K, 1st, and 2nd grade. Spring over 4,000 students.
Who Can Give the Test?	Test may be administered by teachers or other professionals with experience administering tests, such as speech-language pathologists.
Strengths	The connection between understanding basic concepts and early school success remains a primary concern, lending credibility to this test.
Concerns	Because is it newly developed, the Spanish edition lacks the breadth and depth of reliability and validity evidence that supports the English edition; only assesses receptive skills.

Table A–44. Boehm Test of Basic Concepts–Preschool Version

Author	Ann Boehm
Publisher	PsychCorp, Harcourt Assessment
Contact Information	Pearson Attn: Inbound Sales & Customer Support 19500 Bulverde Road San Antonio, TX 78259-3701 Phone: 800.627.7271 Fax: 800.232.1223 ClinicalCustomerSupport@Pearson.com
Cost	$198.00 *(Price current as of April 2014)*
Purpose	To measure a child's knowledge of 26 basic relational concepts considered necessary for achievement in the beginning years of school; designed to assess knowledge of basic relational concepts such as up-down, tallest-shortest.
Age Range	3:0 to 5:11
Time	20 to 30 minutes
Scores or Subtests	Total score only. Test consists of 76 items with different starting points for 3- and 4-year-olds.
Description	Research shows child's knowledge of basic concepts related to kindergarten readiness, school achievement, and performance on psychoeducational test instruments. The test can help identify a child's specific concept weaknesses, which can be relevant for teachers. The test looks at 26 concepts, two questions for each = 56 test items. The child can earn either a score of 2, 1, or 0 on each concept. 2 = child is familiar with concept and its meaning, 1 or 0 = need for further instruction on the concept. There are 5 warm-up questions that examiner can "help" with but does not explain level of help that should be provided.
Reliability	Items selected based on careful review of research but manual doesn't describe how test was reduced from 40 to 26 concepts. All items were made sure to be up-to-date and appropriate. The latest version includes more difficult items. Internal consistency coefficient alpha ranged from 0.85 to 0.92. Standard error of measurement ranged from 2.08 to 2.88, indicating low variability. Test-retest coefficients ranged from 0.90 to 0.94.
Validity	Content validity compared concepts covered to other tests and research supports the inclusion of the topics. Concurrent validity between Boehm-P and Boehm-3 correlation was 0.94. Between Boehm-P and Bracken Basic Concept Scale-Revised, 0.80 for 3-year-olds and 0.73 for 5-year-olds.
Norms	660 children representative of US.population in terms of gender, race/ethnicity, region, and parental education. Sampled at 6-month intervals from 3:0–5:11 years old.
Who Can Give the Test?	Test may be administered by teachers or other professionals with experience administering tests, such as speech-language pathologists.
Strengths	This test may be a good screening tool for children prior to entering 1st grade.
Concerns	Should not be only tool used to determine school readiness; only assesses receptive skills.

Table A–45. Bracken Basic Concept Scale, Receptive and Expressive–Revised

Author	Bruce A. Bracken
Publisher	Psychological Corporation/Pearson Assessments
Contact Information	Pearson Phone: 800.627.7271 Attn: Inbound Sales & Customer Support Fax: 800.232.1223 19500 Bulverde Road ClinicalCustomerSupport@Pearson.com San Antonio, TX 78259-3701
Cost	$229.00 (Expressive), $325.00 (Receptive)
Purpose	Designed to assess basic concept development of children. Measures comprehension of 308 foundational and functionally relevant educational concepts in 11 subtests or concept categories.
Age Range	2:6 to 7:11
Time	10 to 15 minutes
Scores or Subtests	Colors, Letters, Numbers/Counting, Sizes, Comparisons, Shapes, Direction/Position, Self/Social Awareness, Texture/Material, Quantity, and Time/Sequence.
Description	Can be used diagnostically or as a screening test by scoring first six subtests, which make up the School Readiness Composite (SRC). Can be used for norm-referenced, criterion-referenced, or curriculum-based assessments. The Bracken is a developmentally sensitive measure of children's basic concept acquisition and receptive language skills. Enables examiner to assess important conceptual and receptive language abilities.
Reliability	Split-half reliability coefficients ranged 0.78–0.98 for the subtests and 0.96–0.99 for the entire test. SEM subtests range from 0.4–1.4, with a median of 0.75. The total test SEMs range from 1.6–2.8, with a median of 1.85. Test-retest reliability: Subtest reliabilities range from 0.78 (Quantity, Time/Sequence) to 0.88 (School Readiness Composite) with a median reliability coefficient of 0.81. Test-retest reliability for total test is 0.94.
Validity	Content Validity: Basic concept content well developed. Criterion validity: Concurrent- BBCS-R and BBCS T-test analyses revealed no significant differences between means on both tests. BBCS-R and WPPSI-R: strong correlations. Predictive validity: SRC achieved between 82%–90% correct classification rates when identifying children who were nominated for retention by their classroom teachers. Construct BBCS-R and PLS-3: age-equivalent correlations ranged from 0.78 (Verbal Ability Age) to 0.86 (Language quotient). Internal validity: Subtest intercorrelations range 0.26–0.79 and subtests correlated with total test ranged 0.68–0.92.
Norms	Standardization sample was representative of general US population and stratified by age, gender, race/ethnicity, region, and parent education level. Children were between the ages of 2:6 and 7:11, able to understand and speak English and able to attend to and take the test in English without modifications.
Who Can Give the Test?	Designed to be administered by professionals knowledgeable in the administration and interpretation of educational instruments. Individuals who are involved with psychoeducational assessment of screening (e.g., school psychologists, educational diagnosticians, speech-language pathologists, and special education teachers); can be administered by paraprofessionals under appropriate supervision.
Strengths	Manual provides information about making adaptations for individuals with special needs; there are two forms: expressive and receptive; available in English and Spanish.
Concerns	May be difficult for preschool children to sit for either test (receptive or expressive) in one session.

Table A–46. Bracken School Readiness Assessment, 3rd Edition (BSRA-3)

Author	Bruce A. Bracken
Publisher	Pearson
Contact Information	Pearson Attn: Inbound Sales & Customer Support 19500 Bulverde Road San Antonio, TX 78259-3701 Phone: 800.627.7271 Fax: 800.232.1223 ClinicalCustomerSupport@Pearson.com
Cost	$175.45 *(Price current as of April 2014)*
Purpose	Designed to assess a child's readiness for school by examining concept knowledge and receptive language skills.
Age Range	2:6 to 7:11
Time	10 to 15 minutes
Scores or Subtests	School Readiness Composite (SRC) Total Composite score and descriptive classification; Subtests: percent mastery for colors, letters, numbers/counting, size/comparison, and shapes.
Description	Designed to measure the academic readiness of young children by assessing their understanding of basic concepts in the following six areas: Colors, Letters, Numbers/Counting, Sizes, Comparisons, and Shapes. Can be used as a preschool or kindergarten screener.
Reliability	Split-half reliability (Spearman-Brown) ranged from .78 to .97 and test-retest reliability was .88, which is good.
Validity	Concurrent validity with the revised Bracken Basic Concepts Scale is high (corrected r of .81). Correlation coefficients, using the Wechsler Preschool and Primary Scale of Intelligence-Revised (WPPSI-R) ranged from .76 to .88 and .69 to .79 using the Differential Ability Scales. The correlations with scores with the Peabody Picture Vocabulary Test (3rd edition) and Preschool Language Scales-3 (PLS-3) were adequate.
Norms	Standardization in 1997 involved a sample of 1,100 children representative of the 1995 US Census, including small groups of individuals with disabilities (4%) and gifts/talents (1.7%).
Who Can Give the Test?	Designed to be administered by professionals knowledgeable in the administration and interpretation of educational instruments including classroom teachers, school psychologists, educational diagnosticians, speech-language pathologists, or teacher aides under supervision.
Strengths	The protocols and manual user-friendly.
Concerns	Consider only using for younger children, due to an insufficient ceiling, lower reliability, and a larger standard error of measurement when used with 7-year-old children. The BSRA was developed and normed in 1997, making it less current than the 2002 publication date would otherwise indicate.

Table A–47. Brigance Diagnostic Inventory of Basic Skills, 2nd Edition (CIBS II)

Author	Albert Brigance
Publisher	Curriculum Associates, Inc.
Contact Information	Curriculum Associates Corporate Headquarters P.O. Box 2001 North Billerica, MA 01862-9914 — Phone: 800.255.0248 978.667.8000 Fax: 800.366.1158 978.667.5706 http://www.curriculumassociates.com
Cost	$339.00 *(Price current as of April 2014)*
Purpose	Designed to assess basic readiness and academic skills.
Age Range	Grades K to 6
Time	Specific time limits are listed on many tests, others are untimed.
Scores or Subtests	Readiness, Reading, Word Recognition, Oral Reading, Word Analysis, Vocabulary, Language Arts, Handwriting, Grammar Mechanics, Spelling, Reference Skills, Mathematics, Numbers, Operations, Measurement, Geometry.
Description	Criterion-referenced test designed to measure readiness, reading, language arts, and mathematics. It can be used to assess the presence or absence of specific learning skills within learning hierarchies. The second edition, 2010 Copyright, includes normative information.
Reliability	The manual reports internal consistency score reliability (high: composites ranged from 0.45 [graphomotor and writing skills] to 0.97), standard errors of measurement (appropriate for making score bands: composites ranged from 0.65 to 7.46 SEM), test-retest score reliability (high; expected differences in young children and tasks expected to be demonstrated inconsistently [i.e. motor skills]: .63 to .99), and alternative-forms score reliability (high: .70 to .99).
Validity	The manual reports test content validity (based on extensive academic and sequence studies), construct validity (high correlations between some of the subtests, but some professionals do not test all of the assessment, therefore, they remain included), and positive correlations with other academic assessments, among other data. Information about future performance validity, however, is limited to data gathered from previous versions of this assessment.
Norms	The normative information for the 2010 copyright version originates from a study completed in 2008 using 97 sites within 22 states. The study balanced the number of participants from high, middle, and lower socioeconomic backgrounds. Teachers were recruited to give the assessment from four geographic areas (Northeast, Midwest, South, and West). 383 students participated for the readiness sample and 1,411 children participated for the testing of 1st–6th grade. Participants were categorized according to gender, ethnicity, parents' education levels, and family income (participation in federal free/reduced lunch program). The manual attests that the sample reflects the US population, citing the US Bureau of the Census's American Community Survey and the US Department of Education's National Center for Education Statistics, but it does not specify what year these data were collected. Education level is slightly overrepresented in this sample; however, this indicator was projected to increase according to US census data.
Who Can Give the Test?	Manual recommends using teacher aids or other paraprofessionals to administer test.
Strengths	Highlights specific instructional objectives, helps identify what has and has not been learned.
Concerns	Guidelines on where to begin testing are imprecise. Very limited information about reliability, validity, and norms, unless using 2010 copyright edition. Reliability information based on a relatively small sample.

Table A–48. Brigance Diagnostic Inventory of Early Development—II

Author	Albert H. Brigance and Frances Page Glascoe
Publisher	Curriculum Associates, Inc.

Contact Information	Curriculum Associates
	Corporate Headquarters
	P.O. Box 2001
	North Billerica, MA 01862-9914 Phone: 800.255.0248
	                978.667.8000
	Fax: 800.366.1158
	      978.667.5706
	http://www.curriculumassociates.com

Cost	$299.00 *(Price current as of April 2014)*
Purpose	Designed to "determine readiness for school; track developmental progress; provide a range of scores needed for documenting eligibility for special education service; enable a comparison of children's skills within and across developmental domains in order to view strengths and weaknesses; determine entry points for instruction; and assist with program evaluation."
Age Range	Developmental ages birth to 7 years
Time	20 to 35 minutes
Scores or Subtests	24: Fine Motor (Drawing/Visual Motor, Writing, Total), Gross Motor (Nonlocomotor, Locomotor, Total), Total Motor, Receptive Language (Nouns and Early Listening, Actions, Total), Expressive Language (Isolated Skills, Contextual Skills, Total), Total Language, Academic/Cognitive (Quantitative/General, Prereading/Reading, Total), Daily Living (Self-Help, Prevocational, Total), Social-Emotional (Play Skills and Behaviors, Engagement and Initiative, Total), Total Adaptive Behavior.
Description	Criterion-referenced and norm-referenced. Criterion-referenced and norm-referenced components are administered via a combination of parent and teacher interviews, observations, or from an examiner/examinee interaction. Optional class record book.
Reliability	Data regarding the internal consistency for the five domains, subdomains, and the Total Adaptive Behavior scale are provided. The values of alpha range from a low of .34 to a high of 1.00, with the majority being greater than .80. The test-retest reliability was explored with 36 children from birth to 12 months (test was administered twice within 1 week), and the author also reports the results from a study in 1991 that had 1,156 students (interval between test and retest was not provided). Coefficients for these two studies ranged from .68 to 1.00. Inter-rater reliability, is reported from two different studies, with percentages ranging from .82 to .98.
Validity	The validity of the norm-referenced component of the IED-II was assessed in a number of ways, including measures of content, construct, concurrent, and discriminant validity. The content validity of the IED-II was established by extensive reviews of the literature and with help from child development experts. There is also a study that shows that the raw scores increase as children of increasing ages are tested (which should happen for a test that assesses the progression of developmental skills). The construct validity was determined by examining intercorrelations among all of the IED-II subtests and through factor analysis. The correlations among the subtests were generally adequate, though the results consist primarily of a very large table with very little explanatory text. The correlations presented in the table range from below 0.2 to nearly 1.0. The concurrent validity was assessed with a sample of 484 children who were part of the standardization sample. The children were administered comprehensive measures of cognitive, achievement, language, motor, social-emotional, and adaptive behavior skills. The reported correlations are mostly significant. Discriminant validity was assessed in four different analyses, where children were categorized based on separate criteria. The results of the analyses showed that in all four cases, the groups of children were significantly different on at least some of the IED-II subtests.

continues

Norms	Standardization data for the norm-referenced component: 1,171 children ranging in age from birth to 7 years old. The sample is somewhat representative of the US population for ethnic background, parents' level of education, parents' marital status, and family income, though a disproportionate percent of the participants were recruited from healthcare settings. Data collected from 24 states and territories with participants being about evenly split between males and females. Information not provided regarding the neurological or psychiatric status of the normative sample, including no base rates of occurrence for any identifiable disorders. A large number of normative tables, stratified by ages, are available to provide normative data for domains and subdomains. More scores are available for older children to account for a wider range of measurable abilities.
Who Can Give the Test?	Teacher, developmental/school psychologist, or other early childhood professionals.
Strengths	Criterion and norm-referenced, can estimate skill development and mastery and track changes in short intervals, multiple purposes.
Concerns	Needs additional psychometric validation data.

Table A–49. Kaufman Brief Intelligence Test, 2nd Edition (KBIT-2)

Author	Alan S. Kaufman and Nadeen L. Kaufman
Publisher	PsychCorp/Pearson
Contact Information	Pearson Attn: Inbound Sales & Customer Support 19500 Bulverde Road San Antonio, TX 78259-3701 Phone: 800.627.7271 Fax: 800.232.1223 ClinicalCustomerSupport@Pearson.com
Cost	$250.00 complete kit *(Price current as of April 2014)*
Purpose	Intended as a brief measure of verbal and nonverbal intelligence.
Age Range	Ages 4 to 90
Time	15 to 30 minutes
Scores or Subtests	Verbal, Nonverbal, IQ Composite.
Description	The KBIT-2 is designed for traditional brief assessment purposes such as screening, conducting periodic cognitive re-evaluations, and assessing cognitive functioning when it is a secondary consideration.
Reliability	The KBIT-2's IQ Composite internal consistency coefficient of .93 across ages (.89 to .96) is quite good, with reliabilities increasing with age. The Verbal (.91) and Nonverbal (.88) coefficients are somewhat lower but within acceptable ranges, although the Nonverbal scale coefficients are only .78 at ages 4 and 5. IQ Composite test-retest stability was .90 over mean intervals of 22.5 to 30.8 days, with a mean performance increase of 4 points. The Verbal ($r = .91$) and Nonverbal ($r = .83$) scales each showed similar increases on retesting. Coefficients at different ages were adequate (.83 or higher) except for the Nonverbal scale for the 4- through 12-year age groups (.76).
Validity	Construct validity was demonstrated by showing no meaningful differences across gender as well as showing increases in raw scores across age groups. Gifted children showed higher scores that those with intellectual difficulties. Concurrent validity was demonstrated by comparing the KBIT-2 with the K-BIT, the WASI, and the WISC-III.
Norms	The KBIT-2 standardization sample of 2,120 individuals was stratified on race/ethnicity, geographic region, and educational level using the March 2001 Current Population Survey. A close match was obtained except for region, where the South was overrepresented (44.2% versus 36.0%) and the Northeast was under sampled (11.4% versus 19.8%).
Who Can Give the Test?	The test may be administered by trained technicians or paraprofessionals as well as qualified professionals, but results should always be interpreted by a properly qualified professional.
Strengths	Well-designed screening test.
Concerns	The Nonverbal scale requires some interpretive caution for preschool and primary-age children.

Table A–50. Kaufman Survey of Early Academic and Language Skills (K-SEALS)

Author	Alan S. Kaufman and Nadeen L. Kaufman
Publisher	PsychCorp/Pearson
Contact Information	Pearson Attn: Inbound Sales & Customer Support 19500 Bulverde Road San Antonio, TX 78259-3701 Phone: 800.627.7271 Fax: 800.232.1223 ClinicalCustomerSupport@Pearson.com
Cost	$304.95 complete kit *(Price current as of April 2014)*
Purpose	Measure children's language, preacademic skills, and articulation.
Age Range	3:0 to 6:11
Time	15 to 25 minutes
Scores or Subtests	Eight subtests: Vocabulary, Numbers/Letters and Words, Articulation Survey, Early Academic and Language Skills Composite, Language Scales (Expressive Skills, Receptive Skills), Early Academic Scales (Number Skills, Letter and Word Skills).
Description	Can be used for assessment in day care centers, schools, and clinic situations. Targeted to be "more in tune with the curriculum used for intervention or enrichment programs" than intelligence tests.
Reliability	Test-retest: values range from .94 (total composite) to .87 (vocabulary subtests). Internal consistency: – Subtests: .88 to .94 – Scales: .81 to .94 – Composite: .94
Validity	Validation sample: Three subtests show range of intercorrelations from .47 to .67, with Expressive Skills and Receptive Skills Composites showing intercorrelations from .91 to .91. Lack of differentiation among composite scores and lack of meaningful differences among subtests, suggesting overall composite only generally useful score. K-SEALS composite score correlates well with teacher ratings of ability, $r = 0.60$.
Norms	1,000 children, diverse sample across age, gender, race/ethnic, and geographic groups. Norms presented by age. No data presented to describe gender and race/ethnic group differences in scores for subtests or composite scores.
Who Can Give the Test?	The examiner should be trained in administering standardized tests and have speech/language knowledge (for articulation test).
Strengths	Easy to administer, short general intelligence test.
Concerns	Little to offer for differential diagnosis. Lack of validation data to support differential interventions on basis of relative differences between scores and composites. 30% of standardization sample 2:0 to 5:11 had statistically significant differences between Vocabulary and Numbers/Letters and Words Subtests, but test does not explain how to interpret such differences.

Table A–51. Learning Accomplishment Profile, Diagnostic Edition, 3rd Edition (LAP-D, LAP-D Screen, LAP-R, E-LAP)

Author	Aubrey D. Nehring, Elma F. Nehring, John R. Bruni, Patricia L. Randolph, Kaplan Press, Anne R. Sanford, Janet G. Zelman, Elayne M. Golver, and Jodi L. Preminger
Publisher	Kaplan Early Learning Company
Contact Information	Kaplan Early Learning Company 1310 Lewisville Clemmons Rd. Lewisville, NC 27023 Phone: 800.334.2014 336.766.7374 Fax: 800.452.7526 info@kaplanco.com
Cost	$799.95 *(Price current as of April 2014)*
Purpose	Designed to provide the teacher of the young child with a simple criterion-referenced tool for systematic assessment of the child's existing skills.
Age Range	LAP-D 30 to 72 months; LAP-R: 36 to 72 months; Early LAP: birth to 36 months
Time	45 to 90 minutes
Scores or Subtests	Fine Motor (Writing, Manipulation), Language (Comprehension, Naming), Gross Motor (Body Movement, Object Movement), Cognitive (Counting, Matching), Pre-Writing, Self-Help, Personal/Social, Social/Emotional.
Description	4 tests available: Learning Accomplishment Profile Diagnostic Edition, Learning Accomplishment Profile Diagnostic Edition Normed Screen, Learning Accomplishment Profile-Revised Edition, Early Learning Accomplishment Profile. LAP-D Screen, Early LAP, LAP-R are Criterion-Referenced and LAP-D is norm-referenced. Designed "to assist in making relevant educational decisions with regard to young children and to enable the teacher to develop instructional objectives and strategies that are developmentally appropriate."
Reliability	The test manual reports reliability through examination of the correlations with age (strong, .73 to .90), internal consistency (very strong for each subscale and domain, .89 to .97 and .69 to .92 for age groups), standard errors of measurement (fairly small, which indicates that scores can be reflective of true performance), test-retest reliability (very good: .95 to .97 for domain and .88 to .96 for subscale), and inter-rater reliability (high: .90 to .93 for domain and .82 to .93 for subscale).
Validity	The test manual reports that the test's study of construct validity resulted in high positive correlations between subsets, but different performance across ages. This result suggests that while the test might measure similar a similar construct across subscales and domains, it captures information about separate aspects of development. Criterion/concurrent validity is also reported, comparing performance to the Dial-3 or WJ-R (for English examinees) and the Dial-3 and the Batería-R (for Spanish examinees). The LAP-D and Dial-3 showed moderate-very strong correlations (.50 to .92). Correlations were .50 to .79 for LAP-D and WJ-R/Batería-R. Strong correlations (.52 to .83) were also reported between the LAP-D and PPVT-III/TVIP.

continues

Norms	Normed on 2,099 children between 30 and 72 months of age. 77 of these children had diagnosed disabilities; these children were included to examine the test's appropriateness for use with this population. Stratified sample based on language, geographic region, age, race, gender, and type of setting (day care, public school, private school, etc.). Chosen based on 2000 US Census data. Four geographic regions were selected for sampling: Northeast, South, Central, and Southwest (the test manual lists the specific locations which are representative of these regions).
Who Can Give the Test?	Teachers, psychometrists, psychologists, or others who have been trained in its administration. Does not require a special educational level, licensure, or certification.
Strengths	Can be used as part of a multidisciplinary assessment to determine eligibility or to plan and monitor a child's progress. Various tests available based on child's age/assessment desired.
Concerns	Individual objectives linked directly to test items, concern that teacher may "teach to the test." Items narrow in focus and don't always address very functional skills. Norms could be updated.

Table A–52. Leiter International Performance Scale, Revised (Leiter-R)

Author	Gale H. Roid and Lucy J. Miller
Publisher	Stoelting Co.
Contact Information	Stoelting Co. 620 Wheat Lane Wood Dale, Illinois 60191 Phone: 800.860.9775 630.860.9700 Fax: 630.860.9775 Info@StoeltingCo.com
Cost	$925.00 *(Price current as of April 2014)*
Purpose	Constructed as a nonverbal cognitive assessment.
Age Range	Ages 2:0 to 20:11
Time	90 minutes
Scores or Subtests	31 subtests: – Visualization and Reasoning (Figure Ground, Design Analogies, Form Completion, Matching, Sequential Order, Repeated Patterns, Picture Context, Classification, Paper Folding, Figure Rotation); – VR Composite (Fluid Reasoning, Brief IQ, Fundamental Visualization, Spatial Visualization, Full IQ); – Attention and Memory Associated Pairs, Immediate Recognition, Forward Memory, Attention Sustained, Reverse Memory, Visual Coding, Spatial Memory, Delayed Pairs, Delayed Recognition, Attention Divided; and – AM Composite (Memory Screen, Associative Memory, Memory Span, Attention, Memory Process, Recognition Memory).
Description	The Leiter International Performance Scale has recently been updated and standardized on over 2,000 children and adolescents. Its primary purpose continues to be nonverbally assessing the cognitive development of special populations of individuals aged 2 years up to 21 years for whom the usual tests of cognitive abilities are inappropriate. Examples of these populations include those who are deaf, mentally handicapped, speech and language impaired, learning disabled, brain injured, and ESL populations.
Reliability	Average coefficients range from .69 to .90 for internal consistency reliabilities and retest reliabilities. Scores on the AM Battery subtests and composite scores were less stable than scores on the VR Battery.
Validity	Content validity evidence for the test comes from ratings provided by 60 examiners involved in the tryout phase and 114 examiners involved in the standardization phase of data collection. Criterion-related measures were derived by comparing the Leiter-R to other tests of intelligibility, including the WISC-III, Stanford-Binet Intelligence Scale-Fourth Edition, the Wide Range Assessment of Learning and Memory, and the Test of Memory and Learning. Correlations were high enough to suggest that similar abilities are being tested.
Norms	Two samples were used for standardization, a VR Battery sample of 1719 children and an AM Battery sample of 763 children. The test was also administered to 701 atypically developing children with various disabilities. Representation of the samples in terms of region, SES, gender, race, and other variables was slightly nonrepresentative in some cases, but adequate.

continues

Table A–52. *continued*

Who Can Give the Test?	This test should be given by a professional trained in standardized assessment of children, including but not limited to speech-language pathologists and teachers. Examiners should practice giving this test before actually using it, due to the inability to give verbal instructions. Special training in administering the test battery is available through the test publisher as well as college and university courses.
Strengths	Carefully developed test battery.
Concerns	Reliability/Validity scores were partially based on the 1995 standardization administration and have small sample sizes. New scores based on the final edition of the Leiter-R would be preferable.

Table A–53. Mainstream Assessment of Readiness for Children Over Five (MARCOF)

Author	Cynthia S. Robinson
Publisher	Med-El Corporation (North America)
Contact Information	Med-El Corporation Phone: 888.633.3524 2511 Old Cornwallis Road, Suite 100 919.572.2222 Durham, NC 27713 Fax: 919.484.9229 usaeducators@medel.com
Cost	$25.00 *(Price current as of May 26, 2011)*
Purpose	Designed to provide an analysis of the readiness of children with hearing loss to enter mainstream education with hearing peers.
Age Range	5 years+
Time	Information not available.
Scores or Subtests	Audiogram-Access to Sound; Standardized Criteria; Nonstandardized Criteria; Listening Behaviors in Classroom; Spoken Language Skills; Written Language; Overall Academic Considerations; Repair Strategies; Self-advocacy; Test-taking Skills; Independent Work Habits; Social/Emotional Behaviors; Life Experiences; Receiving School-Audiological Considerations; Receiving School-General; Parental Support; Total Score.
Description	MARCOF is a tool for educators and families designed to evaluate the strengths and weaknesses of children with hearing loss who are being considered for mainstream placement. Scores from standardized and nonstandardized assessments should be used to complete this worksheet.
Reliability	N/A
Validity	N/A
Norms	N/A
Who Can Give the Test?	Professionals familiar with the child's strengths and weaknesses should work with the child's parents to complete the worksheet.
Strengths	Good measure for families and professionals to evaluate a child's overall strengths and readiness for mainstream education.
Concerns	Scores may differ depending on who is filling out the worksheet.

Table A–54. Peabody Individual Achievement Test, Revised (PIAT-R)

Author	Frederick C. Markwardt, Jr.
Publisher	PsychCorp/Pearson
Contact Information	Pearson Attn: Inbound Sales & Customer Support 19500 Bulverde Road San Antonio, TX 78259-3701 Phone: 800.627.7271 Fax: 800.232.1223 ClinicalCustomerSupport@Pearson.com
Cost	$522.00 *(Price current as of April 2014)*
Purpose	Designed to measure academic achievement.
Age Range	Ages 5 to 22:11, Grades K to 12
Time	60 minutes
Scores or Subtests	Nine subtests: General Information, Reading Recognition, Reading Comprehension, Total Reading, Mathematics, Spelling, Total Test, Written Expression, Written Language.
Description	The 1998 edition of the Peabody Individual Achievement Test–Revised/Normative Update (PIAT-R/NU) is identical to the 1989 edition but with new norms. The PIAT-R is an individually administered achievement battery that provides wide-range assessment in six content areas including General Information, Reading Recognition, Reading Comprehension, Mathematics, Spelling, and Written Expression.
Reliability	The PIAT-R reports four types of reliability: split-half, Kuder-Richardson, test-retest, and item response theory. Split-Half reliability for the composites ranges from .95 to .99. The lowest coefficient, .83, occurred in Mathematics at the lowest age tested. Test-retest reliability is fairly good, with correlations ranging from the lower to upper .90s for the composites.
Validity	The PIAT-R reports both content and construct validity. Correlations with the PPVT suggest a verbal-conceptual component to this test, not just reading proficiency alone. Because this validity data is so old, newer validity data (correlated with other updated assessments) would be beneficial.
Norms	The new norm tables were developed on a representative sample of 3,184 students in kindergarten through 12th grade in 129 sites in 40 states. The researchers used a stratified multistage sampling procedure to ensure selection of a nationally representative group at each grade. Sampling targets were based on the March 1994 US Census Bureau data.
Who Can Give the Test?	This test should be administered by someone skilled in standardized assessment of children, including but not limited to speech-language pathologists and teachers.
Strengths	Good, broad test of educational achievement.
Concerns	Reliability and validity evidence is the result of studies completed in the 1970s and 1980s, and could be updated.

Table A–55. Stanford Achievement Test Series, 10th Edition (SAT 10)

Author	Harcourt Assessment, Inc.
Publisher	Harcourt Assessment, Inc., PsychCorp/Pearson
Contact Information	Pearson Phone: 800.627.7271 Attn: Inbound Sales & Customer Support Fax: 800.232.1223 19500 Bulverde Road ClinicalCustomerSupport@Pearson.com San Antonio, TX 78259-3701
Cost	$60.00 (per exam) *(Price current as of April 2014)*
Purpose	Measures student achievement in reading, language, spelling, listening, mathematics, science, and social science.
Age Range	Grades K.0 through 12.9
Time	105 to 295 minutes for Basic Battery 135 to 330 minutes for Complete Battery 160 to 212 minutes for Abbreviated Battery
Scores or Subtests	Sounds and Letters, Word Study Skills, Word Reading, Sentence Reading, Reading Comprehension, Total Reading, Mathematics, Mathematics Problem Solving, Mathematics Procedures, Total Mathematics, Language, Spelling, Listening to Words and Stories, Listening, Environment, Science, Social Science.
Description	The Stanford Achievement Test, 10th Edition (Stanford 10) is the latest in a long line of distinguished achievement test batteries dating back to 1923. The Stanford 10 can be administered as either the Full-Length Battery or the Abbreviated Battery. Braille and large print editions are available. The Stanford 10 is untimed. The directions indicate that students be allowed to continue working on a test as long as they are working productively. Suggested times are for planning only. The Stanford 10 consists of 13 test levels that cover kindergarten through Grade 12.
Reliability	The technical report states that the battery exhibits a 'high degree' of internal consistency reliability. Indeed, a review of the multitude of tables of KR20 coefficients for the full-length test (Forms A and B) shows the majority of them to be in the mid-.80s to .90s-certainly satisfactory for the purposes of this test. As would be expected, the coefficients for the abbreviated test tend to be a bit lower, with the majority falling in the .80s. For Forms A and B, correlations across the various tables ranged from .53 to .93, but were usually in the .80s for the various tests composing Forms A and B. Composite scores, such as Total Reading and Total Mathematics were generally close to .90.
Validity	Internal-consistency reliability was determined to be good. Content validity has been built into the test through the well-defined test blueprint and the careful development process. An appendix in the technical data report provides numerous correlations between the various subtests and totals of the Stanford 10 levels with the subtests of the Stanford 9. These correlations, which range from .70s-.80s, provide evidence of convergent validity. Also, correlations between the Stanford 10 and the OLSAT 8 provide additional evidence of construct validation.

Norms	Norms for the Stanford 10 reflect the K–12 population (2002). Both spring and fall norms are provided. The spring standardization involved 250,000 students, and the fall standardization involved 110,000. School districts were chosen based on a stratified cluster sampling design that included variables such as geographic region, SES, urbanicity, and ethnicity. Stratification variables reflected the 2000 Census of Population and Housing and the 2000–2001 National Center for Education Statistics. Special education students who would routinely be tested were included in the standardization samples. The norms are presented in the Spring Multilevel Norms book and the Fall Multilevel Norms book.
Who Can Give the Test	This test is typically administered by teachers in a classroom/group setting.
Strengths	Comprehensive achievement test with solid history; Carefully developed according to high measurement standards; Untimed to reduce test anxiety.
Concerns	It is up to the user to determine that the content of the test matches the curricula and goals of the particular school.

Table A–56. Test of Nonverbal Intelligence, 3rd Edition (TONI-3)

Author	Linda Brown, Rita J. Sherbenou, and Susan K. Johnson
Publisher	Pro-Ed

Contact Information	Pro-Ed, Inc.
	8700 Shoal Creek Boulevard
	Austin, Texas 78757-6897 Customer Service:
	   Phone: 800.897.3202
	   Fax: 800.397.7633
	
	   Publishing Team:
	   Phone: 800.897.3202
	   Fax: 800.397.7633
	
	   info@proedinc.com

Cost	$376.00 complete kit *(Price current as of April 2014)*
Purpose	Developed to assess aptitude, intelligence, abstract reasoning, and problem solving in a completely language-free format.
Age Range	Ages 6:0 through 89:11
Time	15 to 20 minutes
Scores or Subtests	Total score only.
Description	The 3rd edition of the Test of Nonverbal Intelligence (TONI-3) is described as "a language-free measure of cognitive ability." It is designed to assess the aptitude of those whose cognitive, linguistic, or motor skills would interfere with optimal performance on traditional tests of intelligence.
Reliability	Alpha coefficients and standard errors of measurement (SEMs) were calculated for 20 age intervals, delineated by whole years until age 19 and by decades thereafter. The average coefficient for both forms was .93, and the ranges were .89 to .97. SEMs ranged from 3 to 5. Alpha coefficients were: .96 on both forms for males; .95 on both forms for females, Hispanic examinees, and for deaf examinees; .94 on both forms for African Americans and for learning-disabled examinees; and .92 on both forms for gifted examinees. test-retest correlations with a one-week separation ranged from .89 to .94 for both forms for 13-year-olds, 15-year-olds, and 19–40-year-olds. Rescoring of test protocols from the normative sample by staff members of Pro-Ed's research department yielded .99 correlations for each form of the test, providing strong evidence of interrater reliability for trained scorers.
Validity	Correlations between the TONI-3 and the WISC-III range from .53 to .63. The authors base their arguments for content validity on rationales for format and items, classical item analysis, and differential item functioning (DIF) analysis. The argument for content validity rests heavily on the fidelity of the test items to the domain.
Norms	The TONI-3 was administered in 1995 to 2,060 individuals and again in 1996 to another 1,391 individuals, for a total of 3,451 examinees chosen to represent the United States population geographically, and by gender, community type, ethnicity and races, disabling condition, and socioeconomic status.
Who Can Give the Test?	This test should be administered by someone skilled in standardized assessment of children, including but not limited to speech-language pathologists and teachers.
Strengths	Good test of intelligence for those who do not speak English or who have sensory deficits.
Concerns	Only moderately correlated with the WISC-III.

Test of Nonverbal Intelligence, 4th Edition (TONI-4)

The TONI-4 is now available, which contains updated normative information based on a sample of 2,272 people representing 33 different states. With the updated normative information, newer reliability and validity information is available. This updated version also eliminates floor effects.

Table A–57. Universal Nonverbal Intelligence Test (UNIT)

Author	Bruce A. Bracken and R. Steve McCallum
Publisher	Riverside Publishing
Contact Information	Riverside Publishing 3800 Golf Road, Suite 100 Rolling Meadows, IL 60008 Phone: 800.323.9540 630.467.7000 (outside US) Fax: 630.467.7192 RPC_Customer_Service@hmhpub.com
Cost	$618.00 *(Price current as of May 19, 2011)*
Purpose	Designed to provide a more fair measure of the general intelligence and cognitive abilities of children and adolescents who may be disadvantaged by traditional verbal and language-loaded measures.
Age Range	Ages 5 to 17:11, Grades K to 12
Time	10 to 15 minutes: Abbreviated Battery 30 minutes: Standard Battery 45 minutes: Extended Battery
Scores or Subtests	11: Symbolic Memory, Cube Design, Spatial Memory, Analogic Reasoning, Object Memory, Mazes, Memory Quotient, Reasoning Quotient, Symbolic Quotient, Nonsymbolic Quotient, Full Scale IQ.
Description	The UNIT was designed to provide an accurate assessment of intellectual functioning for children and adolescents for whom traditional language-loaded measures may not be appropriate due to speech, language, or hearing impairments, differences in cultural background, or certain psychiatric disorders. The UNIT measures two components of intelligence: memory and reasoning.
Reliability	For the standardization sample, reliability estimates for the full scale range from .84 to .94 for the Abbreviated Battery, from .89 to .95 for the Standard Battery, and from .91 to .94 for the Extended Battery, with the majority of the coefficients in the higher end of each range. The estimates for the clinical/exceptional sample are slightly higher at .96, .98, and .98 for the Abbreviated, Standard, and Extended Batteries, respectively. Subtest reliabilities were somewhat lower, as would be expected. Averaged across all ages, these ranged from .64 for the Mazes subtest to .91 for Cube Design. Test retest reliability was estimated over a 3-week time interval for a sample of 197 children. After correction for restriction of range, these coefficients range from .78 to .91 for the Standard and Extended Battery full scale scores; values for the Abbreviated Battery are only slightly lower, ranging from .74 to .89.

continues

Validity	Evidence of concurrent validity was presented through correlations of the UNIT with the Wechsler Intelligence Scale for Children, 3rd Edition (WISC-III), the Woodcock-Johnson Psycho-Educational Battery,Revised (WJ-R), the Kaufman Brief Intelligence Test (K-BIT), and the Test of Nonverbal Intelligence, 2nd Edition (TONI-2), among others. Although these studies were based on small samples of children, the evidence obtained from them is generally supportive of the validity of the UNIT as a measure of intelligence that shares considerable variance with these commonly used scales. Correlations of the UNIT with measures of academic achievement such as the Tests of Achievement of the WJ-R, the Spanish form of the Woodcock Language Proficiency Battery, Revised (WLPB-R), the Wechsler Individual Achievement Test (WIAT), and the Peabody Individual Achievement Test,Revised (PIAT-R) were presented as evidence of predictive validity. These correlations were typically much lower than those of the UNIT with other measures of intelligence, and varied somewhat widely across the different studies.
Norms	The UNIT was standardized on a carefully chosen, nationally representative sample of 2,100 children aged 5 years, 0 months to 17 years, 11 months, and 30 days. The sample was stratified on the following variables: gender, race, Hispanic origin, region, parental educational attainment, community setting, classroom placement (regular or special education), special education services received (learning disability, speech and language impairments, serious emotional disturbance, mental retardation, giftedness, English as a second language and bilingual education, and regular education).
Who Can Give the Test?	This test should be given by a professional trained in standardized assessment of children, including but not limited to speech-language pathologists and teachers.
Strengths	Provides a much-needed means of obtaining reliable and valid assessments of intelligence for children with a wide array of disabilities who cannot be tested accurately with existing instruments.
Concerns	Validity evidence based on larger groups, as well as studies of predictive validity for school-related measures would be desirable.

Table A–58. Wechsler Individual Achievement Test, 3rd Edition (WIAT-III)

Author	Pearson
Publisher	Pearson
Contact Information	Pearson Attn: Inbound Sales & Customer Support 19500 Bulverde Road San Antonio, TX 78259-3701 Phone: 800.627.7271 Fax: 800.232.1223 ClinicalCustomerSupport@Pearson.com
Cost	$665.00 complete kit *(Price current as of April 2014)*
Purpose	Designed to identify a student's academic strengths and weaknesses, to help make decisions for educational services eligibility, to make educational placements, to diagnosis a specific learning disability, and to plan learning objectives and interventions.
Age Range	4:0 to 19:11 (although norms are also available for ages 20:0–50:11)
Time	Varies greatly, depending on age of examinee and the number of administered subtests. Average administration time: 1 to 17 minutes.
Scores or Subtests	24 total scores (16 subtests and 8 composite scores): Subtests: Listening Comprehension, Early Reading Skills, Reading Comprehension, Math Problem Solving, Alphabet Writing Fluency, Sentence Composition, Word Reading, Essay Composition, Pseudoword Decoding, Numerical Operations, Oral Expression, Oral Reading Fluency, Spelling, Math Fluency–Addition, Math Fluency–Subtraction, and Math Fluency–Multiplication. Composite Scores: Oral Language, Total Reading, Basic Reading, Reading Comprehension & Fluency, Written Expression, Math Fluency, and Total Achievement (raw scores can also be converted into Standard Score, Percentile Rank, Age or Grade Equivalent, Normal Curve Equivalent, Stanine, and Growth Scale Value).
Description	Examiner can administer one, some, or all of the subtests; not all subtests contribute to the Total Achievement composite. The revision of this test is a result of an effort to align with recent state regulations and federal mandates. The Math Fluency and Oral Reading Fluency subtests are new to this edition and were added to identify learning disabilities within the specifications of federal law. This comprehensive assessment of academic ability has value for diagnostic and objective purposes. The test can be scored either by hand or by using the Scoring Assistant software (for Windows only).
Reliability	The manual provides reliability information for each subscale and composite and for each grade level or age. Test-retest estimates for subtests were adequate for the subtests (range: .83–.97) with the exception of the Alphabet Fluency section, with a reported reliability estimate of less than .70. Interscorer agreement is also adequate, with reported reliability for objective tests as 98%–99% and subjective tests as 91%–99%. The reliability information included with the WIAT-III is comprehensive, and it even includes information often left out of assessment manuals.
Validity	The technical manual cites three studies to illustrate three types of validity: content, convergent, and special group. Content correlations between similar subtests of WIAT-II and WIAT-III ranged from .62–.86. The moderate-to-high correlations suggest strong convergent validity for the interpretation of subtests/composites.
Norms	Normative information was obtained using a stratified sample of 2,775 students grades PK–12, based on US Census data from 2005. Student characteristics categorized within this sample are Grade, Age, Sex, Race/Ethnicity, (parent) Education Level, and Geographic Region.

continues

Table A–58. *continued*

Who Can Give the Test?	Professionals trained in administering individually administered psychological or educational assessments.
Strengths	Well constructed assessment which provides strong reliability and validity information, based on representative norms.
Concerns	Even though the test makers promote the test's usage for planning instruction and intervention, the manual provides not reliability or validity information for this purpose. Also, the test manual does not provide evidence regarding differences in test use and interpretation between race/ethnicity or age groups.

Table A–59. Wechsler Intelligence Scale for Children, 4th Edition (WISC-IV)

Author	David Wechsler
Publisher	PsychCorp/Pearson
Contact Information	Pearson Phone: 800.627.7271 Attn: Inbound Sales & Customer Support Fax: 800.232.1223 19500 Bulverde Road ClinicalCustomerSupport@Pearson.com San Antonio, TX 78259-3701
Cost	$1,069.00 complete kit *(Price current as of April 2014)*
Purpose	Designed to assess the cognitive ability of children.
Age Range	Ages 6:0 to 16:11
Time	Core Subtests: 65 to 80 minutes Supplemental: 10 to 15 minutes
Scores or Subtests	• Verbal Comprehension (Similarities, Vocabulary, Comprehension, Information, Word Reasoning, Total); • Perceptual Reasoning (Block Design, Picture Concepts, Matrix Reasoning, Picture Completion, Total); • Working Memory (Digit Span, Letter-Number Sequencing, Arithmetic, Total); • Processing Speed (Coding, Symbol Search, Cancellation, Total); and • Total.
Description	The WISC-IV is the latest revision of Wechsler's intelligence tests for children and adolescents. It is an individually administered intelligence test designed for children 6 years 0 months to 16 years 11 months.
Reliability	Average coefficients across age groups ranged from .79 to .90 for core subtests and .79 to .88 for supplemental subtests. Except for Processing Speed coefficients, all Index coefficients were at or above .90 at all ages. FSIQ reliability was greater than .96 for all ages. Test-retest reliability coefficients present evidence of score stability.
Validity	Content validity was demonstrated. Abundant correlation coefficients are presented as evidence for score validity. In addition to correlations of WISC-IV subtests with each other, also reported are correlations of WISC-IV scores with WISC-III, WPPSI-III, WAIS-III, WASI, WIAT-II, CMS, GRS, BarOn EQ, and ABAS-II scores. All correlation scores were acceptable or better. See technical manual for more detailed information.
Norms	The standardization sample included 2200 examinees, representative of the March 2000 US Census data in regards to age, gender, race, ethnicity, parent education level, and four geographical regions.
Who Can Give the Test?	Examiners should be familiar with the Standards for Educational and Psychological Testing (AERA, APA, & NCME, 1999), have completed graduate training in assessment or be supervised by such a person, and have specialized training when testing persons from unique linguistic, cultural, or clinical backgrounds.
Strengths	A well-developed upgrade of the WISC-III, with improved correlation coefficients. User-friendly and developmentally appropriate.
Concerns	Updated psychometric methods would have been preferred.

Table A–60. Wechsler Preschool and Primary Scale of Intelligence, 3rd Edition (WPPSI-III)

Author	David Wechsler
Publisher	PsychCorp/Pearson
Contact Information	Pearson Attn: Inbound Sales & Customer Support 19500 Bulverde Road San Antonio, TX 78259-3701 Phone: 800.627.7271 Fax: 800.232.1223 ClinicalCustomerSupport@Pearson.com
Cost	$1,086.00 complete kit *(Price current as of APRIL 2014)*
Purpose	Developed for assessing the intelligence of children
Age Range	2:6 to 7:3
Time	30 to 45 minutes for ages 2:6 to 3:11. 60 minutes for ages 4 to 7:3
Scores or Subtests	• Verbal (Receptive Vocabulary, Information, Picture Naming, Vocabulary, Word Reasoning, Comprehension, Similarities); • Performance (Block Design, Object Assembly, Matrix Reasoning, Picture Concepts, Picture Completion); • Processing Speed (Coding, Symbol Search); and • Global Language Composite.
Description	Designed to measure the intelligence of children between the ages of 2 years 6 months to 7 years 3 months. The test kit comes with two manuals, two stimulus books, manipulatives, a scoring template, and an initial supply of test booklets. There are two sets of core subtests for two different age groups. The lower age group has four core subtests and the older age group has seven core subtests.
Reliability	Split-half reliability estimates are acceptable at the subtest level across ages (.83–.95), with only a few subtests being less than .80 at specific ages. Full Scale internal consistency coefficient of .96 is excellent, with all age groups having an internal consistency of .95 or higher. Remaining composites show internal consistency coefficients between .89 and .95 across ages. Interscorer agreement is high. Test-retest reliability ranged from .86 to .92 over an average of 26 days.
Validity	Validity is extensively covered in the test manual. When the WPPSI-R and WPPSI-III were administered to 176 children the results supported the view that the scales measure similar constructs. Corrected correlations were .86, .70, and .85 for Verbal, Performance, and FSIQs respectively. The lower correlation for Performance was thought to be from the WPPSI-III's increased emphasis on fluid ability over visual-spatial tasks on the WPPSI-R. The WPPSI-III was also compared to the WISC-III, the Bayley, the Differential Ability Scales, the Children's Memory Scale, and the WIAT-II. All showed acceptable correlations.
Norms	This test was normed on a sample of 1700 children divided into 9 age groups. The group is comparable to the 2000 US Census data for race/ethnicity and parental education level, as well as other common variables. Geographic sampling is not as well stratified.
Who Can Give the Test	This test should be given by a professional trained in standardized assessment of children, including but not limited to speech-language pathologists and teachers.
Strengths	This new, updated version of the test is more user-friendly, more consistent with current research, and more child-friendly.
Concerns	There is some debate over whether a test of processing speed should be included in a test of intelligence.

Table A–61. Wide Range Achievement Test, 4th Edition (WRAT4)

Author	Gary S. Wilkinson and Gary J. Robertson
Publisher	Psychological Assessment Resources, Inc.
Contact Information	PAR, Inc. 16204 North Florida Avenue Lutz, FL 33549 Phone: 800.331.8378 813.449.4065 Fax: 800.727.9329 http://www4.parinc.com
Cost	$315.00 complete kit *(Price current as of April 2014)*
Purpose	Designed to measure the basic academic skills of reading, spelling, and math computation.
Age Range	Ages 5 to 94
Time	15 to 45 minutes
Scores or Subtests	Five subtests: Word Reading, Sentence Comprehension, Spelling, Math Computation, Reading Composite.
Description	The Wide Range Achievement Test: Fourth Edition (WRAT4) is a norm-referenced achievement test designed to measure the core academic skills of Math Computation, Spelling, Word Reading, and Sentence Comprehension. Uses of the WRAT4 include collecting initial evaluation data, screening individuals to identify persons who might need a more in-depth academic assessment, as part of a re-evaluation of individuals diagnosed with learning and/or cognitive disorders and evaluating achievement-ability discrepancies to identify specific learning disabilities, determining minimal proficiency levels needed to perform in particular educational or vocational settings, for progress monitoring purposes, or using test results as part of a re-evaluation or a comprehensive evaluation for individuals with learning and/or cognitive disorders.
Reliability	Internal consistency reliability coefficients (coefficient alpha) were presented for single ages 5–12, 2-year age groupings 13–18, 6-year groupings at ages 19–24, and 10-year groups ages 25–94+. The reliability estimates for the four subtests and Reading Composite are excellent for screening purposes and good for individual decision making across most age groups. Median corrected alpha reliability coefficients on the four subtests ranged from .87–.93 by age group and .83–.93 by grade level. Reliability coefficients for the Reading Composite ranged from .95–.96 by age and grade. Alternate form retest reliability data were collected 1 month later on average, and corrected stability coefficients ranged from .68 (Sentence Comprehension for ages 19–94) to .92 (Spelling for ages 19–94) for the age-based sample and ranged from .75 (Math Computation) to .90 (Reading Composite) for the grade level sample.
Validity	Minimal evidence for internal validity is presented. There is not an in-depth discussion regarding the development of the test items, criteria for item selection, or relevancy of items. As evidence of content validity, the authors indicate that 77% of the WRAT4 items were retained from the previous WRAT3 (and earlier test editions), which had reportedly undergone thorough statistical analysis during the WRAT3 standardization and review by outside experts (to ensure freedom from ethnic or gender bias and current relevance). Construct validity is demonstrated by increasing raw scores as age and grade increases. Convergent validity was assessed by correlating WRAT4 subtests with similar subtests from a number of well-established achievement tests and cognitive ability measures. The authors also provide data on the relationship between the WRAT4 subtests and the corresponding subtests of the WRAT-Expanded edition. Results indicate moderate to moderately high convergent validity and demonstrate the predicted patterns of relationships.

continues

Norms	The normative sample is based on 3,021 individuals between 5 and 94 years of age. The authors state that the "normative sample was selected according to a stratified national sampling procedure with proportionate allocation controlled for age, gender, ethnicity, geographic region, and educational attainment as an index of socioeconomic status" (professional manual, p. 2).
Who Can Give the Test?	All parts of the WRAT4 require individual administration by either a trained assessor or a paraprofessional, with the exception of Part 2 of the Spelling and Math Computation subtests which, reportedly, can be administered in a small-group format to participants 8 years or older.
Strengths	Relatively brief measure that is easy to administer.
Concerns	Basal and ceiling rules are complex.

Table A-62. Woodcock-Johnson Tests of Achievement (WJ III)

Author	Richard W. Woodcock, Kevin S. McGrew, and Nancy Mather
Publisher	Riverside Publishing
Contact Information	Riverside Publishing 3800 Golf Road, Suite 100 Rolling Meadows, IL 60008 Phone: 800.323.9540 630.467.7000 (outside US) Fax: 630.467.7192 RPC_Customer_Service@hmhpub.com
Cost	$608.00 *(Price current as of May 25, 2011)*
Purpose	Measures academic achievement across several subject areas.
Age Range	2 to 90+ years
Time	Varies, about 5 minutes per test
Scores or Subtests	The WJ III NU Tests of Achievement has two parallel forms (A and B) that are divided into two batteries—Standard and Extended. The Standard Battery includes tests 1 through 12 that provide a broad set of scores. The 10 tests in the Extended Battery provide more in-depth diagnostic information on specific academic strengths and weaknesses. Examiners can administer the Standard Battery either alone or with the Extended Battery.
Description	Practitioners use the WJ III NU Tests of Achievement to help assess students for learning disabilities and to determine if they need special services. The WJ III NU Tests of Achievement include tests and clusters that directly parallel those outlined by IDEA and provide sound procedures for determining learning variances between abilities and achievement. **Subject areas tested include:** Oral Expression Listening Comprehension Written Expression Basic Reading Skills Reading Comprehension Reading Fluency Math Calculation Skills Math Reasoning
Reliability	Most of the WJ III NU tests show strong reliabilities of .80 or higher; several are .90 or higher. The WJ III NU interpretive plan is based on cluster interpretation. The WJ III NU clusters show strong reliabilities, most at .90 or higher. The reliability characteristics of the WJ III NU meet or exceed basic standards for both individual placement and programming decisions.
Validity	Content validity has been demonstrated in relation to the Cattell-Horn-Carroll theory of cognitive abilities. Internal validity was demonstrated with high correlations, and concurrent validity was tested again the Wechsler Preschool and Primary Test of Intelligence–Revised. Correlations ranged from .66–.73.

continues

Norms	Normative data for the test were gathered from 8,818 subjects in over 100 geographically diverse communities in the United States. Individuals were randomly selected within the stratified sampling design that controlled for 10 specific community and individual variables and 13 socioeconomic status variables. The sample consisted of 1,143 preschool subjects; 4,784 kindergarten to twelfth-grade subjects; 1,165 college and university subjects; and 1,843 adult subjects. The WJ III NU uses continuous-year norms to yield normative data at 10 points in each grade. It provides age-based norms by month from ages 24 months to 19 years and by year from ages 2 to 90+ years. And it provides grade-based norms for kindergarten through 12th grade, 2-year college, and 4-year college, including graduate school.
Who Can Give the Test?	Any person administering the WJ III ACH needs thorough knowledge of the exact administration and scoring procedures and an understanding of the importance of adhering to these standardized procedures. Competent interpretation of the WJ III ACH requires a higher degree of knowledge and experience than is required for administering and scoring the tests. Graduate-level training in educational assessment and a background in diagnostic decision-making are recommended. Only trained and knowledgeable professionals who are sensitive to the conditions that may compromise, or even invalidate, standardized test results should make interpretations and decisions. The level of formal education recommended to interpret the WJ III ACH is typically documented by successful completion of an applicable graduate-level program of study that includes, at a minimum, a practicum-type course covering administration and interpretation of tests of academic achievement.
Strengths	Good measure of general achievement.
Concerns	Test time can be quite long when all subtests are administered at once.

Table A–63. Young Children's Achievement Test (YCAT)

Author	Wayne P. Hresko, Pamela K. Peak, Shelley R. Herron, and Deanna L. Bridges
Publisher	Pro-Ed
Contact Information	Pro-Ed, Inc. 8700 Shoal Creek Boulevard Austin, Texas 78757-6897 — Customer Service: Phone: 800.897.3202 Fax: 800.397.7633 Publishing Team: Phone: 800.897.3202 Fax: 800.397.7633 info@proedinc.com
Cost	$250.00 *(Price current as of April 2014)*
Purpose	Designed to help determine early academic abilities
Age Range	4:0 to 7:11
Time	25 to 45 minutes
Scores or Subtests	General Information, Reading, Mathematics, Writing, Spoken Language, Early Achievement Composite; Provides Standard Scores, Age Equivalents, and Percentiles.
Description	The Y-CAT measures early academic abilities to help identify young children who are at risk for school failure. It is designed for English-speaking preschoolers, kindergarteners, and first-graders.
Reliability	Internal consistency values ranged from .74 (General Information, Age 7) to .92 (Reading, Age 4). Most subtest values in the mid- to high .80s. Early Achievement Composite Score had high internal consistency values: .95 to .97. Alphas calculated for nine subgroups, almost all were in .90s for various subtests and ranged from .97 to .99 for composite score. Test-retest reliability calculated using sample of 190 children from two different schools, high scores ranging from .97 to .99 (approximately 2-week interval). Interscorer reliability: correlations between two graduate students scores ranged from .97 to .99, indicating high degree of agreement.
Validity	Content validity: authors reviewed early childhood tests and curriculum materials. Criterion-related validity: Concurrent validity measured by correlating YCAT performance with Comprehensive Scales of Student Abilities, Kaufman Survey of Early Academic and Language Skills, the Metropolitan Readiness Tests, and the Gates-MacGinitie Reading Tests. Most correlations show concurrent validity. Construct Validity: six premises—age differentiation, group differentiation, YCAT's relationship to academic ability, YCAT's relationship to intelligence, subtest interrelationships, and item validity. Does differentiate between students on basis of age. Subgroups (Whites, Blacks, Hispanics, individuals with ADHD) performed identical, though individuals with learning disabilities and mental retardation performed lower, as was expected. Subtests all intercorrelated, with values ranging from .57 to .71. Items of subtest correlated well with total score on subtest.
Norms	Based on 1,224 children sampled from 32 states. Sample designed to be representative of nation and census for geographic region, gender, race, residence, ethnicity, family income, parents' educational attainment, and disability status.

continues

Table A–63. *continued*

Who Can Give the Test?	Should be administered by a person with formal training in administering and interpreting results from assessments. Manual cites guidelines suggested by Anastasi and Urbina (1997) and also recommends examiner has supervised training in using screening tests and practiced administering YCAT several times.
Strengths	Simple administration, colorful easel display format, reliability, validity, well-written test manual.
Concerns	Differential item functioning using Delta Pilot approach (some research says flawed approach).

Table A–64. Expressive One-Word Picture Vocabulary Test (EOWPVT)

Author	Rick Brownell (editor)
Publisher	Academic Therapy Publications
Contact Information	Academic Therapy Publicaitons Phone: 800.422.7249 20 Commercial Blvd. Fax: 888.287.9975 Novato, CA 94949 sales@academictherapy.com
Cost	$175 for the complete kit; $40.00 for the record forms (*(Price current as of October 2014)*.
Purpose	Designed to assess an individual's single-word expressive vocabulary.
Age Range	2:0 to 70+
Time	15 to 25 minutes
Scores or Subtests	Total score only.
Description	The child is shown a picture and is asked to label it.
Reliability	Coefficient alpha to assess homogeneity of test items, median coefficient was 0.96 with range of 0.93 to 0.98. Split-half coefficients reflected median of 0.98 → good internal consistency; Test-retest: only 20 days in between but strong test-retest correlations; Inter-rater reliability: strong confidence level for inter-rater reliability.
Validity	Content-test: simplicity doesn't test other language skills; correlated with 12 other vocabulary measures but correlations not high, median 0.79; Construct: does not correlate well with tests of other domains.
Norms	Normed on 2,327 individuals, norms reflect use of broad demographic characteristics.
Who Can Give the Test?	This test should be administered by a professional trained in standardized assessment of children, including but not limited to speech-language pathologists.
Strengths	Colorful illustrations; directions included on record form along with prompts; speed of administration; can be used in conjunction with ROWPVT to assess receptive and expressive vocabulary. Spanish-Bilingual (2012) version is available.
Concerns	Limited scope of test; only assesses child's ability to label.

Table A–65. Expressive Vocabulary Test–2 (EVT-2)

Author	Kathleen T. Williams
Publisher	Pearson Assessments
Contact Information	Pearson Attn: Inbound Sales & Customer Support 19500 Bulverde Road San Antonio, TX 78259-3701 Phone: 800.627.7271 Fax: 800.232.1223 ClinicalCustomerSupport@Pearson.com
Cost	$441.65 (for both Forms and scoring software) *(Price current as of April 2014)*
Purpose	Designed to assess an individual's single-word expressive vocabulary.
Age Range	2:6 to 90
Time	10 to 20 minutes
Scores or Subtests	Total score only.
Description	Some of the test items require the child to label items while others require the child to produce a synonym. (e.g. The child is shown a picture and the examiner says, "Tell me another word for *below*.") Some other items require the child to produce a word when given a definition. (e.g., The child is shown a picture and the examiner says, "Tell me a word that means a trip by sea.")
Reliability	Internal consistency reliability By Age: Split-Half • Form A: M = .94 • Form B: M = .93 Standard Error of Measurement • Form A: 3.8 • Form B: 3.9 By Grade: Split-Half • Form A: M = .93 • Form B: M = .93 Standard Error of Measurement • Form A: 4.0 • Form B: 4.0 Alternate-form reliability By Age: M = .87 Test–retest reliability By Age: M = .95

Validity	EVT–2 With the PPVT–4 Scale (N = 3,540): Average *r* = .82
	EVT–2 With the CASL:
	Ages 3–5 years (N = 68)
	• Basic Concepts: *r* = .59 • Antonyms: *r* = .67 • Sentence Completion: *r* = .51
	Ages 8–12 years (N = 62)
	• Synonyms: *r* = .50 • Antonyms: *r* = .84 • Sentence Completion: *r* = .72 • Lexical/Semantic Composite: *r* = .80
	EVT–2 With the CELF-4 Scale:
	Ages 5–8 years (N = 55)
	• Core Language: *r* = .80 • Receptive Language: *r* = .68 • Expressive Language: *r* = .79
	Ages 9–12 years (N = 56)
	• Core Language: *r* = .75 • Receptive Language: *r* = .69 • Expressive Language: *r* = .77
	EVT–2 With the GRADE (Total Test score):
	• K, Fall (Level P, N = 50): *r* = .76
	• K, Spring (Level K, N = 65): *r* = .59
	• 1 (N = 52): *r* = .60
	• 2 (N = 48): *r* = .57
	• 3 (N = 63): *r* = .79
	• 4 (N = 61): *r* = .72
	• 6 (N = 49): *r* = .64
	• 8 (N = 47): *r* = .67
	• 10–11 (N = 52): *r* = .64
	EVT–2 With EVT (N = 377): Average *r* = .81
Norms	Data from 4,000 individuals were used for the norm sample. This sample was matched to the U.S. population for sex, race/ethnicity, geographic region, SES, and clinical diagnosis or special ed. placement. Standardization occurred in fall 2005 and spring 2006.
Who Can Give the Test	This test should be administered by a professional trained in standardized assessment of children, including but not limited to speech-language pathologists.
Strengths	Easy to administer, age appropriate starting points are tabbed in the test book; Quick evaluation of expressive vocabulary and word retrieval; assesses more than ability to label; can be used in conjunction with PPVT to assess receptive and expressive vocabulary.
Concerns	Interscorer consistency has not been demonstrated; criterion-related validity is limited.

Table A–66. Peabody Picture Vocabulary Test–4 (PPVT–4)

Author	Lloyd M. Dunn and Douglas M. Dunn
Publisher	Pearson Assessments
Contact Information	Pearson Attn: Inbound Sales & Customer Support 19500 Bulverde Road San Antonio, TX 78259-3701 Phone: 800.627.7271 Fax: 800.232.1223 ClinicalCustomerSupport@Pearson.com
Cost	$441.00 (for both Forms and scoring software) or $238.70 (for one form) *(Price current as of April 2014)*
Purpose	Designed to assess an individual's single-word receptive vocabulary.
Age Range	2:6 to 90 years and older
Time	10 to 15 minutes
Scores or Subtests	No subtests. Can be used along with a test of expressive vocabulary if desired. Scores: Raw scores converted to standard scores, can be converted to percentile ranks, normal curve equivalents, stanines, and age and grade equivalents.
Description	The PPVT-4 is an individually administered, untimed measure of receptive vocabulary. There are two forms, Form A and Form B. Both forms consist of 228 items, each containing four colored pictures arranged on a single space. The examinee points to the picture that best describes the meaning of a word spoken verbally by the examiner.
Reliability	Internal consistency reliability By Age: Split-Half • Form A: M = .94 • Form B: M = .94 Standard Error of Measurement • Form A: 3.6 • Form B: 3.6 By Grade: Split-Half • Form A: M = .95 • Form B: M = .94 Standard Error of Measurement • Form A: 3.6 • Form B: 3.7 Alternate-form reliability By Age: M = .89 Test–retest reliability By Age: M = .93

Table A–66. *continued*

Validity	• Validity: Correlations The PPVT–4 Scale With the EVT–2 (N = 3,540): Average $r = .82$ The PPVT–4 Scale With the CASL: Ages 3–5 years (N = 68) • Basic Concepts: $r = .50$ • Antonyms: $r = .41$ • Sentence Completion: $r = .54$ Ages 8–12 years (N = 62) • Synonyms: $r = .65$ • Antonyms: $r = .78$ • Sentence Completion: $r = .63$ • Lexical/Semantic Composite: $r = .79$ The PPVT–4 Scale With the CELF-4 Scale: Ages 5–8 years (N = 55) • Core Language: $r = .73$ • Receptive Language: $r = .67$ • Expressive Language: $r = .72$ Ages 9–12 years (N = 56) • Core Language: $r = .72$ • Receptive Language: $r = .75$ • Expressive Language: $r = .68$ The PPVT–4 Scale With the GRADE (Total Test score): • K, Fall (Level P, N = 50): $r = .71$ • K, Spring (Level K, N = 65): $r = .40$ • 1 (N = 52): $r = .58$ • 2 (N = 48): $r = .43$ • 3 (N = 63): $r = .65$ • 4 (N = 61): $r = .66$ • 6 (N = 49): $r = .71$ • 8 (N = 47): $r = .79$ • 10–11 (N = 52): $r = .59$ The PPVT–4 Scale With the PPVT–III Scale (N = 322): Average $r = .84$.
Norms	Data from 4,000 individuals were used for the norm sample. This sample was matched to the US population for sex, race/ethnicity, geographic region, SES, and clinical diagnosis or special ed. placement. Standardization occurred in fall 2005 and spring 2006.
Who Can Give the Test?	The PPVT-4 is designed to be administered by a Level B examiner (i.e., Bachelors degree with coursework in principles of measurement, administration, interpretation of tests, and formal training in the content area).
Strengths	Easy to administer with short test administration time; can be used in conjunction with EVT to assess expressive and receptive vocabulary.
Concerns	Somewhat restrictive means of assessing receptive vocabulary due to single-word only format.

Table A–67. Receptive One-Word Picture Vocabulary Test (ROWPVT)

Author	Rick Brownell (editor)
Publisher	Academic Therapy Publications
Contact Information	Academic Therapy Publications 20 Commercial Blvd. Novato, CA 94949 Phone: 800.422.7249 Fax: 888.287.9975 sales@academictherapy.com
Cost	$175 for the complete kit; $40.00 for the record forms *(Price current as of October 2014)*
Purpose	Assesses receptive vocabulary by asking examinee to match object's concept with name.
Age Range	2:0 to 70+
Time	15 to 25 minutes
Scores or Subtests	Total score only.
Description	170-item multiple choice test that assesses an individual's English-hearing vocabulary, reflecting the extent of his or her understanding of single words. Not a timed test; has basal and ceiling rules.
Reliability	Internal consistency-coefficient alpha range 0.97–0.99. Test-retest correlations ranged from 0.78–0.93, coefficient of 0.84 for entire sample, not good stability. Inter-rater reliability 100% agreement but small sample size (30).
Validity	Criterion-compared to 12 other tests that measure receptive language, correlation coefficients ranged from 0.44–0.97.
Norms	Derived from random international sample of 2,327 (all primarily English speakers at school and home).
Who Can Give the Test?	Speech/language pathologists, psychologists, counselors, learning specialists, physicians, occupational therapists, and other personnel who are under the supervision of a professional familiar with assessment and interpretation most often administer the test.
Strengths	Easy to administer with short test administration time; can be used in conjunction with EOWPVT to assess expressive and receptive vocabulary. Spanish-Bilingual (2012) version available.
Concerns	Somewhat restrictive means of assessing receptive vocabulary due to single-word-only format.

APPENDIX B

Resources

Alexander Graham Bell Academy for Listening and Spoken Language

http://www.listeningandspokenlanguage.org/AGBellAcademy/

A website for professional seeking certification or currently certified Listening and Spoken Language Specialists (LSLS™) that work with infants and children who are deaf or hard of hearing and their families.

Address: 3417 Volta Place, NW, Washington, DC 20007

(202) 204-4700 – (Voice)
(202) 337-8314 – (Fax)

E-mail: academy@agbell.org

Alexander Graham Bell Association for the Deaf & Hard of Hearing

http://www.agbell.org

International nonprofit membership organization, support network, and resource center on pediatric hearing loss and spoken language approaches and related issues.

Address: 3417 Volta Place, NW, Washington, DC 20007

(202) 337-5220 – (Voice)
(202) 337-5221 – (TTY)
(202) 337-8314 – (Fax)

Email: info@agbell.org

American Auditory Society

http://www.amauditorysoc.org

Purpose is to increase the knowledge and understanding of the ear, hearing, and balance; their disorders and how to prevent them; and habilitation and rehabilitation of individuals with hearing and balance dysfuntion.

Address: 352 Sundial Ridge Circle, Dammeron Valley, UT 84783-5196

(435) 574-0062 – Voice

American Speech-Language-Hearing Association (ASHA)

http://www.asha.org/

http://www.asha.org/practice-portal/

http://www.asha.org/Advocacy/
state/Performance-Assessment-of-Contributions-and-Effectiveness/?utm_source=
asha&utm_medium=enewsletter&utm_campaign=accessschools032114

Provides information on newborn hearing screening guidelines, current legislation, continuing education, and a special interest group, SIG 9–Hearing and Hearing Disorders in Childhood.

Address: 10801 Rockville Pike, Rockville, MD 20852

(800) 638-8255 – (Voice, TTY)

E-mail: actioncenter@asha.org

American Society for Deaf Children (ASDC)

http://www.deafchildren.org

A national organization of families and professionals that helps create opportunities for children who are deaf and hard of hearing to gain full communication access, particularly through the use of sign language.

Address: 3820 Hartzdale Drive, Camp Hill, PA 17011

(800) 942-2732 – (Voice Hotline, Toll-free)
(866) 895-4206 – (Voice)
(717) 703-0073 – (Voice)
(717) 909-5599 – (Fax)

E-mail: asdc@deafchildren.org

Beginnings For Parents of Children Who Are Deaf or Hard of Hearing, Inc.

https://www.ncbegin.org/

Provides emotional support and access to information as a central resource for families with children who are deaf or hard of hearing, age birth through 21 years of age.

Address: P.O. Box 17646, Raleigh, NC 27619

(800) 541-HEAR – (Toll-free for NC only, Voice, TTY)
(919) 850-2746 – (Voice, TTY)

Boys Town National Research Hospital

http://www.boystownhospital.org/Pages/default.aspx

http://www.babyhearing.org/Parent2Parent/index.asp

Provides parents with a variety of helpful information related to hearing loss in children and information about how some parents have responded to their child's hearing loss and how they have learned to better cope with it.

Address: 555 N 30th St., Omaha, NE 68131

(402) 452-5000 – (Voice)
(800) 448-3000 – (Voice, Toll-free, 24 hours a day)
(800) 448-1833 – (TTY, Toll-free, 24 hours a day)

Centers for Disease Control and Prevention (CDC)

http://www.cdc.gov/ncbddd/hearingloss/index.html

Provides information on hearing screenings and diagnoses, treatments, and research. The site also provides free downloadable resources and materials, available at http://www.cdc.gov/ncbddd/hearingloss/freematerials.html. The CDC Early Hearing 411 app (EHDI411) has been designed and developed by the Early Hearing Detection and Intervention (EHDI) team, National Center for Birth Defects and Developmental Disabilities (NCBDDD), the CDC. The main purpose of this app is to provide a way for parents to manage their children's early hearing care information and share on-line medical and public health resources on infant and/or child hearing loss. The EHDI App is available on iTunes.

Center for Hearing and Communication

http://www.chchearing.org

Works to improve the quality of life for people with all degrees of hearing loss and to offer comprehensive services regardless of age or mode of communication.

Address: 50 Broadway, New York, NY 10004

(917) 305-7700 – (Voice)
(917) 305-79999 – (TYY)

Center for Parent Information and Resources (Formerly known as National Dissemination Center Information Center for Children & Youth with Disabilities [NICHCY])

http://www.parentcenterhub.org

National information and referral center that provides information on disabilities and related issues, with a focus on children from birth through 22 years of age.

Address: Center for Parent Information and Resources, c/o Statewide Parent Advocacy Network, 35 Halsey St., Fourth Floor, Newark, NJ 07102

(973) 642-8100 – (Voice)

E-mail: malizo@parentcenterhub.org

Early Hearing Detection & Intervention–Pediatric Audiology

http://ehdipals.org/

Provides links to services, information, resources, and services for children with hearing loss. Also provides information about local audiology facilities and professional resources.

Family Voices

http://www.familyvoices.org

A national, grassroots organization that is a clearinghouse for information and education concerning the health care of children with special health needs.

Address: 2340 Alamo SE, Ste. 102, Albuquerque, NM 87106

(505) 872-4774 – (Voice)
(888) 835-5669 – (Voice, Toll-free)
(505) 872-4780 – (Fax)

E-mail: kidshealth@familyvoices.org

Hands & Voices

http://www.handsandvoices.org

Hands and Voices is a parent driven, nonprofit organization dedicated to providing unbiased support to families with children with hearing loss.

Address: Families For Hands & Voices, PO Box 3093, Boulder, CO 80307

(217) 357-3647 – (Voice)
(866) 422-0422 – (Voice, Toll-free)

E-mail: parentadvocate@handsandvoices.org

Healthy Children

http://www.healthychildren.org

This website provides links and information about child development, healthy living, safety, and new research. There are links to healthcare sites and tips and tools to educate parents and caregivers. Developed from the American Academy of Pediatrics.

Hear Me Foundation

http://www.hearmefoundation.org

Promotes positive life experiences via camp activities and year-round events primarily for oral-deaf and hard-of-hearing children, their siblings, and their families.

Address: 4814 Woodstream Village Drive, Kingwood, TX 77345

(281) 359-6725 – (Voice)

Hereditary Hearing Loss

http://hereditaryhearingloss.org/

The Hereditary Hearing loss Homepage aims to give an up-to-date overview of the genetics of hereditary hearing impairment for researchers and clinicians.

John Tracy Clinic

http://www.jtc.org

A website for families with a child who is deaf or hard of hearing and the professionals that provide intervention including parent education course and services to children who are deaf or hard of hearing.

Address: 806 West Adams Boulevard, Los Angeles, CA 90007

(213) 748-5481 – (Voice)
(213) 747-2924 – (TYY)

Listen-Up Web!

http://www.listen-up.org/

Provides resources and information geared to the special needs of children who are deaf and hard of hearing, and their families.

E-mail: kay@listen-up.org

National Association for the Deaf

http://www.nad.org

This is a federation of state associations, organization and corporate affiliates, and individuals advocating for the civil rights of deaf and hard of hearing Americans.

Address: 8630 Fenton Street, Suite 820, Silver Spring, MD 20910-4500

(301) 587-1788 – (Voice)
(301) 587-1789 – (TYY)

National Center for Hearing Assessment & Management (NCHAM)

http://www.infanthearing.org/

Provides information on newborn hearing screening programs, legislation, equipment, and other related issues.

Address: Utah State University, 2880 Old Main Hill, Logan, UT 84322

(435) 797-3584 – (Voice)

E-mail: mail@infanthearing.org

FAMILY RESOURCES

Colorado Families for Hands & Voices

http://cohandsandvoices.org/rmap/roadmap/

This organization is designed to: arm families with the knowledge of "next steps" following a referral on the hearing screen and/or diagnosis of hearing loss; help families get the support they need well before the 1, 3, and 6 month EHDI guidelines; keep babies safe from the risks of unnecessary sedation for diagnostic hearing testing by using natural sleep before three months of age; and encourage an ongoing discussion of hearing screening at birth as well as throughout a child's developing years.

Hardofhearingchildren.com

http://www.hardofhearingchildren.com

Information and advocacy for people interested in hard of hearing children. Comprehensive source of information, resources, and support for parents and children.

Address: PAMC Inc., 353 Gordon St, Guelph Ontario, Canada N1G 1X8

(519) 780-0843 – (Voice)

E-mail: candlish@hardofhearingchildren.com

Hearing Journey–Cochlear Implant Forum

http://hearingjourney.com/Listening_Room

A website that provides the opportunities to meet other families that have a child with cochlear implants or hearing aids, as well as activities designed for children with a hearing loss in the journey of learning language.

Magic Keys–ABC Fast Phonics and Children's Storybooks Online

http://magickeys.com

A website that provides resources to families with a child who is deaf or hard of hearing and professionals who provide interventions services including phonics teaching resources and children's stories.

Minnesota Early Hearing Detection and Intervention Program

http://www.improveehdi.org/mn/roadmap.cfm

The MN EHDI Program roadmap outlines how to develop a care plan for the first year of life for the child identified with hearing loss.

INFORMATION FOR FAMILIES AND PROFESSIONALS

Parents as Teachers National Center, Inc. (PAT)

http://www.patnc.org

PAT is an international early childhood parent education and family support program. PAT serves families throughout pregnancy until their child enters kindergarten, usually age 5. The program is designed to enhance child development and school achievement through parent education accessible to all families. It is a universal access model.

Address: 2228 Ball Drive, St. Louis, MO 63146

(314) 432-4330 – (Voice)
(314) 432-8963 – (Fax)
(866) PAT4YOU; (866) 728-4968 – (Toll-free)

Raising Deaf Kids

http://www.raisingdeafkids.org

Website provides information and resources on hearing loss for parents.

Address: 3440 Market St., 4th floor, Philadelphia, PA 19104

E-mail: info@raisingdeafkids.org

Sound Foundation for Babies

http://www.cochlear.com/wps/wcm/connect/in/home/support/rehabilitation-resources/early-intervention/sound-foundation-for-babies/sound-foundation-for-babies

A website for families with a child who is deaf or hard of hearing and professionals that provided weekly activities for listening and learning spoken language.

PROFESSIONAL RESOURCES

American Academy of Audiology

http://www.audiology.org/resources/documentlibrary/Documents/
PediatricAmplificationGuidelines.pdf

2013 Pediatric Amplification Guideline.

Boys Town National Research Hospital

http://babyhearing.org/Audiologists/verification/index.asp

Verification resources and videos.

Champion Program

http://www.aap.org/en-us/advocacy-and-policy/aap-health-initiatives/PEHDIC/
Pages/Early-Hearing-Detection-and-Intervention-by-State.aspx

This website also includes information specifically to supporting children with hearing loss, including information on state EHDI programs, the American of Academy State Chapter.

Medical Home

http://www.medicalhomeinfo.org/

National Center for Medical Home Implementation through the American Academy of Pediatrics. This resource is for health professionals, families, and anyone interested in creating a medical home for all children and youth.

National Institute on Deafness & Other Communication Disorders

http://www.nidcd.nih.gov

The National Institute on Deafness and Other Communication Disorders (NIDCD), part of the National Institutes of Health (NIH), conducts and supports research in the normal and disordered processes of hearing, balance, taste, smell, voice, speech, and language.

Oberkotter Foundation

http://oberkotterfoundation.org

A website for families with a child who is deaf or hard of hearing and professionals that offer resources, parent guidance, public awareness, and professional learning opportunities provided by LSLogic™.

Purdue Ear Lab Frequency Lowering Resources

http://web.ics.purdue.edu/~alexan14/fittingassistants.html

Frequency lowering fitting assistants for Phonak, Unitron, Widex, Siemens, and ReSound.

Supporting Success for Children with Hearing Loss

http://successforkidswithhearingloss.com/

Our mission is to help YOU to improve the futures of children who are hard of hearing or deaf via Resources, Products, Continuing Education, and Membership Networking. Resources developed and presented by Karen L. Anderson, PhD.

The Situational Hearing Aid Response Profile

http://audres.org/rc/sharp/

SHARP is short for Situational Hearing Aid Response Profile and was developed at the Boys Town National Research Hospital to characterize the audibility of speech signals across a wide range of realistic listening situations with varying acoustics.

University of Western Ontario PedAMP Protocol

http://www.dslio.com/page/en/pedamp/manual.html

The University of Western Ontario Pediatric Audiological Monitoring Protocol Version 1.0 (UWO PedAMP v1.0) consists of a battery of outcome evaluation tools and aims to systematically evaluate several auditory-related outcomes of infants and children with PCHI who may or may not wear hearing aids.

ZERO TO THREE: National Center for Infants, Toddlers and Families

http://www.zerotothree.org

A national nonprofit organization that promotes the healthy development of infants and toddlers by supporting and strengthening families, communities, and those who work on their behalf. Dedicated to advancing current knowledge; promoting beneficial policies and practices; communicating research and best practices to a wide variety of audiences; and providing training, technical assistance, and leadership development.

Address: 2000 M Street, NW, Suite 200, Washington, DC 20036

(202) 638-1144 – (Voice)

BOOKS AND RESOURCES

Apel, K., & Masterson, J. (2013). *Beyond baby talk: From speaking to spelling: A guide to language and literacy: Development for parents and caregivers.* New York, NY: Three Rivers Press.

Cochlear Limited. (2003). *Listen, learn, and talk* [Videos and Printed Materials]. Alexandria, NSW, Australia: Author.

Estabrooks, W. (Ed.). (2012). *101 Frequently asked questions about auditory-verbal practice.* Washington, DC: Alexander Graham Bell Association for the Deaf and Hard of Hearing.

Estabrooks, W., & Birkenshaw-Fleming, L. (2006). *Hear and listen! Talk and sing, songs for young children who are deaf or hard of hearing and others who need help in learning to talk* (2nd ed.). Washington, DC: Alexander Graham Bell Association for the Deaf and Hard of Hearing.

Gleason, J. B., & Ratner, N. B. (2012). *The development of language* (8th ed.). Boston, MA: Allyn & Bacon.

Hoff, E. (2012). *Language development* (5th ed.). Belmont, CA: Thomson Wadsworth.

Hollinger, P., & Doner, K. (2003). *What babies say before they can talk.* New York, NY: Simon & Schuster.

Hulit, L. M., Howard, M. R., & Fahey, K. P. (2011*). Born to talk: An introduction to speech and language development* (5th ed.). Toronto, Canada: Pearson Education.

Human development: The first two-and-one-half years: Program 7—Language and Program 4—Infant communication concept media. (n.d.). [Videos showing stages of language development]. Irvine, CA: Concept Media.

Ling, D. (2002). *Speech and the hearing-impaired child: Theory and practice* (2nd ed.). Washington, DC: Alexander Graham Bell Association for the Deaf and Hard of Hearing.

Otto, B. W. (2009). *Language development in early childhood education* (3rd ed.). Boston, MA: Merrill

Owens, R. E. (2008). *Language development: An introduction* (7th ed.). Boston, MA: Allyn & Bacon.

Paul, R. (2006). *Language disorders from infancy through adolescence* (3rd ed.). St. Louis, MO: Mosby Elsevier.

Pepper, J., & Weitzman, E. (2004). *It takes two to talk: A practical guide for parents of children with language delays* (3rd ed.). Toronto, Canada: The Hanen Centre.

Poland, C., & Chouinard, A. (2008). *Let's talk together: Home activities for early speech and language development.* Maple Grove, MN: Talking Child, LLC.

Pollack, D., Goldberg, D., & Caleffe-Schenck, N. (1997). *Educational audiology for the limited-hearing infant and preschooler: An auditory-verbal program.* Springfield, IL: Charles C. Thomas.

Rossi, K. (2005). *Let's learn around the clock: A professional's early intervention toolbox.* Washington, DC: Alexander Graham Bell Association for the Deaf and Hard of Hearing.

Glossary

1-3-6. Screen hearing before 1 month of age, diagnosed hearing loss before 3 months, and intervene for children with identified hearing loss before 6 months.

Accommodation. An alteration of environment, format, or equipment that allows an individual with a disability to gain access to content.

Acoustic accessibility. Refers to the behavior of sound in a room (any room—home, school or community-based), its impact on children, and its effect on the ability of a child to extract meaning from sound.

Acoustic highlighting. Slightly exaggerating the targeted speech sounds.

Amplitude compression. Automated systems that adjust the amount of amplification provided by the hearing aid based on the input level of sound received at the hearing aid microphone.

Ancillary examiner. One who has received in-depth training in the measure(s) to be used and who administers testing in the native language in the presence of a licensed professional.

ANSD. Auditory Neuropathy Spectrum Disorder is a clinical syndrome characterized by electrophysiological evidence of normal or near normal cochlear function and absent or abnormal auditory pathway transduction.

Assessment. The act of making a judgment about something.

Audibility. How much of the speech signal can be heard.

Auditory-verbal therapy. Therapeutic method in which a hearing-impaired child is taught to use available hearing; lip reading is discouraged to maximize attention to sound and hearing.

Bell curve. A graph that shows the normal distribution of variables. Most of the values cluster around the mean.

Bilateral listener. A listener who receives cochlear implants in both ears.

Bilingual. The ability to understand and use a majority and minority language.

Bimodal listener. A listener who has a hearing aid in one ear and a cochlear implant in the other ear.

Bound morphemes. Units that cannot stand alone; they must be attached to a free morpheme (e.g., pre-, -ing).

Bundled payments for care improvement (BPCI). An initiative in which organizations enter into payment agreements with Medicare and Medicaid that include financial and performance accountability for episodes of care.

Cerumen. Wax; normal, protective secretion of the ear canal.

Classroom Audio Distribution Systems (CADS; also called sound field systems). Similar to a wireless public address system, but designed specifically to ensure that the entire speech signal, including the weak high-frequency consonants, reaches every child in the room using infrared or FM transmission.

Confidence interval. Range for what this score actually represents.

Congenital. Before or at birth.

Connectivity. The connection of the child's personal hearing assistance technology (HAT) to various educational technologies such as tablets and computers.

Construct validity. The extent to which a test measures the concept or construct that it is intended to measure.

Content validity. The extent to which a variable measures what it is intended to measure.

Correlation coefficient. Measures the degree of association between two sets of numbers; correlation coefficient ranges from −1 to 1, with the numbers closest to 1 indicating a strong association between the two sets of test scores. The negative numbers refer to an inverse relationship: that is, as the score on one measure increases, the other decreases.

Criterion referenced. Tests that determine whether the test taker has mastered the material. Such tests do not compare one test taker to another.

Criterion-referenced measures. Assessments that compare an individual's performance to a predetermined age or grade-level benchmark.

Crystallized intelligence. The individual's store of acquired knowledge and ability to reason and communicate verbally.

Culturally and linguistically diverse (CLD). A person who is exposed to, and/or immersed in more than one set of cultural beliefs, values, and attitudes. These beliefs, values, and attitudes may be influenced by race/ethnicity, sexual orientation, religious or political beliefs, or gender identification. A person who has had significant exposure to more than one language or dialect.

Curriculum-based measures. Assessments developed for a specific intervention that allow a child's progress to be closely monitored throughout the intervention.

Data-driven decisions. Using the scores on standardized tests to make educational decisions.

Decibel (dB). The standard unit for measuring and describing the intensity of a sound; the logarithmic unit of sound intensity or sound pressure; one-tenth of a Bel.

Digital noise reduction. Signal processing strategy designed to limit the impact of noise on hearing aid users.

Digital RF systems (also called DM— digital modulation systems). These provide a higher level of analysis and control over the signal received by the microphone; and then the signal is delivered to the listener using a carrier frequency that "hops"—a feature that makes these systems less susceptible to interference from nearby radio frequency (RF) devices.

Diphthong. Sequence of two vowels within the same syllable that forms a single sound /eɪ, aɪ, aʊ, oʊ, ɔɪ/ as in the words *rate*, *hide*, *how*, *hope*, and *boy*.

Directional microphones. Maintain or enhance amplification for sounds arriving from the front of the listener and reduce amplification for sounds arriving from behind the listener or from the sides.

Dysgraphia. Writing impairment characterized by difficulties in single-word spelling in the absence of written expression deficits.

Dyslexia. Reading impairment characterized by difficulties in accurate and/or fluent word recognition in the absence of listening comprehension deficits.

Early intervention (EI). Services provided to children who have or at risk of developing a handicapping condition or special need that may affect their development. Services are begun between birth and school age. These services may be preventative or be remediation.

Early interventionist. A specialist who coordinates the services for a birth to age 3 child who is disabled or delayed. These services may be academic, social, and/or psychological.

Educational accessibility. The child with hearing loss should have access to curriculum and instruction in the classroom at the same level and rate as typically hearing peers.

Educational streaming. The mode of delivery of videos from YouTube, websites and other online educational programming to the child's and/or classroom's computer system.

Effective. Providing services based on scientific knowledge to all who could benefit and refraining from providing services to those not likely to benefit.

Efficient. Avoiding waste, including waste of equipment, supplies, ideas, and energy.

EHDI. Early hearing detection and intervention programs are located in states and U.S. territories. These programs are designed to identify infants and newborns with hearing loss by universal hearing screening and diagnostic testing which allows them to be enrolled in an early intervention program.

Electromagnetic interference. Disturbance that affects an electrical circuit.

Episode of care (EOC). All services provided for a specific illness during a specific time period.

Equitable care. Care that does not vary in quality because of personal characteristics such as gender, ethnicity, geographic location, and socioeconomic status.

Family-centered and culturally effective care. Care that involves the whole family and not just the child, is culturally appropriate for that family, and is effective.

Feedback suppression systems. Automatically limit the amount of gain that can be provided in the hearing aid to decrease the whistling or buzzing sound that occurs when amplified sound from the hearing aid is picked up by the microphone and amplified again.

Fluid reasoning. The ability to recognize patterns and use inductive and deductive reasoning to solve novel problems not taught in school.

Free morphemes. Units that can stand alone (most words).

Frequency. The number of times that a regularly repeated event, such as sound vibration, occurs in a specified amount of time, usually cycles per second. On an audiogram it may be called pitch and is measured in hertz (Hz).

Frequency lowering. Hearing aid signal processing strategies that relocate high-frequency speech information to lower frequencies where hearing thresholds may be better or the hearing aid may provide more gain.

Garden variety poor reading. Reading impairment characterized by deficits in word recognition as well as comprehension.

Garden variety poor writing. Writing impairment characterized by deficits in single-word spelling as well as written expression.

HAT. Hearing Assistance Technology, for example, personal FM systems.

Head shadow effect. Limits the audibility of sounds originating from the same side as the impaired ear. The head shadow effect can result in 10 to 20 dB attenuation for sounds that originate from the opposite side of the head.

Healthy People. A government program that provides science-based, 10-year national objectives for improving the health of all Americans.

Hearing age (HA). The time difference between the date of the examination and the date that the child received a hearing aid or his or her cochlear implant was activated.

HL. Hearing Level is the decibel scale used to convert to an audiometric zero from the decibel sound pressure level (dB SPL).

Inter-judge reliability. The extent to which the test yields the same results when two or more clinicians administer the test.

Intervention age (IA). The time difference between the date of the examination and the date that the child received consistently appropriate, auditory-based intervention.

LENA system. A system in which the child carries a device to record the language environment. The device is then plugged into the computer and the audio is automatically uploaded, processed, and analyzed.

Limited English proficient. Description of an individual whose primary language is not English and who has a limited ability to read, write, speak, or understand English.

Listening map. A construct to illustrate the complexity of a child's acoustic navigational demands inside and outside of school.

Long-term average speech spectrum (LTASS). The frequency range and level for a speech signal averaged over time and plotted with the hearing thresholds in dB SPL to estimate audibility.

Majority language. The language spoken by the majority population in any one country.

Medical home. A way of organizing the primary care of a patient that emphasizes coordination and communication.

Metalinguistics. Conscious awareness of the form and structure of language and how these factors relate to and produce meaning.

Metaphonologic. Ability to manipulate speech sounds auditorily.

Minority language. Any other language spoken in a country that is not that country's majority language (e.g., Mandarin in the United States).

Modification. A change in the administration or actual content of the test in such a way that both students with disabilities and typical students would potentially benefit.

Morphologic. Units of meaning.

Morphology. Study of word structure and how words are formed.

Motherese. The way that many mothers and other caregivers talk with small children.

Motivational interviewing. Technique that can be used to help engage the family in the assessment and therapeutic process.

Norm-referenced. Tests that were given to a group of students that formed the basis of comparison for the test items. It compares the test taker to other similar test takers.

Norm-referenced measures. Assessments that compare an individual's performance to a normative sample.

Oral language. The foundation of learning to read and write. Speaking and listening skills learned in the preschool years are crucial to future reading and writing achievement and school success.

Orthographic. Related to written language and includes spelling rules, punctuation, and capitalization.

Otitis media. Middle-ear infection; most common cause of conductive hearing loss in children; an inflammation of the middle ear, typically with fluid present in the normally air-filled middle-ear space.

Patient-centered care. Care that is respectful of and responsive to individual patient preferences, needs, and values and ensuring that patient values guide all clinical decisions.

Percent agreement. A metric that is employed when qualitative aspects of the tests require replicability.

Personal FM. A wireless personal listening device that includes a remote microphone placed near the desired sound source, usually the speaker's mouth, and a receiver for the listener, who can be positioned anywhere within approximately 50 feet of the person talking.

Phoneme. The smallest meaningful unit of sound in a language.

Phonologic. The production of speech sounds, sound patterns, and rules of sound organization in meaningful language.

Phonological awareness. The ability to recognize that words are made up of a variety of sounds.

Phonological memory. Working memory as it relates to phonology; refers to a process of receiving, analyzing, and processing sound elements in language.

Phonological processes. Patterns of speech errors that typically developing children use when learning to talk.

Phonological processing. A processing skill that includes the ability to see or hear a word, break it down into sounds, and then associate the sounds with the letters that make up the word.

Phonological recoding. Using reading skills to change written symbols into sounds.

Phonology. Study of speech sounds.

Poor comprehension. Reading impairment characterized by difficulties in understanding what one reads in spite of adequate word recognition skills.

Pragmatics. The social aspects of language (e.g., eye contact, turn-taking); how language is used.

Prescriptive methods. Determine the amount of amplification needed.

Print knowledge. Alphabet knowledge, print concepts, written word concepts.

Probe-microphone systems. These measure or estimate the output of the hearing aid in the ear canal, taking into account the individual acoustic characteristics of the hearing aid fitting and ear.

Processing speed. The ability to perform simple cognitive tasks quickly and accurately, requiring focused attention and concentration.

Prosody. The melody and rhythm of speaking, including pitch, intonation, intensity, and duration.

Psychometrics. Field of study where psychological responses are measured; may include responses such as intelligence, skills, abilities, educational achievement, and emotions.

Red flag. Term used to signal a concern, problem, or an undesirable characteristic that demands attention and should be addressed or corrected.

Reliability. The ability to repeat or replicate the measures included in the test.

Reverberation (RT—Reverberation Time). The amount of time it takes for a steady state sound to decrease 60 dB from its peak amplitude.

Safe. Avoiding injuries to patients from the care that is intended to help them.

Sample. A group of test subjects that is representative of the whole population being studied or normed.

Semantics. The meaning of words or groups of words in a language system.

Sensitivity. The proportion of actual positives that are correctly identified as positives. It is also known as the true positive rate.

Sequential language learners. Those who have learned one language before the age of 3 and will begin, or have begun, exposure and learning of the second language after the age of 3.

Short-term/working memory. The ability to hold information in mind while using it to solve problems.

Signal-to-noise ratio (SNR). The relationship between a primary signal such as the teacher's or parent's speech, and background noise.

Simultaneous language learners. Those who will be or have been exposed to, or have learned, more than one language before the age of 3.

SNHL. Sensorineural hearing loss; there is damage to the inner ear (cochlea), or to the nerve pathways from the inner ear to the brain. SNHL cannot be medically or surgically corrected in most cases. This is the most common type of permanent hearing loss.

Specificity. The proportion of actual negatives that are correctly identified as negatives. It is also known as the true negative rate.

Speech banana. The speech banana is a term used to describe the area where phonemes appear on an audiogram. Even though there are other sounds outside of the speech banana, audiologists and interventionists are most concerned with the frequencies and audibility of those phonemes within the speech banana because a hearing loss in those frequencies can affect a child's ability to learn language.

Speech intelligibility index (SII). The idea that different frequency regions of the speech signal carry different amounts of importance for understanding speech. The SII is expressed as a proportion (between 0 and 1) or percentage (between 0 and 100), where higher values represent greater audibility of the speech signal.

Speech perception. Process by which the sounds of speech are heard, interpreted as meaningful speech, and understood.

Speech production. Process by which the sounds of speech that a speaker intends to say are formulated and articulated.

Standard error of measurement. A statistical estimate of the amount of random error in the assessment of results or scores. It measures the accuracy with which a sample represents a population.

Standard scores. The score in a norm-referenced assessment to compare one student's test performance to another.

Strategic seating. Customized seating in the dynamic environment of a classroom in order to give the student educational accessibility.

Suprasegmental patterns. The prosodic aspect of speech production including pitch, loudness, rate, and duration of speech patterns.

Syntax. The rules governing grammatical constellation of language units.

Timely. Reduced waits and sometimes harmful delays for both those who receive and those who give care.

UNHS. Universal newborn hearing screening; infants screened for hearing loss, preferably prior to hospital discharge.

Validity. The extent to which a test measures what it is designed to assess.

Visual-spatial processing. The ability to perceive, analyze, and think with visual patterns, including the ability to mentally manipulate, store, and recall visual representations.

Written expression impairment. Writing impairment characterized by difficulties in planning, translating, and/or reviewing a written composition in the absence of single-word spelling deficits.

Index